11/23 $2

Mental Health and Addiction Services
(902) 679-2870
(902) 825-4825

Dissemination and Implementation of Evidence-Based Psychological Interventions

Dissemination and Implementation of Evidence-Based Psychological Interventions

Edited by R. Kathryn McHugh
and
David H. Barlow

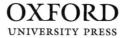

OXFORD
UNIVERSITY PRESS

Oxford University Press, Inc., publishes works that further
Oxford University's objective of excellence
in research, scholarship, and education.

Oxford New York
Auckland   Cape Town   Dar es Salaam   Hong Kong   Karachi
Kuala Lumpur   Madrid   Melbourne   Mexico City   Nairobi
New Delhi   Shanghai   Taipei   Toronto

With offices in
Argentina   Austria   Brazil   Chile   Czech Republic   France   Greece
Guatemala   Hungary   Italy   Japan   Poland   Portugal   Singapore
South Korea   Switzerland   Thailand   Turkey   Ukraine   Vietnam

Copyright © 2012 by Oxford University Press

Published by Oxford University Press, Inc.
198 Madison Avenue, New York, New York 10016
www.oup.com

Oxford is a registered trademark of Oxford University Press

Library of Congress Cataloging-in-Publication Data
Dissemination and implementation of evidence-based psychological
interventions / edited by R. Kathryn McHugh and David H. Barlow.
   p. ; cm.
 Includes bibliographical references and index.
 ISBN 978-0-19-538905-0 (alk. paper)
 I. McHugh, R. Kathryn (Rebecca Kathryn) II. Barlow, David H.
 [DNLM: 1. Mental Disorders—prevention & control.
2. Mental Disorders—therapy. 3. Evidence-Based Medicine—methods.
4. Information Dissemination—methods. 5. Psychotherapy—methods. WM 400]
 LC classification not assigned
 616.89—dc23   2011031967

9 8 7 6 5 4 3 2 1

Printed in the United States of America on acid-free paper

{CONTENTS}

{PREFACE}

Successes in basic and clinical psychological science have yielded highly efficacious, effective, and durable interventions for psychological disorders. However, excitement about the potential for improved clinical outcomes and cost benefits of evidence-based psychological interventions (EBPIs) has been mitigated by the spotty transfer of these interventions to service provision settings. Few children and adults with psychological disorders receive any treatment; even fewer receive evidence-based treatment. Recognition of this public health need has resulted in not only a commitment but also an urgent mandate to increase access to EBPIs (Institute of Medicine, 2001; President's New Freedom Commission on Mental Health, 2003; U.S. Department of Health and Human Services, 1999).

In attempting to meet this public health need, it has become increasingly clear that traditional methods for the spread of interventions (e.g., academic publications, 1- to 2-day workshops) are not sufficient to achieve widespread adoption and successful implementation. Accordingly, there is a need for more proactive strategies for the dissemination and implementation of EBPIs toward the eventual establishment of evidence-based procedures for transporting interventions. Internationally, stakeholders have begun to respond to this need and several billion dollars have been committed to these efforts thus far.

Our aim for this volume is to characterize the current status and future directions of the rapidly expanding area of dissemination and implementation (D&I) in mental health care. Among our motivations for this volume was that many D&I efforts developed independently under different motivating circumstances. For these efforts, the urgency to proceed rapidly often prevented systematic collaboration and communication among groups on the best practices for D&I (McHugh & Barlow, 2010). We are fortunate to have contributors from many of the largest and most innovative D&I efforts in mental health care providing the latest information on the practices and outcomes of their programs.

This volume is written in two parts. The first three chapters set the stage for the descriptions of D&I efforts and include discussion of the history of EBPIs and the need for D&I, an overview of D&I science, and a review of the effectiveness of methods for clinician training in EBPIs. The second part of the volume includes detailed descriptions of leading D&I programs internationally, written by leaders of these efforts. Each of these chapters includes descriptions of the motivating circumstances for the effort, the procedures and practices utilized, and available outcomes data.

The D&I programs represented in this volume range in aims and scope and include both national and local efforts. Several large national efforts are described in Chapters 4 through 7. Efforts to implement evidence-based treatments by the National Health Service in the United Kingdom and the Veterans Health Administration (VHA) in the United States are among the largest efforts internationally. In Chapter 4, David M. Clark describes the Improving Access to Psychological Therapies Program in the United Kingdom, a sweeping national effort to ensure availability of evidence-based treatments by providing intensive training and utilizing a stepped-care model consistent with best-practice recommendations for the treatment of anxiety and depression. In Chapter 5, Josef I. Rusek, Bradley E. Karlin, and Antonette Zeiss describe the innovative approaches taken to facilitate implementation and maintenance of best practices for anxiety, depression, and severe mental illness in the VHA, the largest integrated health care system in the United States. In Chapter 6, Lori Ebert, Lisa Amaya-Jackson, Jan Markiewicz, and John A. Fairbank describe a comprehensive model for implementing EBPIs for child traumatic stress. The Learning Collaborative Model was developed through efforts of the National Child Traumatic Stress Network—a national academic–community collaboration funded by the Substance Abuse and Mental Health Services Administration—that has been implemented widely to improve access to effective care among traumatized children. Finally, in Chapter 7, Susan M. Wilczynski, Dennis C. Russo, and Walter P. Christian describe the National Standards Project of the National Autism Center and the efforts to integrate the literature on evidence-based interventions for autism spectrum disorders and to disseminate this information to care systems, including both treatment facilities and schools.

Efforts at the state level are described in Chapters 8 and 9. Jeanne C. Rivard, Vijay K. Ganju, Kristin A. Roberts, and G. Michael Lane provide an overview of state efforts initiated at both the federal and state levels to improve access to EBPIs. Several novel strategies for facilitating implementation, such as university–state mental health system collaborations, as well as the importance of the development of financial infrastructure for the initiation and maintenance of these efforts are described. Efforts to improve evidence-based mental health care in the state of Hawaii have represented a particular success of D&I. Brad J. Nakamura, Charmaine K. Higa-McMillan, and Bruce F. Chorpita describe the impetus for and implementation of these efforts with a particular focus on sustaining and maintaining the significant advances achieved in recent years in improving access to care for children and adolescents in Hawaii.

Chapters 10 through 12 highlight efforts to implement three specific EBPIs: Dialectical Behavior Therapy (DBT), the Triple P—Positive Parenting Program (Triple P), and Multisystemic Therapy (MST). The treatment developers for each of these three interventions have demonstrated particular success in providing support for intervention transport to service provision settings. Sara J. Landes and Marsha M. Linehan describe the implementation of the DBT Intensive Training Model developed in response to the lack of effectiveness of standard training workshops.

The dissemination and implementation of the Triple P program is unique relative to the other interventions in this volume given the population-based approach taken by its developers. Matthew R. Sanders and Rachel Calam describe the unique challenges and strategies of utilizing a universal approach to disseminating an intervention, including a number of direct-to-consumer strategies, such as the use of mass media. Sonja K. Schoenwald describes the many factors that have played a role in the diffusion and implementation of MST, considering policy as well as service provision demands for the intervention, and the development and refinement of procedures to most effectively transport and maintain the adherent administration of this treatment.

It is of note that the programs and efforts described in this volume are only a sampling of the D&I efforts ongoing internationally to improve access to EBPIs. As these programs continue to develop and expand, communication and collaboration will be critical to the rapid advancement of knowledge on the best practices for transporting EBPIs to routine practice. In Chapter 13, we look toward the future of this area, providing our best approximation of 10 important future directions for the science and practice of D&I in mental health care.

Effective interventions have been established for a wide range of psychological disorders for children and adults. Yet, low access to mental health care generally, and evidence-based care specifically, has limited the public health impact of these innovations. Achievement of a greater public health benefit of psychological interventions will require not only significant resource commitment to both applied and research agendas but also collaboration among varied stakeholder groups to address this complex challenge. The field has reached widespread success in the development of highly effective treatments and now must discover how to translate this success to the reduction of the societal burden of mental illness.

REFERENCES

Institute of Medicine. (2001). *Crossing the quality chasm: A new health system for the 21st Century*. Washington, DC: Author.

McHugh, R. K., & Barlow, D. H. (2010). Dissemination and implementation of evidence-based psychological interventions: A review of current efforts. *American Psychologist, 65*, 73–84.

President's New Freedom Commission on Mental Health. (2003). *Achieving the promise: Transforming mental health care in America*. Retrieved October 12, 2011, from http://govinfo.library.unt.edu/mentalhealthcommission/reports/reports.htm

U.S. Department of Health and Human Services. (1999). *Mental health: A report of the Surgeon General*. Rockville, MD: Author.

{ACKNOWLEDGMENTS}

The editors gratefully acknowledge the contributors to this volume for sharing their experiences and expertise in this fledgling area of research and practice and for their dedication to achieving a greater public health impact for the field. We also would like to express our gratitude to the editorial staff at Oxford University Press, especially Sarah Harrington and Pamela Hanley, for their support of this volume and guidance throughout the process.

{CONTRIBUTORS}

Lisa Amaya-Jackson, MD, MPH, Department of Psychiatry and Behavioral Sciences, Duke University School of Medicine, Durham, North Carolina

David H. Barlow, PhD, ABPP, Department of Psychology, Boston University, Boston, Massachusetts

Rachel Calam, PhD, School of Psychological Sciences, University of Manchester, Manchester, United Kingdom

Bruce F. Chorpita, PhD, Department of Psychology, University of California, Los Angeles, Los Angeles, California

Walter P. Christian, PhD, ABBP, ABPP, May Institute, Randolph, Massachusetts

David M. Clark, DPhil, FBA, FMedSci, Department of Experimental Psychology, University of Oxford, Oxford, United Kingdom

Lori Ebert, PhD, Department of Psychiatry and Behavioral Sciences, Duke University Medical Center, Durham, North Carolina

John A. Fairbank, PhD, Department of Psychiatry and Behavioral Sciences, Duke University Medical Center and VA Mid-Atlantic (VISN6) Mental Illness Research, Education and Clinical Center (MIRECC), Durham, North Carolina

Vijay K. Ganju, PhD, Consultant, Austin, Texas

Charmaine K. Higa-McMillan, PhD, Department Psychology, University of Hawaii at Hilo, Hilo, Hawaii

Bradley E. Karlin, PhD, Office of Mental Health Services, Veterans Administration Central Office, Washington, District of Columbia

Sara J. Landes, PhD, National Center for PTSD, Veterans Affairs Palo Alto Health Care System, Palo Alto, California; Department of Psychiatry and Behavioral Sciences, University of Washington, Seattle, Washington

G. Michael Lane Jr, MA, MPH, National Association of State Mental Health Program Directors Research Institute, Inc. Falls Church, Virginia

Marsha M. Linehan, PhD, Department of Psychology, University of Washington, Seattle, Washington

Jan Markiewicz, MEd, Department of Psychiatry and Behavioral Sciences, Duke University Medical Center, Durham, North Carolina

R. Kathryn McHugh, PhD, Division of Alcohol and Drug Abuse, McLean Hospital, Belmont, Massachusetts; Department of Psychiatry, Harvard Medical School, Boston, Massachusetts

Brad J. Nakamura, PhD, Department of Psychology, University of Hawaii at Manoa, Honolulu, Hawaii

Jeanne C. Rivard, PhD, Division of Behavioral and Social Sciences and Education, National Research Council, The National Academies, Washington, District of Columbia

Kristin A. Roberts, MA, National Association of State Mental Health Program Directors Research Institute, Inc. Falls Church, Virginia

Dennis C. Russo, PhD, ABPP, Departments of Family Medicine and Psychology, Brody School of Medicine and East Carolina University, Greenville, North Carolina

Josef I. Ruzek, PhD, National Center for PTSD, Veterans Affairs Palo Alto Health Care System, Palo Alto, California

Matthew R. Sanders, PhD, Parenting and Family Support Centre, School of Psychology, The University of Queensland, Brisbane, Queensland, Australia

Sonja K. Schoenwald, PhD, Department of Psychiatry and Behavioral Sciences, Medical University of South Carolina, Charleston, South Carolina

Susan M. Wilczynski, PhD, BCBA, National Autism Center, Randolph, Massachusetts

Antonette Zeiss, PhD, Office of Mental Health Services, Veterans Administration Central Office, Washington, District of Columbia

PART I

Background

The Reach of Evidence-Based Psychological Interventions

R. Kathryn McHugh and David H. Barlow

In recent years, the mental health field has increasingly emphasized scientific evidence as a core element of its practice. This shift from a prioritization of clinical expertise and anecdotal evidence to that of scientific evidence is similar to that seen in medicine at the turn of the 20th century (see Baker, McFall, & Shoham, 2008). As the field has increasingly accepted the notion that science must undergird practice and evidence supporting the efficacy and effectiveness of psychological treatments has grown, the challenge of how to transport these findings to service provision settings emerged. This chapter provides an overview of the movement toward evidence-based mental health care, including a description of the brief history of evidence-based psychological interventions (EBPIs) and the current status of the research–practice gap. As such, this chapter will serve as a backdrop for subsequent chapters highlighting state-of-the-art efforts to disseminate and implement EBPIs. Our definition of evidence-based psychological interventions encompasses both treatment and preventive interventions targeting psychological disorders and is distinguished from those targeting wellness or personal growth (psychotherapy; see Barlow, 2006).

THE EMERGENCE OF EVIDENCE-BASED PSYCHOLOGICAL INTERVENTIONS

The movement toward a greater standardization of psychological interventions arose in the 1960s as an attempt to improve operational definitions of key concepts in psychotherapy research (Barlow, 2011; Bergin & Strupp, 1972). The development of manuals to guide the application of interventions—which originated with brief psychodynamic approaches (Luborksy & DeRubeis, 1984)—provided a framework to define these interventions more clearly and to facilitate their empirical evaluation through increasing reliability of administration and replicability (Barlow, 2011). Although studies of the efficacy of psychological interventions were conducted prior to the development of manualized therapies (see Barlow, 2011; Bergin & Strupp, 1972; Luborsky, Singer, & Luborsky, 1975), the shift to more standardization provided the conditions necessary to facilitate major advances in the empirical investigation of treatment effects.

In subsequent years, there has been a proliferation of research on intervention efficacy and effectiveness. With concurrent advances in methods for evaluating EBPIs and research on the etiology and nature of psychological disorders, the success of the intervention outcome research agenda has grown. At this time, evidence from large-scale outcome trials and quantitative reviews suggest that psychological interventions are robust and durable for a range of psychological disorders often with outcomes similar to—if not superior to—front-line pharmacotherapy for these conditions (e.g., Barlow, 2004; Barlow, Gorman, Shear, & Woods, 2000; Butler, Chapman, Forman, & Beck, 2006; Coldwell & Bender, 2007; Dutra et al., 2008; Fairburn et al., 2009; Hofmann & Smits, 2008; Keller et al., 2000; Linehan et al., 2006; Nathan & Gorman, 2007; Roth & Fonagy, 2005; Safren et al., 2010; Silverman, Pina, & Viswesvaran, 2008; Weisz, Jenson-Doss, & Hawley, 2006). Moreover, EBPIs are associated with favorable cost efficacy/effectiveness and cost offset (e.g., Byford et al., 2007; The Centre for Economic Performance's Mental Health Policy Group, 2006; Domino et al., 2009; McHugh et al., 2007; Miklowitz & Scott, 2009). Patients also consistently report a preference for psychological treatments over pharmacotherapy (e.g., Feeny, Zoellner, Mavissakalian, & Roy-Byrne, 2009; Hazlett-Stevens et al., 2002; Hofmann et al., 1998; Mitchell et al., 1990; van Schaik et al., 2004), with a meta-analytic review of preference studies finding that patients were three times more likely to report preference for psychological relative to pharmacological treatment (McHugh, Whitton, Peckham, Welge, & Otto, 2011).

Although the majority of outcomes research has occurred in the context of efficacy trials, studies of treatment effectiveness also support the use of EBPIs. These studies have demonstrated that EBPIs administered to heterogeneous patient groups in clinical settings achieve treatment outcomes comparable to those reported in highly controlled efficacy trials (e.g., Farrell, Schlup, & Boschen, 2010; Franklin, Abramowitz, Kozak, Levitt, & Foa, 2000; Houghton, Saxon, Bradburn, Ricketts, & Hardy, 2009; Morrison et al., 2004; Persons, Bostrom, & Bertagnolli, 1999; Stewart & Chambless, 2007; Stuart, Treat, & Wade, 2000). For example, in a large effectiveness trial of cognitive behavioral therapy (CBT) for panic disorder in primary care settings, Roy-Byrne and colleagues (2005) randomized 232 patients to treatment as usual or a combination of evidence-based psychological (CBT) and pharmacological treatment (an algorithm-based program, beginning with selective serotonin reuptake inhibitors). The evidence-based treatment group experienced significantly greater symptom (e.g., panic attack frequency) and functional/quality-of-life improvement which was durable over a year of follow-up.

Despite these successes, mitigated outcomes relative to efficacy trials have also been noted (e.g., Addis et al., 2006; Curtis, Ronan, & Borduin, 2004; Westbrook & Kirk, 2005). However, failures to achieve comparable outcomes of EBPIs in service provision settings may be attributable to failed implementation, not necessarily a failure of the intervention (e.g., Henggeler, Melton, Brondino, Scherer, & Hanley, 1997). For example, failure to reach outcomes benefits of the same magnitude as efficacy trials may be attributable to insufficient treatment fidelity (see Henggeler, 2004; McHugh, Murray, & Barlow, 2009). Thus, the evidence accruing at this time supporting the outcomes benefits seen with EBPIs—with implementation being the potential key variable in this success—suggests that the transport of these interventions to service provision settings results in similar benefits to those seen in controlled trials. However, more evaluation of the effectiveness of interventions as administered in service provision settings is still needed.

EVALUATING THE EVIDENCE: DEFINING AND IDENTIFYING EVIDENCE-BASED PSYCHOLOGICAL INTERVENTIONS

With the proliferation of treatment development and outcome research, a need for procedures to identify the level of empirical support for specific treatments emerged to facilitate the selection and use of these treatments by clinical systems and providers. The overabundance of treatments available with varying degrees of empirical support gave rise to a body of information difficult for any individual clinician or clinical setting to navigate. Relative to D&I efforts, this issue resulted in a major challenge to clinicians and dissemination effort leaders alike; how should treatments be selected for a specific setting?

Two major approaches to this question have been introduced. One approach has been to provide clinicians with skills for the interpretation and consolidation of the empirical literature to guide decision making. This approach has been used in other health fields to facilitate evidence-based practice (Sackett, Straus, Richardson, Rosenberg, & Haynes, 2000). Drawing from this previous work in medicine, Norcross, Hogan, and Koocher (2008) proposed a process for the utilization of evidence-based practice by mental health clinicians. The steps of this process include (a) asking a clinical question; (b) identifying the best research; (c) evaluating this research; (d) utilizing this research with a patient; (e) integrating clinician expertise, patient preference, and individual difference variables (e.g., age, race, sex) with this evidence; and (f) evaluating the effectiveness of the approach. This strategy for utilizing and administering evidence-based treatment focuses on the development of a skill set used to consume, interpret, and apply the research evidence within the context of clinician experience and patient factors. This approach has been used in developing competency in the practice of evidence-based behavioral medicine (Council for Training in Evidence-Based Practice, 2008; Spring, 2007).

The second approach has been the development of guidelines for treatment selection based on consolidation of the literature on treatment efficacy/effectiveness to facilitate identification of interventions for providers and systems. Both government agencies and professional organizations have spearheaded efforts to develop such clinical practice guidelines in mental health. For example, the Agency for Healthcare Policy and Research (now called the Agency for Healthcare and

Research Quality; AHRQ) in the United States and the National Institute for Health and Clinical Excellence (NICE) in the United Kingdom are government agencies that evaluate research evidence in health and provide guidance on effective and cost-effective treatments. Other government organizations such as the Substance Abuse and Mental Health Administration (SAMHSA) and the Veterans Affairs/ Department of Defense (VA/DoD) also have developed their own practice guidelines based on evidence reviews. Professional organizations, such as the American Psychiatric Association, have also consolidated research evidence into best practice guidelines, and the American Psychological Association has recently decided to do the same. In addition to formal practice guidelines, many resources are available as guides to evidence-based intervention (e.g., Barlow, 2007; Nathan & Gorman, 2007; Roth & Fonagy, 2005). The number of guidelines has expanded such that resources compiling available guidelines have been developed (e.g., the National Guideline Clearinghouse, www.ngc.gov). Table 1.1 provides examples of some of the major guideline resources for EBPIs. These efforts from agencies, groups, and investigators vary in the standards utilized for evaluating evidence to establish best practices and likewise vary in their categorization of treatments (see Chambless & Ollendick, 2001). For example, the American Psychological Association in 1995 (Barlow, 1996) and in a later revision in 2002 (American Psychological Association, 2002) argued

TABLE 1.1 Practice Guideline Resources

Organization	Website
AHRQ National Guideline Clearinghouse	www.guideline.gov
American Psychiatric Association	http://www.psych.org/psych_pract/treatg/pg/ prac_guide.cfm
American Psychological Association, Division 12	www.psychologicaltreatments.org
ABCT/American Psychological Association, Division 53	http://www.abct.org/SCCAP/
Canadian Medical Association	http://www.cma.ca/index.php/ci_id/54316/ la_id/1.htm
Canadian Psychiatric Association	http://publications.cpa-apc.org/browse/ documents/67
Department of Veterans Affairs/ Department of Defense	http://www.healthquality.va.gov/
National Health Service, National Institute for Clinical Excellence	http://guidance.nice.org.uk/
Royal Australian and New Zealand College of Psychiatrists	http://www.ranzcp.org/resources/ practice-guidelines.html
SAMHSA National Registry of Evidence-based Programs and Practices	www.nrepp.samhsa.gov

Note. ABCT = Association for Behavioral and Cognitive Therapies; AHRQ = Agency for Healthcare and Research Quality; SAMHSA = Substance Abuse and Mental Health Services Administration.

that consideration for the inclusion of a treatment in best practice guidelines should involve evaluation of evidence for both the efficacy (i.e., internal validity) and effectiveness (i.e., utility in service provision settings) of treatments.

The specific process for distilling the treatment literature and identifying the level of support for interventions has been complex and controversial. For example, the American Psychological Association Division 12 Task Force on Promotion and Dissemination of Psychological Procedures (Chambless et al., 1998) developed an algorithm for evaluating available evidence to identify the level of empirical support for specific psychological treatments. Three categories were developed: (a) well-established treatments, (b) probably efficacious treatments, and (c) experimental treatments. For a treatment to reach the "well-established" category, it must meet the following criteria according to Chambless and colleagues (1998): (a) two or more controlled clinical trials yielding efficacy greater than placebo (or an active treatment) or equivalent efficacy to an existing evidence-based treatment, or (b) more than nine high quality single case design studies supporting the treatment's efficacy relative to placebo (or other active treatment). In addition, the studies must have used treatment manuals for standardization of delivery, must have utilized specified patient samples, and must be replicated by two or more investigators (or groups of investigators).

Although practice guidelines can potentially be abused by payor systems in attempts to reduce cost and have been criticized in the methods by which they are derived (see Barlow, 1996), the need for syntheses of the empirical literature on treatment efficacy and effectiveness is clearly needed for these results to be successfully disseminated. Particularly for systems without the time and financial resources to be active consumers of the research literature (as suggested by the Norcross et al., 2008 model), the need for an easily accessed and interpreted guideline is crucial to the ability to identify EBPIs. Moreover, this allows for greater standardization within and across systems, facilitating ongoing evaluation and quality improvement in service provision settings.

THE RESEARCH–PRACTICE GAP

As the empirical support for psychological interventions has built over time, there has been a notable lack of widespread transport of these treatments outside of academic research settings. The research–practice gap has been highlighted as a major public health problem in both medicine generally and psychology specifically. In a 2001 report on the status of health care in the United States, the Institute of Medicine characterized the disconnect between research and practice as "not just a gap, but a chasm" (2001, p. 1). Indeed, the poor adoption of evidence-based mental health care in service provision settings has been supported by several large-scale reports (e.g., President's New Freedom Commission on Mental Health, 2003; U.S. Department of Health and Human Services, 1999).

These reports are further supported by empirical studies that consistently suggest that EBPIs are not well incorporated in routine practice. It is important to note that not only is access to evidence-based services limited but also many individuals in need do not receive *any* mental health services (Young, Klap, Sherbourne, & Wells, 2001). For example, an estimate based on rates of psychological disorders, treatment receipt, and treatment dropout noted that only an estimated 17% of children in need of services receive a full dose of any mental health treatment regardless of evidence base (Kazdin, 2008). Studies of clinical practice have identified low usage rates of evidence-based treatments for eating disorders (Crow, Mussell, Peterson, Knopke, & Mitchell, 1999; Haas & Clopton, 2003; Mussell et al., 2000), anxiety disorders (Becker, Zayfert, & Anderson, 2004; Goisman, Warshaw, & Keller, 1999), and substance use disorders (Santa Ana et al., 2008), among others (Stewart & Chambless, 2007). Similarly, rates of adherence to practice guidelines are low (Phillips & Brandon, 2004). The utilization of EBPIs in graduate and internship psychology training programs has also lagged (Crits-Christoph, Frank, Chambless, Brody, & Karp, 1995; Weissman et al., 2006; Woody, Weisz, & McLean, 2005).

The factors contributing to this gap are heterogeneous and complex, further highlighting the challenge of targeting this problem. Considering the complex and nuanced nature of many EBPIs, their transport into service provision settings involves a variety of potential barriers at the level of patients, providers, and organizations. Barriers to adoption and utilization of EBPIs have been discussed extensively (see Addis, 2002; Barlow, Levitt, & Bufka, 1999; McHugh & Barlow, 2010; Stirman, Crits-Christoph, & DeRubeis, 2004). Three major categories of barriers have been highlighted: motivation of providers to adopt new procedures, training barriers, and organizational/systems barriers.

As with any paradigm-shifting change, the movement toward evidence-based care has met with resistance. A range of criticisms have been aimed at the evidence-based care movement, such as the limitations of the randomized controlled trial design, the proscribed nature of treatment manuals, and the lack of accounting for the therapeutic relationship as a mechanism of change. For example, in a discussion of the implementation of EBPIs for children in Hawaii, Chorpita and colleagues (2002) wrote that "clinical reluctance remained a primary obstacle to dissemination" (p. 167). Such negative perceptions of evidence-based practices have been widely reported (see Addis & Krasnow, 2000; Addis, Wade, & Hatgis, 1999; Barlow et al., 1999) and cited as the primary barrier to adoption by clinicians (Pagoto et al., 2007). Many of these attitudes may be fueled by popular myths about EBPIs (Barlow et al., 1999), such as the belief that EBPIs are rigid treatments that cannot be applied flexibly (Borntrager, Chorpita, Higa-McMillan, & Weisz, 2009). These concerns stem from the core issue of the applicability of scientific methods to the study of psychological treatment and the dichotomy between the "art" and "science" of psychological treatment which has consistently characterized the movement toward evidence-based medicine.

Once a decision has been made to adopt an intervention, training service providers to use EBPIs is a major challenge. Training in the utilization of treatments and the ongoing supervision, monitoring, and consultation necessary to maintain high fidelity and positive outcomes require the commitment of significant financial and time resources. Moreover, research on the best training strategies and measures for evaluating training outcomes is in the very early stages (McHugh & Barlow, 2010). The process of training and the challenges that efforts face with respect to training are discussed in detail in Chapter 3.

Finally, the transport of an intervention that is developed and tested in a controlled research setting into an already established system with specific needs and existing infrastructure can be exceptionally challenging. For example, lack of funding and institutional support for efforts can serve as a barrier at the planning stages and throughout the implementation process. The availability/accessibility of information, fit of intervention (e.g., session length, duration, frequency) to the system's needs and characteristics (e.g., prevalence of problems, cultural considerations), and cost of adoption are all important factors for individual clinicians and organizations to consider when weighing the decision of whether to implement an EBPI. Treatment settings are often taxed and may not have infrastructure that is supportive of the training necessary to adopt EBPIs. Limited time and funding for such efforts and lack of mandates or incentives present major challenges to adoption.

Despite these barriers, the reliable demonstration of outcome benefits has driven the field closer to consensus regarding the need for EBPIs. As Kazdin (2008) argued: "Debates internal to the field about [evidence-based treatments] and their applicability ignore arguably the most critical question—how can we get our treatments to the many people in need of services" (p. 202). This issue—of how to successfully transport interventions to service provision settings—is the focus of this volume.

MOVING TOWARD DISSEMINATION AND IMPLEMENTATION

The evidence identifying the limited availability of EBPIs in service provision settings implies a failure of traditionally utilized dissemination and implementation strategies to overcome barriers to adopting these practices. Moreover, results from empirical studies provide further support for this implication (see Chapter 2, this volume). Historically, the field has assumed the potential for *diffusion* (the spread of treatments passively without directed efforts) through strategies such as the publication of research results in academic journals, the availability of treatment manuals for purchase, and presentation at professional conferences for which clinicians self-select. However, it has become increasingly evident that more active and targeted strategies are necessary for successful transport. Such principles and program exemplars will be discussed in this volume.

The development and evaluation of psychological interventions has resulted in groundbreaking changes in our understanding of psychological disorders and their prevention and treatment. The next great challenge of the field is to determine how to allow these advances to achieve their potential public health impact. At this time, there is a need for a shift of priorities from the development and testing of prevention and treatment interventions to the development and testing of dissemination and implementation interventions. Research on the procedures by which EBPIs are spread to service provision settings is in the early stages of development and validation. The next chapter provides a broad overview of theories of dissemination and implementation drawn from both health/mental health and other disciplines.

REFERENCES

Addis, M. E. (2002). Methods for disseminating research products and increasing evidence-based practice: Promises, obstacles, and future directions. *Clinical Psychology: Science and Practice, 9*, 367–378.

Addis, M. E., Hatgis, C., Cardemil, E., Jacob, K., Krasnow, A. D., & Mansfield, A. (2006). Effectiveness of cognitive-behavioral treatment for panic disorder versus treatment as usual in a managed care setting: 2-year follow-up. *Journal of Consulting and Clinical Psychology, 74*, 377–385.

Addis, M. E., & Krasnow, A. D. (2000). A national survey of practicing psychologists' attitudes toward psychotherapy treatment manuals. *Journal of Consulting and Clinical Psychology, 68*, 331–339.

Addis, M. E., Wade, W. A., & Hatgis, C. (1999). Barriers to the dissemination of evidence-based practices: Addressing practitioners' concerns about manual-based psychotherapies. *Clinical Psychology: Science and Practice, 6*, 430–441.

American Psychological Association. (2002). Criteria for evaluating treatment guidelines. *American Psychologist, 57*, 1052–1059.

Baker, T. B., McFall, R. M., & Shoham, V. (2008). Current status and future prospects of clinical psychology: Toward a scientifically principled approach to mental and behavioral health care. *Psychological Science in the Public Interest, 9*, 67–103.

Barlow, D. H. (1996). Health care policy, psychotherapy research, and the future of psychotherapy. *American Psychology, 51*, 1050–1058.

Barlow, D. H. (2004). Psychological treatments. *American Psychologist, 59*, 869–878.

Barlow, D. H. (2006). Psychotherapy and psychological treatments: The future. *Clinical Psychology: Science and Practice, 13*, 216–220.

Barlow, D. H. (2007). *Clinical handbook of psychological disorders* (4th ed.). New York: Guilford.

Barlow, D. H. (2011). A prolegomenon to clinical psychology: Two 40-year odysseys. In D. H. Barlow (Ed.), *The Oxford handbook of clinical psychology.* (pp. 3–20). New York, NY: Oxford University Press.

Barlow, D. H., Gorman, J. M, Shear, M. K., & Woods, S. W. (2000). Cognitive-behavioral therapy, imipramine, or their combination for panic disorder: A randomized controlled trial. *Journal of the American Medical Association, 283*, 2529–2536.

Barlow, D. H., Levitt, J. T., & Bufka, L. F. (1999). The dissemination of empirically supported treatments: A view to the future. *Behaviour Research and Therapy, 37*(Suppl. 1), 147–162.

Becker, C. B., Zayfert, C., & Anderson, E. (2004). A survey of psychologists' attitudes towards and utilization of exposure therapy for PTSD. *Behaviour Research and Therapy, 42*, 277–292.

Bergin, A. E., & Strupp, H. H. (1972). *Changing frontiers in the science of psychotherapy.* Chicago, IL: Aldine Atherton Inc.

Borntrager, C. F., Chorpita, B. F., Higa-McMillan, C., & Weisz, J. R. (2009). Provider attitudes toward evidence-based practices: Are the concerns with the evidence or with the manuals. *Psychiatric Services, 60,* 677–681.

Butler, A. C., Chapman, J. E., Forman, E. M., & Beck, A. T. (2006). The empirical status of cognitive-behavioral therapy: A review of meta-analyses. *Clinical Psychology Review, 26,* 17–31.

Byford, S., Barrett, B., Roberts, C., Wilkinson, P., Dubicka, B., Kelvin, R. G., et al. (2007). Cost-effectiveness of selective serotonin reuptake inhibitors and routine specialist care with and without cognitive behavioural therapy in adolescents with major depression. *British Journal of Psychiatry, 191,* 521–527.

The Centre for Economic Performance's Mental Health Policy Group. (2006). *The depression report: A new deal for depression and anxiety disorders.* London, England: London School of Economics and Political Science.

Chambless, D. L., Baker, M. J., Baucom, D. H., Beutler, L. E., Calhoun, K. S., Crits-Christoph, P., et al. (1998). Update on empirically validated therapies II. *The Clinical Psychologist, 51,* 3–15.

Chambless, D. L., & Ollendick, T. H. (2001). Empirically supported psychological interventions: Controversies and evidence. *Annual Review of Psychology, 52,* 685–716.

Chorpita, B. F., Yim, L. M., Donkervoet, J. C., Arensdorf, A., Amundsen, M. J., McGee, C., et al. (2002). Toward large-scale implementation of empirically supported treatments for children: A review and observations by the Hawaii Empirical Basis to Services Task Force. *Clinical Psychology: Science and Practice, 9,* 165–190.

Coldwell, C. M., & Bender, W. S. (2007). The effectiveness of assertive community treatment for homeless populations with severe mental illness: A meta-analysis. *American Journal of Psychiatry, 164,* 393–394.

Council for Training in Evidence-Based Behavioral Practice. (2008). *Definition and competencies for evidence-based behavioral practice (EBBP).* Retrieved May 10, 2011, from http://www.ebbp.org/documents/EBBP_Competencies.pdf

Crits-Christoph, P., Frank, E., Chambless, D. L., Brody, C., & Karp, J. F. (1995) Training in empirically validated treatments: What are clinical psychology students learning? *Professional Psychology: Science and Practice, 26,* 514–522.

Crow, S., Mussell, M. P., Peterson, C., Knopke, A., & Mitchell, J. (1999). Prior treatment received by patients with bulimia nervosa. *International Journal of Eating Disorders, 25,* 39–44.

Curtis, N. M., Ronan, K. R., & Borduin, C. M. (2004). Multisystemic treatment: A meta-analysis of outcome studies. *Journal of Family Psychology, 18,* 411–419.

Domino, M. E., Foster, E. M., Vitiello, B., Kratochvil, C. J., Burns, B. J., Silva, S. G., et al. (2009). Relative cost-effectiveness of treatments for adolescent depression: 36-week results from the TADS randomized trial. *Journal of the American Academy of Child and Adolescent Psychiatry, 48,* 711–720.

Dutra, L., Stathopoulou, G., Basden, S. L., Leyro, T. M., Powers, M. B., & Otto, M. W. (2008). A meta-analytic review of psychosocial interventions for substance use disorders. *American Journal of Psychiatry, 165,* 179–187.

Fairburn, C. G., Cooper, Z., Doll, H. A., O'Connor, M. E., Bohn, K., Hawker, D. M., et al. (2009). Transdiagnostic cognitive-behavioral therapy for patients with eating disorders: A two-site trial with 60-week follow-up. *American Journal Psychiatry, 166,* 311–319.

Farrell, L. J., Schlup, B., & Boschen, M. J. (2010). Cognitive-behavioral treatment of child-hood obsessive-compulsive disorder in community-based clinical practice: Clinical significance and benchmarking against efficacy. *Behavior Research and Therapy, 48*, 409–417.

Feeny, N. C., Zoellner, L. A., Mavissakalian, M. R., & Roy-Byrne, P. P. (2009). What would you choose? Sertraline or prolonged exposure in community and PTSD treatment seek-ing women. *Depression and Anxiety, 26*, 724–731.

Franklin, M. E., Abramowitz, J. S., Kozak, M. J., Levitt, J. T., & Foa, E. B. (2000). Effectiveness of exposure and ritual prevention for obsessive-compulsive disorder: Randomized compared with nonrandomized samples. *Journal of Consulting and Clinical Psychology, 68*, 594–602.

Goisman, R. M., Warshaw, M. G., & Keller, M. B. (1999). Psychosocial treatment prescrip-tions for generalized anxiety disorder, panic disorder and social phobia, 1991-1996. *American Journal of Psychiatry, 156*, 1819-1821.

Haas, H. L., & Clopton, J. R. (2003). Comparing clinical and research treatments for eating disorders. *International Journal of Eating Disorders, 33*, 412–420.

Hazlett-Stevens, H., Craske, M. G., Roy-Byrne, P. P., Sherbourne, C. D., Stein, M. B., & Bystritsky, A. (2002). Predictors of willingness to consider medication and psychosocial treatment for panic disorder in primary care patients. *General Hospital Psychiatry, 24*, 316–321.

Henggeler, S. W. (2004). Decreasing effect sizes for effectiveness studies-implications for the transport of evidence-based treatments: Comment on Curtis, Ronan, and Borduin (2004). *Journal of Family Psychology, 18*, 420–423.

Henggeler, S. W., Melton, G. B., Brondino, M. J., Scherer, D. G., & Hanley, J. H. (1997). Multisystemic therapy with violent and chronic juvenile offenders and their families: The role of treatment fidelity in successful dissemination. *Journal of Consulting and Clinical Psychology, 65*, 821–833.

Hofmann, S. G., Barlow, D. H., Papp, L. A., Betweiler, M. D., Ray, S. E., Shear, M. K., et al. (1998). Pretreatment attrition in a comparative treatment outcome study on panic disorder. *American Journal of Psychiatry, 155*, 43–47.

Hofmann, S. G., & Smits, J. A. J. (2008). Cognitive-behavioral therapy for adult anxiety disorders: A meta-analysis of randomized placebo-controlled trials. *Journal of Clinical Psychiatry, 69*, 621–632.

Houghton, S., Saxon, D., Bradburn, M., Ricketts, T., & Hardy, G. (2009). The effectiveness of routinely delivered cognitive behavioural therapy for obsessive-compulsive disorder: A benchmarking study. *British Journal of Clinical Psychology, 49*, 473–489.

Institute of Medicine. (2001). *Crossing the quality chasm: A new health system for the 21st Century*. Washington, DC: Author.

Kazdin, A. E. (2008). Evidence-based treatments and delivery of psychological services: Shifting our emphases to increase impact. *Psychological Services, 5*, 201–215.

Keller, M. B., McCullough, J. P., Klein, D. N., Arnow, B., Dunner, D. L., Gelenberg, A. J., et al. (2000). A comparison of nefazodone, the cognitive behavioral-analysis system of psychotherapy, and their combination for the treatment of chronic depression. *New England Journal of Medicine, 342*, 1462–1470.

Linehan, M. M., Comtois, K. A., Murray, A. M., Brown, M. Z., Gallop, R. J., Heard, H. L., et al. (2006). Two-year randomized controlled trial and follow-up of dialectical behavior therapy vs therapy by experts for suicidal behaviors and borderline personality disorder. *Archives of General Psychiatry, 63*, 757–766.

Luborsky, L., & DeRubeis, R. J. (1984). The use of psychotherapy treatment manuals: A small revolution in psychotherapy research style. *Clinical Psychology Review, 4*, 5–14.

Luborsky, L., Singer, B., & Luborsky, L. (1975). Comparative studies of psychotherapies: Is it true that 'everybody has won and all must have prizes?' *Archives of General Psychiatry, 32*, 996–1008.

McHugh, R. K., & Barlow, D. H. (2010). Dissemination and implementation of evidence-based psychological interventions: A review of current efforts. *American Psychologist, 65*, 73–84.

McHugh, R. K., Murray, H. W., & Barlow, D. H. (2009). Balancing fidelity and adaptation in the dissemination of empirically-supported treatments: The promise of transdiagnostic interventions. *Behaviour Research and Therapy, 47*, 946–953.

McHugh, R. K., Otto, M. W., Barlow, D. H., Gorman, J. M., Shear, M. K., & Woods, S. W. (2007). Cost-efficacy of individual and combined treatments for panic disorder. *Journal of Clinical Psychiatry, 68*, 1038–1044.

McHugh, R. K., Whitton, S. W., Peckham, A. D., Welge, J. A., & Otto, M. W. (2011). Patient preference for for the treatment of psychiatric disorders: A meta-analytic review. Manuscript under editorial review.

Miklowitz, D. J., & Scott, J. (2009). Psychosocial treatments for bipolar disorder: Cost-effectiveness, mediating mechanisms, and future directions. *Bipolar Disorders, 11*(Suppl. 2), 110–122.

Mitchell, J. E., Pyle, R. L., Eckert, E. D., Hatsukami, D., Pomeroy, C., & Zimmerman, R. (1990). A comparison study of antidepressants and structuring intensive group psychotherapy in the treatment of bulimia nervosa. *Archives of General Psychiatry, 47*, 149–157.

Morrison, A. P., Renton, J. C., Williams, S., Dunn, H., Knight, A., Kreutz, M., et al. (2004). Delivering cognitive therapy to people with psychosis in a community mental health setting: An effectiveness study. *Acta Psychiatrica Scandinavica, 110*, 36–44.

Mussell, M. P., Crosby, R. D., Crow, S. J., Knopke, A. J., Peterson, C. B., Wonderlich, S. A., et al. (2000). Utilization of empirically supported psychotherapy treatments for individuals with eating disorders: A survey of psychologists. *International Journal of Eating Disorders, 27*, 230–237.

Nathan, P. E., & Gorman, J. M. (Eds.). (2007). *A guide to treatments that work* (3rd ed.). New York, NY: Oxford University Press.

Norcross, J. C., Hogan, T. P., & Koocher, G. P. (2008). *Clinician's guide to evidence-based practices: Mental health and the addictions.* New York, NY: Oxford University Press.

Pagoto, S. L., Spring, B., Coups, E. J., Mulvaney, S., Coutu, M. F., & Ozakinci, G. (2007). Barriers and facilitators of evidence-based practice perceived by behavioral science health professionals. *Journal of Clinical Psychology, 63*, 695–705.

Persons, J. B., Bostrom, A., & Bertagnolli, A. (1999). Results of randomized controlled trials of cognitive therapy for depression generalize to private practice. *Cognitive Therapy and Research, 23*, 535–548.

Phillips, K. M., & Brandon, T. H. (2004). Do psychologists adhere to the clinical practice guidelines for tobacco cessation? A survey of practitioners. *Professional Psychology: Research and Practice, 35*, 281–285.

President's New Freedom Commission on Mental Health. (2003). *Achieving the promise: Transforming mental health care in America.* Retrieved October 12, 2011, from http://govinfo.library.unt.edu/mentalhealthcommission/reports/reports.htm

Roth, A., & Fonagy, P. (2005). *What works for whom? A critical review of psychotherapy research.* New York, NY: Guilford Press.

Roy-Byrne, P. P., Craske, M. G., Stein, M. B., Sullivan, G., Bystritsky, A., Katon, W., et al. (2005). A randomized effectiveness trial of cognitive-behavioral therapy and medication for primary care panic disorder. *Archives of General Psychiatry, 62,* 290–298.

Sackett, D. L., Straus, S. E., Richardson, W. S., Rosenberg, W., & Haynes, R. B. (2000). *Evidence-based medicine: How to practice and teach EBM* (3rd ed.). Edinburgh, England, & New York, NY: Churchill Livingstone.

Safren, S. A., Sprich, S., Mimiaga, M. J., Surman, C., Knouse, L., Groves, M., et al. (2010). Cognitive behavioral therapy vs relaxation with educational support for medication-treated adults with ADHD and persistent symptoms: A randomized controlled trial. *Journal of the American Medical Association, 304,* 875–880.

Santa Ana, E. J., Martino, S., Ball, S. A., Nich, C., Frankforter, T. L., & Carroll, K. M. (2008). What is usual about "treatment-as-usual"? Data from two multisite effectiveness trials. *Journal of Substance Abuse Treatment, 35,* 369–379.

Silverman, W. K., Pina, A. A., & Viswesvaran, C. (2008). Evidence-based psychosocial treatments for phobic and anxiety disorders in children and adolescents. *Journal of Clinical Child and Adolescent Psychology, 37,* 105–130.

Spring, B. (2007). Evidence-based practice in clinical psychology: What it is, why it matters; what you need to know. *Journal of Clinical Psychology, 63,* 611–631.

Stewart, R. E., & Chambless, D. L. (2007). Does psychotherapy research inform treatment decision in private practice? *Journal of Clinical Psychology, 63,* 267–281.

Stirman, S. W., Crits-Christoph, P., & DeRubeis, R. J. (2004). Achieving successful dissemination of empirically supported psychotherapies: A synthesis of dissemination theory. *Clinical Psychology: Science and Practice, 11,* 343–359.

Stuart, G. L., Treat, T. A., & Wade, W. A. (2000). Effectiveness of an empirically based treatment for panic disorder delivered in a service clinic setting: 1-year follow-up. *Journal of Consulting and Clinical Psychology, 68,* 506–512.

U.S. Department of Health and Human Services. (1999). *Mental health: A report of the Surgeon General.* Rockville, MD: Author.

van Schaik, D. J., Klijn, A. F., van Hout, H. P., van Marwijk, H. W., Beekman, A. T., de Haan, M., et al. (2004). Patients' preferences in the treatment of depressive disorder in primary care. *General Hospital Psychiatry, 26,* 184–189.

Weissman, M. M., Verdeli, H., Gameroff, M. J., Beldsoe, S. E., Betts, K., Mufson, L., et al. (2006). National survey of psychotherapy training in psychiatry, psychology, and social work. *Archives of General Psychiatry, 63,* 925–934.

Weisz, J. R., Jenson-Doss, A., & Hawley, K. M. (2006). Evidence-based youth psychotherapies versus usual clinical care. *American Psychologist, 61,* 671–689.

Westbrook, D., & Kirk, J. (2005). The clinical effectiveness of cognitive behaviour therapy: Outcome for a large sample of adults treated in routine practice. *Behaviour Research and Therapy, 43,* 1243–1261.

Wolpe, J. (1969). *The practice of behavior therapy.* New York, NY: Pergamon.

Woody, S. R., Weisz, J., & McLean, C. (2005). Empirically supported treatments: 10 years later. *The Clinical Psychologist, 58*, 5–11.

Young, A. S., Klap, R., Sherbourne, C. D., & Wells, K. B. (2001). The quality of care for depressive and anxiety disorders in the United States. *Archives of General Psychiatry, 58*, 55–61.

The Science of Dissemination and Implementation
Sonja K. Schoenwald, R. Kathryn McHugh, and David H. Barlow

Achieving successful uptake of an innovation is not a challenge unique to mental health care or even health care more generally. As the dissemination and implementation of evidence-based psychological interventions is in its relative infancy, the process of developing, testing, and refining effective procedures that reliably facilitate the dissemination and implementation of effective interventions will be enriched by consideration of models drawn from other industries and disciplines. Since 2000, several groups of authors have described and synthesized some of the theoretical frameworks underlying these models and their relevance to research designed to increase the systematic use of effective psychological interventions (see Schoenwald & Hoagwood, 2001; Simpson & Flynn, 2007; Southam-Gerow, Austin, & Marder, 2008; Stirman, Crits-Christoph, & De Rubeis, 2004). Heuristic models of dimensions of the intervention and practice context hypothesized to influence the effectiveness, dissemination, and/or implementation of evidence-based psychological interventions have also been presented (Schoenwald, Kelleher, Weisz, & the Research Network on Youth Mental Health, 2008; Southam-Gerow et al., 2008). In this chapter, we aim to familiarize readers with key constructs from the dominant theories, conceptual frameworks, and heuristic models increasingly informing research on facilitation of the systematic use of evidence-based psychological treatments in routine care. We also highlight factors associated with dissemination or implementation in other fields and, where available, in mental health, and summarize what is known about strategies to support dissemination or implementation. This chapter will serve as a framework for subsequent chapters describing efforts specific to the dissemination and implementation of psychological interventions.

WORKING DEFINITIONS

Prior to reviewing these theories and their application to mental health care, it is necessary to clarify relevant definitions. Indeed, the terminology used in this area has been inconsistent and complicated by the heterogeneity of the industries and disciplines from which it is drawn. *Diffusion* refers to the naturally occurring process of information spread and was the topic of early attempts to characterize the process by which innovations were adopted. Research on the *dissemination* of mental health care interventions has been described as addressing "how information about mental health care interventions is created, packaged, transmitted, and interpreted among various important stakeholder groups," while "research on *implementation* includes a focus on the level to which mental health interventions can fit within real world mental health service systems" (Chambers, Ringeisen, & Hickman, 2005, p. 313). Recent National Institutes of Health research funding announcements note implementation research examines "the use of socio-behavioral strategies to adopt, integrate and scale-up evidence-based health interventions and change practice patterns within specific settings," and, once an intervention is implemented, "implementation research can address whether health interventions are *sustained* in regular, on-going practice and whether they are responsible for public health changes through methods such as impact evaluations" (National Institutes of Health, 2009). These definitions bring clarity to the vagaries of the concepts of diffusion, dissemination, and implementation originally described and investigated in the context of academic disciplines and industries outside of health and mental health. These definitions are not, however, uniformly endorsed within the still-fledgling arena of dissemination and implementation science in treatment and services research; they also, as illustrated in this chapter, vary in the disciplines and literatures from which they are drawn.

DIFFUSION AND DISSEMINATION

Models of diffusion and dissemination emanate from different industries and disciplines and have developed over years of study since early diffusion theorists such as Gabriel Tarde (1903) and George Simmel (1908). Next, we describe some of the major conceptual models of diffusion and dissemination that have emanated from different theories: adopter-based theories, socio-technical theories of technology transfer, social marketing theories, basic behavioral science theories, and other integrated theories. Where available, we discuss applications of these approaches to increasing the use of evidence-based psychological interventions in routine care.

Adopter-Based Theories

Adopter-based theories predominated early research on diffusion (e.g., Tarde, 1903) and focused on factors that influence an individual's or group's decision to adopt an innovation. Although all of the theories reviewed in this chapter acknowledge the importance of potential adopters, the two reviewed in this section—Rogers'

Diffusion of Innovations theory (2003) and Brown's model of diffusion (1995)—
place specific emphasis on the adopter as the core element of their model.

Diffusion of Innovations Theory

Diffusion of Innovations theory (Rogers, 2003) has become arguably the most
influential model of dissemination across fields, including mental health (see Miller,
Sorensen, Selzer, & Brigham, 2006; Stirman et al., 2004). Rogers constructed this
theory through consolidation of research and theory from disparate fields such as
agriculture, communication, and sociology. The four main elements of the diffusion
process according to Diffusion of Innovations theory are (a) the innovation itself,
(b) communication channels, (c) time, and (d) the social system. These processes are
described below.

(a). The adopter focus of Diffusion of Innovations theory is best illustrated
in Rogers' description of five attributes of an innovation that appear to
affect the rate of its adoption. An innovation's relevance is defined by
characteristics as *perceived* by potential adopters. Adopter perceptions of
an innovation are hypothesized to contribute substantially to the rate of
adoption, and in some cases are estimated to predict well over half of the
variance in adoption rates (Rogers, 2003, p. 221). Relevant perceptions of
an innovation are categorized as the *advantages* of the innovation relative
to alternatives; its *compatibility* with the adopter's beliefs, needs, and
experiences; its *complexity*; the opportunity to *try* the innovation before
deciding to adopt; and the degree to which it is *observable* or visible.
In addition to perceptions of an innovation, Rogers argues that the
adaptability of an innovation also is related to adoption. Specifically,
the greater the potential for adaptation of an innovation to better fit
the adopter, the more likely adoption is to occur.

(b). Communication is the process by which information about an
innovation reaches potential adopters. The communication channels by
which information is transmitted are another key component of the
dissemination process. Rogers (2003) suggests that peer communication
is most effective for influencing adoption decisions, whereas mass
media (or other broad-based strategies) are effective for quickly creating
widespread general knowledge about or visibility of an innovation.
Understanding the transmission of information throughout social
networks provides information to facilitate communication about an
innovation. For example, the identification and education of opinion
leaders—individuals within a system who are well connected and may
have particular influence over the attitudes and behaviors of others—has
been used successfully as an intervention for introducing information to
a social system such as the dangers of tobacco use (Valente, Hoffman,
Ritt-Olson, Lichtman, & Johnson, 2003) and HIV prevention

(Sikkema et al., 2000). In addition to the importance of the messenger, the content of messages is also important.

(c). Rogers (2003) describes three elements of dissemination that relate to time: the innovation-decision process, the degree to which an individual or group tends to adopt innovations earlier or later (i.e., innovativeness), and the rate of an innovation's adoption. The innovation-decision process involves stages of gaining knowledge about an innovation, the development of an opinion about the innovation (persuasion), the decision to initiate behavior to adopt or not adopt the innovation (e.g., gathering information or trying an innovation), the use of the new innovation (implementation), and confirmation or reinforcement of the decision (e.g., evaluating pros and cons, communicating with others), leading to a decision whether or not to adopt the innovation.

Some individuals or groups tend to be more innovative and risk taking in adopting new innovations, whereas others tend to be more conservative and adopt later (or not at all) once the innovation has been further vetted. Rogers emphasizes the importance of targeting different adopter groups at different stages of dissemination to maximize success. For example, early efforts may benefit from targeting earlier adopter groups (who may be easier to convince), who can then facilitate communication back to later adopter groups. The rate of the adoption of an innovation is influenced by how quickly more moderate adopter groups elect to adopt. Rogers describes that the rate of adoption often takes the form of an "S-shaped" curve, characterized by slow early adoption, followed by an increased slope, and finally a decrease in the slope as the rate of adoption slows.

(d). The final component of Rogers' theory—the social system—can influence the innovation-decision process depending on the degree to which individual decisions are made independently or by a system. For example, organizations are often the unit making the decision to adopt. In mental health care, this could be a single facility, a group of facilities, or a larger system such as a state mental health care system. As such, the contribution of individual providers to the decision to adopt a new intervention varies widely. Given the importance of individuals within the system to the ultimate utilization of an intervention, ensuring that representatives from relevant stakeholder groups (e.g., upper and lower management, providers, patients/families, community leaders) are contributing to the decision is of particular importance. Moreover, adoption has consequences for the social system as a whole that can influence the system in both intended (e.g., improving productivity) and unintended (e.g., increasing social gaps or disparities) ways. This implication for systems further highlights the importance of considering the range of stakeholders potentially impacted by a decision to adopt an innovation.

Brown's Model of Diffusion

Another adopter-based model that underscores the importance of perceptions of an innovation was described by Brown (1995). Brown identified six relevant perceptions of an innovation influencing the utilization of empirical evidence to inform intervention in drug abuse service provision settings. These include relevance (the degree to which the intervention is a good fit to the particular goals and needs of a system), timeliness (the timing of the intervention relative to the ability of a facility to make the decision to adopt), clarity (the degree to which the information is accessible to and can be understood by relevant consumers), credibility (credibility of the innovation and the person/group communicating about the innovation), replicability (the degree to which an innovation tested in a research setting can achieve similar results and can be feasibly implemented in a setting given its particular structure, funding, and resources), and acceptability (the degree to which the intervention is desirable to stakeholders). Brown (1995) refers to the traditional dissemination strategy of academia—peer-reviewed journals—as a particularly inaccessible and ineffective communication strategy.

Socio-Technical Technology Transfer Theories

The socio-technical theory of technology transfer emphasizes the importance of both the innovation ("content") and social factors ("context") in the dissemination of an innovation. Socio-technical theory differs somewhat from adopter-based models in its emphasis on the context of innovation adoption, but also embodies some constructs similar to those found in adopter-based models. For example, socio-technical theory posits that "boundary spanners" (Aldrich & Herker, 1977)—individuals and organizations familiar with both a specific innovation and the individuals, groups, and organizations in the context targeted for adoption— facilitate adoption; and adopter-based theories posit that social networks or opinion leaders facilitate adoption. Socio-technical theory has been used by organizational researchers to explain the successful (or unsuccessful) implementation of new technologies and emphasizes that the organizations, and sometimes communities, implementing a new technology are as important as the innovation and the individual user to determining the success of the innovation (Rousseau, 1977; Trist, 1985). Socio-technical and adopter-based theories share a conceptualization of innovation adoption as a social process, and one that is likely to be iterative and to involve individual and organizational consumers of the innovation. They differ in the extent to which they emphasize the relative importance to adoption of the end-user and the organizational or community context in which the user is embedded (Berg, Aarts, & van der Lei, 2003). The notions that innovation adoption involves (a) interaction, and even collaboration, among potential adopters, innovation developers, and testers and (b) the work context in which the adopter operates represented a conceptual shift away from dissemination theories that placed more emphasis on the individual adopter as a receiver of innovations in isolation from the context in which the innovation is used. Conceptualizing innovation dissemination as an interactive process that occurs in a work context has been emphasized in mental health care to shift away from unidirectional models of dissemination from "research to practice" (e.g., Chorpita & Nakamura, 2004).

In a review of the behavioral science knowledge base on technology transfer for the National Institute on Drug Abuse, Backer, David, and Soucy (1995) identified four necessary conditions for successful technology transfer: (a) awareness of and access to the relevant information, (b) evidence for the ultimate success of the innovation (including transportability, system readiness, and successful outcomes), (c) available resources, and (d) interventions to overcome barriers to adoption. This review drew from both adopter-based and socio-technical theories to present a model for technology transfer in addictions treatment. Based on the available literature, Backer and colleagues (1995) highlighted six key strategies to success including direct contact between potential adopters and innovation experts, careful planning for adoption, consultation on change, provision of information relevant to the adopter (most notably, whether it will work), presence of opinion leaders and innovation champions, and stakeholder involvement in planning.

Social Marketing Theories

Social marketing involves the application of traditional marketing strategies to public concerns (Andreason, 1995), is adopter oriented, and emphasizes the importance of using messages tailored to specific adopter groups. Social marketing also draws heavily from basic behavioral models (described below). Originally focused primarily on ideas and knowledge related to public concerns (e.g., public health advertising campaigns), the scope of social marketing grew to include medical and social service innovations (Backer & Marston, 1993). Social marketing strategies tailor information and activities related to the knowledge, product, or service of interest to the attitudes, beliefs, and behaviors of distinct groups of potential consumers. The social marketing process is grounded in traditional marketing principles, such as audience segmentation, the "four Ps" (product, price, place, and promotion), and competition (Grier & Bryant, 2005). These approaches emphasize piloting developed materials and conducting continuous monitoring and evaluation to inform efforts. Audience segmentation—consisting of dividing potential consumers into groups based on similarities and then targeting messages to each group—provides a strategy for making messages relevant and accessible to heterogeneous stakeholder groups.

Social marketing approaches have been effective as strategies for disseminating information on varied public health agendas, such as efforts to improve health behaviors (see Grier & Bryant, 2005). An example of the social marketing approach in mental health was reported in a case study of disseminating two evidence-based psychological interventions for substance abuse (Martin, Herie, Turner, & Cunningham, 1998). This effort involved (a) the development of an advisory committee consisting of heterogeneous stakeholder groups to identify system needs, build support for the effort, and begin to recruit champions for later stages of the effort; (b) in the audience segmentation stage, using results from the planning analysis to identify the intervention that would best fit each target group (e.g., the early intervention program was selected for sites that were more likely to serve patients in earlier stages of substance misuse and abuse); and (c) collecting pilot data at trial sites that were then shared with other potential adopter sites. Results of the case study were promising, with more than 70% of sites deciding to offer the treatment 1 year following training and more than 80% of sites trying the intervention at some point (defined as offering the full intervention to at least one patient). These results were then fed back to each of the sites to discuss strategies for maintaining commitment to the intervention.

Basic Behavioral Science Theories

Behavioral science theories posit models of how information, beliefs, and motivation influence decisions and change behavior. Accordingly, these theories provide a framework for examining the behavioral elements of dissemination and implementation, such as the decision to adopt, initiating adoption, and maintaining adoption. Focusing on the behavior of individuals and on factors influencing individual decision making, these models are reminiscent of adopter-based theories. Some examples of basic behavioral science theories include the theory of reasoned action (TRA; Fishbein & Ajzen, 1975) and the related theory of planned behavior (TPB; Ajzen, 1991), social cognitive theory (Bandura, 1986), and the theory of interpersonal behavior (Triandis, 1980). In a review of prospective and cross-sectional studies of the application of behavioral theories (including those listed above) to clinician behaviors and behavioral intentions, the strongest predictor of behavior was TRA/TPB (Godin, Belanger-Gravel, Eccles, & Grimshaw, 2008). TRA/TPB predicted 25% to 34% of the variance in behavior in prospective studies, and 59% of the variance in behavioral intentions in cross-sectional studies. These findings suggest TRA/TPB theories may be particularly applicable to dissemination efforts in health care; however, experimental designs are needed to further evaluate these associations.

TRA/TPB posits that behavioral intentions (and the factors that influence them) are the most important predictor of actual behavior. These theories emphasize three factors that contribute to behavioral intentions: (a) expected value of the behavior, (b) perception of the behavior relative to social norms, and (c) self-efficacy to engage in the behavior. Studies of TRA/TPB as applied to clinician behavior suggest that expected value is most consistently associated with behavioral intentions, but that the relative importance of the three contributors to intentions varies across samples (Perkins et al., 2007).

Because they identify specific factors influencing individual behavior, basic behavioral theories are particularly promising for developing interventions to change behavior. Perkins and colleagues (2007) suggest that TRA/TPB could be used as framework for dissemination efforts by targeting the predictor of behavioral intention (i.e., expected value, norms, and self-efficacy) that is most relevant to the adopter group (e.g., using informational interventions to increase expected value). The ongoing Ontario Printed Education Materials (OPEM) trial—a study of the effect of distribution of printed materials to physicians on adoption of evidence-based practices (see Zwarenstein et al., 2007)—developed both non–model-driven materials (a "standard" message) and materials based on the TPB model to test whether using a theory-derived message would better facilitate behavior change (Francis et al., 2007). The evaluation of this and similar application of behavioral theories to dissemination strategies is needed.

Other Dissemination Theories

Given the relevance of dissemination to varied industries and disciplines, a number of models—and models that integrate aspects of several models—have been posited to explain how dissemination occurs. For example, the Community Organization Model (Bracht, Kingsbury, & Rissel, 1999) is similar to social marketing approaches, but places greater emphasis on a community-based approach in which demonstration sites are emphasized as means to spread an innovation within the community. The five steps of this model are (a) community analysis and assessment, (b) design and initiation, (c) implementation, (d) program maintenance, and (e) dissemination and reassessment. This model emphasizes collaborative partnerships in which investigators work within communities as team members (instead of serving as outside experts bringing a product to the community). Such community partnerships are consistent with other models emphasizing stakeholder group involvement as a core element of successful dissemination.

Several attempts to integrate existing dissemination theories have been made in recent years. For example, Simpson and Flynn (2007) described the revised Texas Christian University (TCU) Program Change Model, which incorporates elements of both dissemination and implementation, with a focus on organizational characteristics influencing change. Within this model the decision to adopt a treatment requires leadership support, quality and utility of the innovation, and adaptability of the innovation. The decision process includes a trial period in which further attitudes toward adoption and development as well as barriers are assessed. Organizational behavior models of implementation are described in more detail below.

Testing Dissemination Strategies

Despite the publication of several commentaries on dissemination theories applied to mental health care (e.g., Miller et al., 2006; Stirman et al., 2004), the systematic testing of models of dissemination and empirical investigation of dissemination strategies have yet to occur on a large scale. The Fairweather Lodge experiment (Fairweather, Sanders, & Tornatzky, 1974) is an early all-too-rare example of an attempt to experimentally evaluate the proactive dissemination of a psychological intervention. The Lodge experiment prospectively examined three strategies to disseminate an alternative to psychiatric hospitalization for adults, all of which had demonstrated promise in a randomized trial. Although significant methodological problems complicate efforts to draw clear conclusions from the study, the original study design was clear: three distinct methods of persuading hospitals to establish a lodge for mentally ill adult patients were deployed; hospitals were randomly assigned to receive one of these methods; and moves to adopt the model were tracked. The three dissemination strategies varied the information and persuasion activities offered to hospital administrators and staff. Nonetheless, fewer than 10% of hospitals attempted to adopt the Lodge model, and many of these did so incompletely.

More recent examples include a randomized trial conducted by Atkins and colleagues (2008) to evaluate the dissemination of recommended practices for teacher management of attention-deficit/hyperactivity disorder in children in school settings. Schools were randomly assigned to either a key opinion leader ($n = 6$) or comparison condition ($n = 4$) to evaluate the influence of teacher opinion leaders on the decision of other teachers to adopt recommended practices through consultation with mental health professionals. Schools in which key opinion leaders were recruited reported greater use of recommended management strategies relative to schools without opinion leaders. This study provided support for the use of key opinion leaders as a strategy for facilitating dissemination strategies and is consistent with studies in medicine supporting the effectiveness of opinion leaders (see Doumit, Gattellari, Grimshaw, & O'Brien, 2007; Lomas et al., 1991); however, the effectiveness of this strategy remains unclear (see implementation section below).

Lock and Kaner (2000) tested social marketing strategies to disseminate a screening and brief intervention program for alcohol misuse to general practitioners in the United Kingdom. General practitioners ($N = 729$) were randomized to one of three marketing strategies: postal marketing, telemarketing, and personal marketing. Results indicated that the postal marketing strategy was least successful in subsequent adoption. Despite yielding the highest adoption rate, the personal marketing strategy was less cost-effective than the telemarketing strategy because of its higher cost. This study highlights the need for consideration of not only effectiveness but also cost-effectiveness of interventions in dissemination research.

In contrast to the experimental studies just described, most dissemination studies in mental health have been correlational, naturalistic, or quasiexperimental in nature. Several of these studies have demonstrated associations between key dissemination concepts and adoption of treatment practices. For example, Bartholomew and colleagues (2007) reported a positive association between perceived relevance of a treatment and organizational support/organizational climate on decisions to adopt substance abuse interventions following a training workshop. Another example is the program developed by the Addiction Technology Transfer Center called the Science to Service Laboratory. This program builds upon many of the central tenets of dissemination theories (particularly Rogers' model) including targeting perceptions of treatment innovations, identifying champions within organizations, and planning with organizations to overcome barriers to adoption and implementation, among others (see Squires, Gumbley, & Storti, 2008). More than 90% of sites involved in training for contingency management report successfully adopting and implementing the intervention. Such studies provide valuable information about the application of proactive dissemination strategies informed by different theories of diffusion and technology transfer. Rigorous testing using experimental rather than correlational designs will be critical to understanding which theory of dissemination or model that integrates diverse theories best advances the dissemination and implementation of effective mental health services.

IMPLEMENTATION

Just as effective strategies can be used to disseminate effective or ineffective products or services (including treatments), so, too, the implementation of an effective product or service can range from effective to ineffective. The study of innovation has a long history in organizational research; and, within the last two decades, implementation failure (rather than innovation failure) has increasingly been scrutinized as a factor underlying an organization's inability to achieve the intended benefits of an adopted innovation (Klein & Sorra, 1996). Among motivating factors for the increased attention to innovation implementation was evidence that, for example, only a small fraction of studies (as few as 4 of 99) of the effects of managerial interventions actually assessed the degree to which the intervention was implemented (Hackman & Wageman, 1995). Indeed, one organizational scholar argued well before this discovery that it is more important to know what an organization *does* than what it *decided* to do (Wolfe, 1994). This proposition is consistent with prominent models of the diffusion of innovation among individuals, in which adoption is conceptualized as a decision, while implementation is conceptualized behaviorally (Rogers, 2003).

Organizational Research on Implementation

A comprehensive review of the conceptualization and measurement of implementation in organizational research (Real & Poole, 2005) suggests that theories of implementation can be categorized in terms of two dichotomies: (a) variance and process theories and (b) a fixed and adaptive nature of innovation. An adaptive innovation is designed to be malleable. Examples include product innovations such as groupware, in which parameters and functions are tailored to different user groups, and process innovations that do not have widely accepted formats, such as voluntary participation employee assistance programs. A fixed innovation is one considered to be a mostly stable program or process to be put into effect. Examples include product innovations such as a spreadsheet software program for individual use, and process innovations such as Total Quality Management that are formulaic and relatively mature in their development and testing. In the fixed-variance approach, implementation is defined as an outcome—the degree to which the innovation is used as intended at the outset. For innovations to be used by individuals, such as the spreadsheet software, the proportion of potential users is a frequent indicator of the effectiveness of implementation. For organizational innovations, such as re-engineering initiatives or continuous quality improvement systems, implementation is often measured as the degree to which the innovation is assimilated as intended into the organization. Phrases such as implementation "roll-out" reflect the fixed-variance conceptualization of implementation. The variance perspective gives rise to definitions of implementation such as the "transition period during which targeted organizational members ideally become increasingly skillful, consistent, and committed in their use of an innovation" (Klein & Sorra, 1996, p. 1057). The majority of implementation research in the organizational literature flows from this conceptualization. This research aims to identify organizational factors that are critical to implementation success (e.g., top management support, centralization, formalization, size, absorptive capacity, user–designer relationships), as summarized in several reviews accessible to readers who are not organizational research experts (see, e.g., Damanpour, 1991, 1996).

Several conceptual models of implementation have been developed on the basis of theory, research, and experience in such diverse arenas as agriculture, business, the military, and medicine. With few exceptions, empirical validation of implementation models is rare. Klein and colleagues (e.g., Klein, Conn, & Sorra, 2001) have found evidence to support relations among several factors and the successful implementation of advanced technology processes and in industry. These factors are (a) the quality and quantity of training, including ongoing technical assistance as needed, rewards for usage, and user-friendliness; (b) positive team or organizational climate; (c) managerial support; (d) financial resources; (e) organizational learning orientation that supports staff skill development, competence, and growth; and (f) patience in enduring short-term stumbling blocks to reach stable and enduring performance gains. Relatively little is known, however, about the extent to which these factors generalize to the implementation of evidence-based psychological treatments in routine clinical care and, conversely, the extent to which factors and processes perceived as unique to the content, process, and practice contexts of psychological treatments in general, or to a particular treatment, affect their implementation and outcomes (Schoenwald & Hoagwood, 2001).

Accordingly, the following sections of this chapter represent a sort of "successive approximation" approach to mapping the implementation literature developed in other industries and academic disciplines onto the enterprise of mental health care and the treatment and services research designed to improve the effectiveness of that care. First, key constructs and findings from research on the implementation of health care are summarized. Then, recently proposed heuristic models of implementation in substance abuse and mental health services are identified, as are examples of findings from studies supporting linkages among elements in these models. Finally, examples are provided of research testing the effects on implementation and outcomes of strategies that manipulate one or more of these elements.

Implementation Research in Health Care

A decade ago, to stimulate the effective implementation of evidence-based medicine, Richard Grol and Jeremy Grimshaw wrote a cogent review of the theoretical perspectives underlying strategies to support such implementation and the evidence regarding the effectiveness of these strategies (Grol & Grimshaw, 1999). The authors identified seven distinct theoretical approaches—educational, epidemiologic, marketing, behaviorist, social influence, organizational, and coercive—and lessons for implementation emanating from each. For example, a behaviorist perspective posits most people seek reinforcement and rewards (e.g., feedback), and thus begets strategies such as practical tools and reminders to make life easier for a target group, whereas an organizational approach holds that the practice setting (i.e., leadership, teamwork, resources, the structure of work) can be a major barrier to implementation, and that strategies to restructure care processes and build innovation into routines are needed. A social influence perspective holds that respected peers are a potential resource to promote the implementation of an innovation, whereas a marketing approach emphasizes the importance of tailoring the message about the innovation, if not the innovation itself, to the needs and perspectives of distinct target groups. Grol and Grimshaw proposed a practical, five-stage framework for changing the practice of medicine to more effectively implement assessment and treatment strategies with empirical evidence of effectiveness. The framework included development of a concrete proposal for change; analysis of the target setting and group to identify obstacles to change; linking interventions to needs, facilitators, and obstacles to change; development of an implementation plan; and monitoring progress with implementation.

Two years later, an overview of 41 systematic reviews of interventions designed to support "professional behavior change interventions" in medicine published prior to 1998 suggested evidence was mixed regarding the various steps in this framework (Grimshaw et al., 2001). The review reaffirmed that passive approaches, such as distribution to practitioners of information about a particular procedure or practice, are generally ineffective in producing behavior change, and noted most other interventions are effective under some circumstances, while none are effective in all circumstances. Specifically, educational outreach approaches such as the use of reminders influenced relatively simple professional behaviors, such as medication-prescribing practices, but only if the prompts did not focus on routine procedures and there were not too many of them. On the other hand, there was no evidence that consensus-based educational approaches (i.e., professionals coming together to tailor guidelines to their local practice conditions) improved implementation of evidence-based guidelines.

More recently, meta-analyses conducted by the Cochrane Collaboration suggest additional nuances. For example, across 15 studies of interventions tailored to context-specific barriers to innovation implementation, results were inconsistent, and there were unanswered questions about the validity of the data on barriers and the extent to which the most significant barriers were targeted by the interventions (Shaw et al., 2005). With respect to the influence of opinion leaders, on the other hand, a substantial number of randomized trials found favorable results with respect to fairly straightforward practices (e.g., use of prescription guidelines), but the vast majority of these were conducted in hospital settings and pertained to physician influence on one another in such settings, thereby leaving open the question of the applicability of the findings to other settings, professionals, and practices (Doumit et al., 2007). A large number of randomized trials of audit and feedback interventions (interventions in which a summary of clinical performance with patients over a specified time is provided to physicians) showed small to moderate effects on physician compliance with a desired practice, with greater effects found for physicians having low baseline adherence to the practice and when the feedback was delivered more intensively (Jamtvedt, Young, Kristoffersen, O'Brien, & Oxman, 2006).

For more complex professional behaviors, multifaceted interventions may be needed, with, for example, coercive interventions (policies about funding, medical necessity requirements to authorize health care) providing a floor and ceiling for local and individual variations in a practice, and a combination of training, organizational strategies, and consumer preference, demand, and satisfaction supporting professional behavior change on the job (Ferlie & Shortell, 2001; Grimshaw et al., 2001; Schoenwald & Henggeler, 2004). Consistent with this proposition, Helfrich and colleagues considered the extent to which models of implementation focused primarily on the behavior of individuals would hold for the implementation in health care of "complex innovations—innovations requiring coordinated use by multiple organizational members" (Helfrich, Weiner, McKinney, & Minasian, 2007, p. 280). They proposed that for such innovations, select attributes of an innovation conceptualized in diffusion theory as pertinent to an individual's adoption of the innovation—namely, fit of the innovation with the practice and values of an individual adopter—could be reframed from an organizational perspective as the fit between the innovation and an organizational and professional mission. In their qualitative study of hospital and clinic implementation of new programs in cancer prevention and control, Helfrich and colleagues found support for the importance of organizational and managerial support, implementation policies and practices, and resources, as the authors had predicted on the basis of the Klein et al. model of implementation. In addition, the fit of the innovation with organizational needs, competencies, and experience was perceived as important to implementation of the new cancer prevention and control programs, a finding echoed in survey data obtained from directors of community-based mental health clinics that serve children (Schoenwald, Chapman et al., 2008). This notion that implementation models for innovations that are complex and require coordinated use by organizational members may differ somewhat from models of implementation for innovations that are less complex and can be carried out by an individual may be particularly pertinent to the design of research on the implementation of psychological interventions. As noted elsewhere (Schoenwald & Hoagwood, 2001), such interventions vary with respect to the degree to which adequate implementation may be accomplished by an individual clinician within previously established service delivery models (e.g., weekly outpatient hour) and organizational and funding structures—as might be the case, for example, in substituting an hour of cognitive-behavioral treatment for depression for an eclectic approach—and those for which implementation requires coordinated actions of team members and alternate models of service delivery and funding, such as Multidimensional Treatment Foster Care (MTFC; Chamberlain, 2003) or Multisystemic Therapy (MST; Henggeler, Schoenwald, Borduin, Rowland, & Cunningham, 2009).

The picture emerging thus far from experimental studies of strategies to facilitate practitioner implementation of technologies in health care (e.g., computerized feedback systems) and protocols or practices (medication algorithms, cancer care protocols) suggests that a kind of titration may be warranted of the intensity and complexity of the implementation strategy to the target behavior. When new practices are relatively complex and/or require conjoint changes in behavior of others within an organization, differentiated strategies may be needed to support implementation at different levels of the practice context. A related speculation is that different theories of technology transfer may align more or less well with the demand characteristics of different types of innovations. For example, the implementation of innovations a physician can execute in relative isolation (i.e., receiving computerized feedback on one's prescription patterns relative to established guidelines) may be effectively supported by strategies focused on adopter-based perceptions (diffusion theory) or adopter motivation and intention (TRA/TPB theory), while the implementation of innovations requiring collaboration and/or organizational accommodation, such as hip replacement surgery or HIV/AIDS management in patients, may require equal focus on the technology, organizational context of work, and individual adopter (socio-technical theory).

Emerging Conceptual Models of Evidence-Based
Treatment Implementation

As noted in the Introduction, mental health treatment and services researchers have increasingly focused on distilling those kernels most likely to pertain to the development of a research agenda from the array of fields and academic disciplines that have produced models and studies of the diffusion, dissemination, and implementation of innovations. Identification of these facts should speed progress toward the successful dissemination and implementation of effective psychological treatments (see, e.g., Fixsen, Naoom, Blase, Friedman, & Wallace, 2005; Schoenwald Kelleher, et al., 2008; Southam-Gerow et al., 2008). To models of implementation of evidence-based practices in mental health, Rhagavan and colleagues (Rhagavan, Bright, & Shadoin, 2008) have added a multilevel conceptualization of the role of policy in supporting implementation. Using examples from medicine and mental health, Rhagavan and colleagues illustrate how policies enacted at the organizational, regulatory and purchasing agency, political (i.e., legislative), and social levels can be more or less well aligned with the demand characteristics of effective implementation of evidence-based practices. One aspect of policy and policymaking not addressed in this conceptualization but potentially quite relevant to the establishment of policies to support the implementation of effective practices is the extent to which policymaking roles are influenced by empirical evidence. This factor has been identified as contributing to the favorable effectiveness of efforts to reduce tobacco use relative to those directed toward reducing violent crime (Biglan & Taylor, 2000). To wit: efforts to reduce tobacco control emerged in the public health field, which has a history of basing its practices on empirical evidence, and political leaders often defer to health care professionals when formulating public policy relevant to health, and are often trained in medicine or related branches of public health themselves. In contrast, the organizations mandated to do something about antisocial behavior do not have the same empirical tradition. Crime control policies are often set by elected officials without training in empirical methods or a command of the evidence related to crime control. Accordingly, research is needed that is designed to understand and increase the use of evidence by policymakers in general, and by the types of policymakers with the greatest influence over treatments for particular target populations, specifically.

Recently, Damschroder and colleagues (2009) proposed a Consolidated Framework for Implementation Research (CFIR) for health services that culls from published theories, models, and evidence. The authors used a snowball sampling approach to identify a pool of published theories characterized by conceptually compelling constructs and/or evidence of influence of those constructs on implementation, consistent definitions of constructs, potential for measurement, and consistency with their own research. The resulting "meta-theoretical framework" (Damschroder et al., 2009, p. 12) reflects five major domains relevant to implementation: the intervention; inner setting (organization, division, department, etc.);

outer setting (socio-political, regulatory, financing context); individuals involved; and processes by which implementation is accomplished. Each domain is further characterized in terms of characteristics and processes found across the models consolidated. The CFIR does contain some constructs whose relations to implementation (in other arenas and in health services) have not yet been demonstrated empirically, and the accompanying text is not entirely clear about the extent to which referenced work reflects empirical support for the salience of the concept. The framework is, however, parsimonious and a useful starting place for the consideration of which variables and processes are most likely to influence the implementation of evidence-based psychological treatments in diverse practice contexts. Applying the CFIR to child mental health and child welfare, Aarons and colleagues have identified particular variables and processes characterizing the outer and inner contexts that are likely to be more or less important at different phases of intervention implementation (Aarons, Hurlburt, & Horwitz, 2011). In so doing, the authors have combined the multilevel models of effective implementation emanating from health care as well as temporal aspects of implementation articulated in dominant models of the diffusion of innovation and some organizational models of implementation to identify leverage points for research on the implementation of effective psychological interventions in public mental health and child welfare.

Research on Implementation of Substance Abuse Interventions

A stage-based approach to implementation of innovations in substance abuse services has also been developed by the substance abuse treatment research program at Texas Christian University (TCU). The TCU Program Change Model for planning and implementing innovations for substance abuse treatment improvement posits three phases reminiscent of the five-step change process outlined by Grol and Grimshaw. The TCU model incorporates elements of the implementation model posited by Klein and colleagues described previously. The TCU model added counselor motivations and perceptions that may, along with organizational attributes, affect some components of some phases of implementation. In the TCU model, the Strategic Planning phase includes assessment of staff needs, organizational functioning, and an integrative review; the Preparation phase includes specifying goals, planning action, and evaluating progress; and the Implementation Process phase includes training, adoption—within which decision and action occur—and implementation, within which effectiveness, feasibility, and sustainability of implementation are demonstrated. Each of these, in turn, is conceived as influenced by somewhat distinctive attributes of the organization. Motivation is conceived as critical to training, whereas organizational resources, staff attributes, and program climate are critical to adoption, and program climate and costs to implementation. In addition, different aspects of the practice context are conceptualized as bearing upon the different phases of the adoption, implementation, and sustainability journey, and a feedback loop connects what is learned from one phase to what is done in the next. To date, the TCU group has established cross-sectional associations among organizational climate (as well as other organizational characteristics) and client engagement, participation, and satisfaction with substance abuse services (Greener, Joe, Simpson, Rowan-Szal, & Lehman, 2007). Linkages with the outcomes of services have not yet been established. In addition, national surveys of substance abuse treatment organizations have identified organizational predictors of the intention to adopt a particular substance abuse treatment (Knudsen & Roman, 2004), although results are mixed regarding actual adoption or implementation at either the clinician or organizational level (Heinrich & Fournier, 2005).

A recently completed prospective, nonexperimental study of the adoption and initial implementation of Contingency Management (CM) procedures statewide among outpatient clinicians in public mental health and substance abuse service sectors examined the effects of treatment, client, clinician, organizational, and service system variables on clinician interest in and adoption and initial implementation of CM (Henggeler et al., 2007, 2008). Findings suggested the differential pertinence to adoption and implementation of variables within these domains. Interest in CM was high, as evidenced by attendance at 1-day CM workshops by 80% of practitioners. Attendance was predicted by organizational motivation and readiness to change, but not by practitioner demographics, professional background, or attitudes toward evidence-based practices. Conversely, practitioner professional experience (greater education and years in current job), service sector (mental health), and attitudes (favorable toward behavior therapy, treatment manuals as a means to enhance positive outcomes, willingness to adopt an innovation if mandated by agency leadership) predicted the odds a practitioner would use CM, while organizational variables did not. The fidelity of practitioner implementation of CM, however, was predicted by a combination of practitioner and organizational characteristics.

Testing Implementation Strategies

Although the evidence base on strategies to increase the adoption and implementation of evidence-based treatments lags considerably behind research on treatment efficacy and effectiveness, noteworthy gains are being made in this regard. This section provides some examples of such research.

CHANGING THE INTERVENTION ITSELF

The Clinic Treatment Project (CTP), undertaken by the MacArthur Foundation–funded Research Network for Youth Mental Health is an example of a study that tests the effects of manipulation of the contours of the treatment itself on implementation and outcomes. The multisite randomized trial is embedded in community treatment settings and tests the effectiveness and implementation of two different ways clinicians might deploy empirically supported treatment procedures, following standard manualized protocols or using the modules from these manuals more flexibly, for highly prevalent problems of school-aged children referred for outpatient treatment. The trial also includes a third condition, provision of routine clinical care for such youth, thereby making possible comparisons of the relative effectiveness of the two different ways of deploying the evidence-based treatments and of both treatment approaches relative to usual care. In addition, a qualitative study describes clinician implementation of the two treatment methods and experiences with the training and clinical supervision required for such implementation (Palinkas et al., 2008). Outcome analyses are currently under way.

CLINICIAN-FOCUSED INTERVENTIONS

There are examples of studies testing the effects of interventions to support the implementation by clinicians of evidence-based treatments in the child welfare, substance abuse, and mental health service sectors. In the child welfare sector, a recently completed randomized effectiveness trial tested the effects of a consultation and fidelity monitoring strategy on the implementation of SafeCare®, an intervention with demonstrated effectiveness in changing parental behaviors proximal to child neglect, and intensive case management services (Aarons, Sommerfeld, Hecht, Silovsky, & Chaffin, 2009). Professionals trained either in SafeCare® or the intensive case management model provided fidelity monitoring in the form of support and consultation to staff in the respective conditions. Support and monitoring was associated with lower staff turnover and lower emotional exhaustion in the SafeCare® condition and higher emotional exhaustion in the case management condition. The authors interpret these findings as suggesting that evidence-based practices and workplace-based support and monitoring of them have a protective effect against staff turnover and staff burnout, while the provision of additional support and monitoring absent the provision of effective intervention tools may be experienced by staff simply as an increase in oversight and a decrease in autonomy (Aarons, Fettes, Flores, & Sommerfeld, 2009).

A few randomized trials have examined variants of training and training plus support on clinician implementation of treatments for substance abuse (Miller, Yahne, Moyers, Martinez, & Pirritano, 2004; Sholomskas et al., 2005). Findings indicate intensive and sustained training efforts are more successful at increasing the adoption and improving the implementation of research-based interventions. Recent findings suggest this is the case even when the clinicians learning a new evidence-based treatment are already implementing another evidence-based treatment. In an experimental study of the effects of varying the intensity of quality assurance strategies on the implementation of a new evidence-based treatment protocol, CM, for adolescent substance abuse by therapists already practicing another evidence-based treatment, MST (Henggeler, Sheidow, Cunningham,

Donohue, & Ford, 2008), more rather than less intensive support was needed to implement the CM protocol.

Within the last decade, "audit and feedback" interventions have been examined in the context of adult psychotherapy in usual care settings, often in multiple baseline studies, but occasionally in randomized trials (see, e.g., Lambert et al., 2003). Results have been mixed, with some studies finding decreases in clinician performance (Bickman, 2009). Based on a comprehensive review of theory and research on individual behavior change and its implication for the receipt and use of performance feedback, Bickman and colleagues developed the Contextualized Feedback Intervention and Training (CFIT) system (Bickman, Riemer, Breda, & Kelly, 2006). In contrast to many feedback systems examined in prior studies that focus solely on the clinician, the CFIT is implemented at the clinician and organizational level. The CFIT model includes organizational assessment, a comprehensive computer-aided system for measuring treatment progress, feedback reports to clinicians and supervisors, and training. Preliminary results from a large randomized trial currently under way suggest that feedback affects the topics clinicians and clients discuss in treatment. In addition, more frequent use of feedback reports by clinicians predicts greater client improvement and reduces treatment length, and clients with greater symptom severity improve more quickly–although clinicians are less likely to read feedback reports for those clients relative to clients with moderate symptoms (Kelley, Vides de Andrade, Sheffer, & Bickman, 2010).

ORGANIZATIONAL AND COMMUNITY INTERVENTIONS

Two experimental studies, one just completed, the other still under way, are examining organizational, community, and local service system influences on the implementation and outcomes of evidence-based treatments in usual care and of strategies designed to leverage positive influences and attenuate negative influences. The recently completed randomized trial tested a two-level strategy for implementing an evidence-based treatment in 14 rural Appalachian counties (Glisson & Schoenwald, 2005). The implementation strategy included (a) the introduction of an MST program for delinquent youth in each county and (b) the ARC (Availability, Responsiveness, and Continuity) organizational intervention that addresses service barriers in the organization and community contexts of the program (Glisson, 2008; Glisson, Dukes, & Green, 2006). The study's rationale is based on evidence that service barriers can be created by organizational and community social contexts through the norms and values that govern expectations about the way things are done, shared beliefs about the cause, prevention and treatment of mental health problems, and existing organizational and community service structures. Within each county, youth were randomly assigned to the new MST program or to usual services programs, yielding four treatment conditions (MST plus ARC, MST only, ARC only, control). Analyses currently under way focus on the behavioral and placement outcomes of youth in all conditions through 18 months postreferral, and on the effects of ARC on MST implementation indicators. The findings from this study will illuminate the independent and combined effects on youth outcomes of an organizational and community development strategy (ARC) and an evidence-based treatment (MST), and the extent to which the organizational and community development intervention affects the implementation of the evidence-based treatment.

A randomized trial currently under way tests two methods of implementing Multidimensional Treatment Foster Care (MTFC) in 40 non–early-adopting California counties (Chamberlain et al., 2008). MTFC was originally developed as a community-based alternative to the incarceration and residential placement of delinquent youth, and has also been found efficacious with youth in foster care at risk of placement disruption. A conceptual model of moderators and mediators of the Community Development Team (CDT) intervention on different stages of MTFC implementation—preimplementation, implementation, and sustainability—guides the study hypotheses. Hypothesized moderators of CDT effects reflect "outer context" variables such as county poverty level, while hypothesized mediators are more dynamic inner context variables such as organizational culture and climate, practitioner attitudes, and therapeutic procedures. Counties are randomly assigned to standard implementation of MTFC, in which protocols designed by the MTFC training organization (TFC Consultants, Inc.) are used to assist one county at a time in developing and implementing MTFC and the CDT condition, in which small groups of counties interested in dealing with a common issue assemble to obtain support and technical assistance. The CDT model was developed in 1993 by the California Institute for Mental Health to encourage counties to collaborate on projects and programs to improve mental health services. This is the first experimental study to our knowledge testing the effects of a specific set of outer and inner context variables on distinct stages of implementation of an evidence-based treatment, and as a function of an experimental manipulation of the process used to support the implementation of that treatment. The findings from this study will shed light on the extent to which knowledge about influences on innovation implementation garnered in other fields (business, health care) generalize to mental health care, and on the effects of two different strategies to support the implementation of such treatments in public service systems.

SUMMARY

This chapter characterizes some of the major theories of dissemination and implementation and conceptual models informed by them drawn from disciplines mostly outside of the area of health care. The scope of these theories and models is broad, as they were derived on the basis of observation, experience, and study of the uptake and implementation of diverse products, services, and types of knowledge.

Initial attempts to apply the models to understanding and manipulating the processes entailed in the dissemination and implementation of evidence-based psychological interventions are under way. Several larger scale experimental studies of the dissemination or implementation of psychological interventions that are informed by one or more of the theories described in this chapter are ongoing and involve numerous organizations, practitioners, and patients. At this time, however, evidence remains limited regarding the effectiveness and cost-effectiveness of strategies designed to enhance uptake or implementation.

The efforts to disseminate and implement psychological interventions described in subsequent chapters are informed by these theoretical frameworks to different degrees, with some explicitly focusing on extant models of dissemination and implementation. The accounts of these efforts provide invaluable information about the nature and impact of these strategies. Complementing these efforts with controlled trials establishing their relative effectiveness and cost-effectiveness will ultimately be necessary to determine the best procedures for disseminating and implementing psychological interventions. It is also important to note that optimal procedures may differ from context to context and intervention to intervention. The heterogeneity of interventions to be transported and the contexts in which they are being introduced will likely necessitate some tailoring of strategies. As evident in subsequent chapters, the approaches to date differ widely depending on the type of intervention (e.g., ranging from self-help computerized therapies in the Improving Access to Psychological Therapies Program to the very intensive treatment models of Dialectical Behavior Therapy and Multisystemic Therapy; see Chapters 4, 9, and 11, this volume) and the system of care.

A component of implementation that is particularly complex in psychological interventions relative to other innovations is the intensity of training needed to facilitate clinical providers' ability to implement treatments with competency and fidelity. Indeed, training may be one of the core challenges to successful implementation (McHugh & Barlow, 2010). The following chapter reviews research on training in evidence-based psychological interventions and discusses models of training and outcomes evaluation for dissemination and implementation efforts.

Acknowledgement

The primary support for this manuscript was provided by NIMH research grants 1P30MH074678 (J. Landsverk, PI) and 1P20MH0784458 (M. Atkins, PI) and by the Annie E. Casey Foundation. The views presented here are those of the authors alone and do not necessarily reflect the opinions of the Anne E. Casey Foundation.

Sonja K. Schoenwald is a Board Member and stockholder in MST Services, LLC, which has the exclusive licensing agreement through the Medical University of South Carolina for the dissemination of MST technology.

REFERENCES

Aarons, G. A., Fettes, D. L., Flores, L. E., & Sommerfeld, D. H. (2009). Evidence-based practice implementation and staff emotional exhaustion in children's services. *Behavior Research and Therapy, 47,* 954–960.

Aarons, G. A., Hurlburt, M., & Horwitz, S.M., (2011). Advancing a conceptual model of evidence-based practice implementation in public service sectors. *Administration and Policy in Mental Health And Mental Health Services Research, 38,* 4–23.

Aarons, G. A., Sommerfeld, D. H., Hecht, D. B., Silovsky, J. F., & Chaffin, M. J. (2009). The impact of evidence-based practice implementation and fidelity monitoring on staff turnover: Evidence for a protective effect. *Journal of Consulting and Clinical Psychology, 77,* 270–280.

Aldrich, H., & Herker, D. (1977). Boundary spanning roles and organization structure. *Academy of Management Review, 2,* 217–230.

Andreasen, A. R. (1995). *Marketing social change: Changing behavior to promote health, social development, and the environment.* San Francisco, CA: Jossey-Bass

Atkins, M. S., Frazier, S. L., Leathers, S. J., Graczyk, P. A., Talbott, E., Jakobsons, L., et al. (2008). Teacher key opinion leaders and mental health consultation in low-income urban schools. *Journal of Consulting and Clinical Psychology, 76,* 905–908.

Ajzen, I. (1991). The theory of planned behavior. *Organizational Behavior and Human Decision Processes, 50,* 179–211.

Backer, T. E., David, S. L., & Soucy, G. (1995). *Reviewing the behavioral science knowledge base on technology transfer* (NIDA Research Monograph 155, NIH Publication No. 95–4035). Rockville, MD: National Institute on Drug Abuse.

Backer, T. E., & Marston, G. (1993). Partnership for a drug-free America: An experiment in social marketing. In T. E. Backer & E. Rogers (Eds.), *Organizational aspects of health communication campaigns: What works?* (pp. 10–24). Newbury Park, CA: Sage.

Bandura, A. (1986). *Social foundations of thought and action: A social cognitive theory.* Englewood Cliffs, NJ: Prentice-Hall.

Bartholomew, N. G., Joe, G. W., Rowan-Szal, G. A., & Simpson, D. D. (2007). Counselor assessments of training and adoption barriers. *Journal of Substance Abuse Treatment, 33,* 193–199.

Berg, M., Aarts, J., & van der Lei, J. (2003). ICT in health care: Sociotechnical approaches. *Methods of Information in Medicine, 42,* 297–301.

Bickman, L. (2009, November). *Lessons learned on how to improve the quality of mental health services with CFIT (Contextualized Feedback Intervention and Training).* Invited presentation, American Evaluation Association Annual Meeting, November 11–14, 2009, Orlando, FL.

Bickman, L., Riemer, M., Breda, C., & Kelly, S. D. (2006). CFIT: A system to provide a continuous quality improvement infrastructure through organizational responsiveness, measurement, training, and feedback. *Report on Emotional & Behavioral Disorders in Youth, 6,* 86–89 .

Biglan, A., & Taylor, T. K. (2000). Why have we been more successful in reducing tobacco use than violent crime? *American Journal of Community Psychology, 28,* 269–302.

Bracht, N., Kingsbury, L., & Rissel, C. (1999). Community organization principles in health promotion: A five-stage model. In N. Bracht (Ed.), *Health promotion at the community level 2: New advances* (pp. 83–104). Thousand Oaks, CA: Sage.

Brown, B. S. (1995). Reducing impediments to technology transfer in drug abuse programming. In T. E. Backer, S. L. David, & G. Soucy (Eds.) *Reviewing the behavioral science knowledge base on technology transfer* (NIDA Research Monograph 155, NIH Publication No. 95–4035) (pp. 169–185). Rockville, MD: National Institute on Drug Abuse.

Chamberlain, P. (2003). The Oregon Treatment Foster Care Model: Features, outcomes, and progress in dissemination. Special Series, Current strategies for moving evidence-based interventions into clinical practice. *Cognitive and Behavioral Practice, 10*, 303–311.

Chamberlain, P., Brown, C. H., Saldana, J., Reid, W., Wang, L., Marsenich, T., et al. (2008). Engaging and recruiting counties in an experiment on implementing evidence-based practice in California. *Administration and Policy in Mental Health and Mental Health Services Research, 35*, 250–260.

Chambers, D. A., Ringeisen, H., & Hickman, E. E. (2005). Federal, state, and foundation initiatives around evidence-based practices for child and adolescent mental health. *Child and Adolescent Psychiatric Clinics of North America, 14*, 307–327.

Chorpita, B. F., & Nakamura, B. J. (2004). Four considerations in the dissemination of intervention innovations. *Clinical Psychology: Science and Practice, 11*, 364–367.

Damanpour, F. (1991). Organizational innovation: A meta-analysis of effects of determinants and moderators. *The Academy of Management Journal*, 34, 555–590.

Damanpour, F. (1996). Organizational complexity and innovation: Developing and testing multiple contingency models. *Management Science, 42*, 693–716.

Damschroder, L. J., Aron, D. C., Keith, R. E., Kirsch, S. R., Alexander, J. A., & Lowery, J. C. (2009). Fostering implementation of health services research findings into practice: A consolidated framework for advancing implementation science. *Implementation Science, 4*, 50. doi:10.1186/1748–5908-4–50

Doumit, G., Gattellari, M., Grimshaw, J., & O'Brien, M. A. (2007). Local opinion leaders: Effects on professional practice and health care outcomes. *Cochrane Database Systematic Reviews, 24*, CD000125.

Fairweather, G. W., Sanders, D. H., & Tornatzky, L. G. (1974). *Creating change in mental health organizations*. Elmsford, NY: Pergamon Press.

Ferlie, E. B., & Shortell, S. M. (2001). Improving the quality of health care in the United Kingdom and the United States: A framework for change. *The Milbank Quarterly, 79*, 281–315.

Fishbein, M., & Ajzen, I. (1975). *Belief, attitude, intention, and behavior: An introduction to theory and research*. Reading, MA: Addison-Wesley.

Fixsen, D. L, Naoom, S. F., Blase, K. A., Friedman, R. M., & Wallace, F. (2005). *Implementation research: A synthesis of the literature*. Tampa, FL: University of South Florida, Louis de la Parte Florida Mental Health Institute, The National Implementation Research Network (FMHI Publication #231).

Francis, J. J., Grimshaw, J. M., Zwarenstein, M., Eccles, M. P., Shiller, S., Godin, G., et al. (2007). Testing a theory-inspired message ("TRY-ME"): A sub-trial within the Ontario Printed Educational Message (OPEM) trial. *Implementation Science, 2*, 39. doi:10.1186/1748–5908-2–39

Glisson, C. (2008). Interventions with organizations: The ARC model. In K. Sowers & C. Dulmus (Eds.), *The comprehensive handbook of social work and social welfare* (Vol. 3, pp. 556–581). Hoboken, NJ: John Wiley & Sons.

Glisson, C., Dukes, D., & Green, P. (2006). The effects of the ARC organizational intervention on caseworker turnover, climate, and culture in children's service systems. *Child Abuse and Neglect, 30*, 855–880.

Glisson, C., & Schoenwald, S. K. (2005). An organizational and community development strategy for implementing evidence-based children's mental health treatments. *Mental Health Services Research, 7*, 1–17.

Godin, G., Belanger-Gravel, A., Eccles, M., & Grimshaw, J. (2008). Healthcare professionals' intentions and behaviours: A systematic review of studies based on social cognitive theories. *Implementation Science, 3*, 36. doi:10.1186/1748–5908-3–36

Greener, J. M., Joe, G. W., Simpson, D. D., Rowan-Szal, G. A., & Lehman, W. E. K. (2007) Influence of organizational functioning on client engagement in treatment. *Journal of Substance Abuse Treatment, 33*, 139–147.

Grier, S., & Bryant, C. A. (2005). Social marketing in public health. *Annual Review of Public Health, 26*, 319–329.

Grimshaw, J. M., Shirran, L., Thomas, R., Mowatt, G., Fraser, C., Bero, L., et al. (2001). Changing provider behavior: An overview of systematic reviews of interventions. *Medical Care, 39*, 8(Suppl. 2), pp. II-2–II-45.

Grol, R., & Grimshaw, J. (1999). Evidence-based implementation of evidence-based medicine. *Journal on Quality Improvement, 25*, 503–513.

Hackman, J. R., & Wageman, R. (1995). Total quality management: Empirical, conceptual, and practical issues. *Administrative Science Quarterly, 40*, 309–342.

Heinrich, C. J., & Fournier, E. (2005). Instruments of policy and administration for improving substance abuse treatment practice and program outcomes. *Journal of Drug Issues, 35*, 481–500.

Helfrich, C. D., Weiner, B. J., McKinney, M. M., & Minasian, L. (2007). Determinants of implementation effectiveness: Adapting a framework for complex interventions. *Medical Care Research and Review, 64*, 279–303.

Henggeler, S. W., Chapman, J. E., Rowland, M. D., Halliday-Boykins, C. A., Randall, J., Shackelford, J., et al. (2007). If you build it, they will come: Statewide practitioner interest in CM for youths. *Journal of Substance Abuse Treatment, 32*, 121–131.

Henggeler, S. W., Chapman, J. E., Rowland, M. D., Halliday-Boykins, C. A., Randall, J., Shackleford, J., et al. (2008). Statewide adoption and initial implementation of contingency management for substance abusing adolescents. *Journal of Consulting and Clinical Psychology, 76*, 556–567.

Henggeler, S. W., Schoenwald, S. K., Borduin, C. M., Rowland, M. D., & Cunningham, P. B. (2009). *Multisystemic therapy for antisocial behavior in children and adolescents* (2nd ed.). New York: The Guilford Press.

Henggeler, S. W., Sheidow, A. J., Cunningham, P. B., Donohue, B. C., & Ford, J. D. (2008). Promoting the implementation of an evidence-based intervention for adolescent marijuana abuse in community settings: Testing the use of intensive quality assurance. *Journal of Clinical Child & Adolescent Psychology, 37*, 682–689.

Jamtvedt, G., Young, J. M., Kristoffersen, D. T., O'Brien, M. A., & Oxman, A. D. (2006). Audit and feedback: Effects on professional practice and health care outcomes. *Cochrane Database of Systematic Reviews, 2*, CD000259

Kelley, S. D., Vides de Andrade, A. R., Sheffer, E., & Bickman, L. (2010). Exploring the black box: Measuring youth treatment process and progress in usual care. *Administration and Policy in Mental Health and Mental Health Services Research.* Advance online publication. doi:10.1007/s10488-010-0298-8

Klein, K. J., Conn, A. B., & Sorra, J. S. (2001). Implementing computerized technology: An organizational analysis. *Journal of Applied Psychology, 86,* 811–824.

Klein, K. J., & Sorra, J. S. (1996). The challenge of innovation implementation. *Academy of Management Review, 21,* 1055–1080.

Knudsen, H. K., & Roman, P. M. (2004). Modeling the use of innovations in private treatment organizations: The role of absorptive capacity. *Journal of Substance Abuse Treatment, 26,* 51–59.

Lambert, M. J., Whipple, J. L., Hawkins, E. J., Vermeersch, D., Nielsen, S. L., & Smart, D. W.(2003). Is it time for clinicians to routinely track patient outcome? A meta-analysis. *Clinical Psychology: Science and Practice, 10*(3), 288–301.

Lock, C. A., & Kaner, E. F. S. (2000). Use of marketing to disseminate brief alcohol intervention to general practitioners: Promoting health care interventions to health promoters. *Journal of Evaluation in Clinical Practice, 6,* 345–357.

Lomas, J., Enkin, M., Anderson, G. M., Hannah, W. J., Vayda, E., & Singer, J. (1991). Opinion leaders vs audit and feedback to implement practice guidelines: Delivery after previous cesarean section. *Journal of the American Medical Association, 265,* 2202–2207.

Martin, G. W., Herie, M. A., Turner, B. J., & Cunningham, J. A. (1998). A social marketing model for disseminating research-based treatments to addictions treatment providers. *Addiction, 93,* 1703–1715.

McHugh, R. K., & Barlow, D. H. (2010). Dissemination and implementation of evidence-based psychological interventions: A review of current efforts. *American Psychology, 65,* 73–84.

Miller, W. R., Sorensen, J. L., Selzer, J. A., & Brigham, G. S. (2006). Disseminating evidence-based practices in substance abuse treatment: A review with suggestions. *Journal of Substance Abuse Treatment, 31,* 25–39.

Miller, W. R., Yahne, C. E. Moyers, T. B., Martinez, J., & Pirritano, M. (2004). A randomized trial of methods to help clinicians learn motivational interviewing. *Journal of Consulting and Clinical Psychology, 72,* 1050–1062.

National Institutes of Health. (2009). *3rd Annual NIH conference on the science of dissemination and implementation: Methods and measurement.* Conference announcement. Bethesda, MD: Author. Retrieved April 18, 2010, from http://conferences.thehillgroup. com/obssr/DI2010/abstracts.html#topics

Palinkas, L. A., Schoenwald, S. K., Hoagwood, K., Landsverk, J., Chorpita, B. F., Weisz, J. R., et al. (2008). An ethnographic study of implementation of evidence-based practice in child mental health: First steps. *Psychiatric Services, 59,* 738–746.

Perkins, M. B., Jensen, P. S., Jaccard, J., Gollwitzer, P., Oettingen, G., Pappadopulos, E., et al. (2007). Applying theory-driven approaches to understanding and modifying clinicians' behavior: What do we know? *Psychiatric Services, 58,* 342–348.

Real, K., & Poole, M. S. (2005). Innovation implementation: Conceptualization and measurement in organizational research. *Research in Organizational Change and Development, 15,* 63–134.

Rhagavan, R., Bright, C. L., & Shadoin, A. L. (2008). Toward a policy ecology of implementation of evidence-based practices in public mental health settings. *Implementation Science, 3,* 26. doi:10.1186/1748-5908-3-26

Rogers, E. M. (2003). *Diffusion of innovations* (5th ed.). New York: Free Press.

Rousseau, D. M. (1977). Technological differences in job characteristics, employee satisfaction, and motivation: A synthesis of job design research and sociotechnical systems theory. *Organizational Behavior and Human Performance, 19*, 18–42.

Schoenwald, S. K., Chapman, J. E., Kelleher, K., Hoagwood, K. E., Landsverk, J., Stevens, J., et al. (2008). A survey of the infrastructure for children's mental health services: Implications for the implementation of empirically supported treatments (ESTs). *Administration and Policy in Mental Health and Mental Health Services Research, 35*, 84–97.

Schoenwald, S. K., & Henggeler, S. W. (2004). A public health perspective on the transport of evidence based practices. *Clinical Science and Practice, 11*, 360–363.

Schoenwald, S. K., & Hoagwood, K. (2001). Effectiveness, transportability, and dissemination of interventions: What matters when? *Psychiatric Services, 52*, 1179–1189.

Schoenwald, S. K., Kelleher, K., Weisz, J. R., & the Research Network on Youth Mental Health. (2008). Building bridges to evidence-based practice: The MacArthur Foundation Child System and Treatment Enhancement Projects (Child STEPs). *Administration and Policy in Mental Health and Mental Health Services Research, 35*, 66–72.

Shaw, B., Cheater, F., Baker, R., Gillies, C. Hearnshaw, H., Flottorp, S., et al. (2005). Tailored interventions to overcome identified barriers to change: Effects on professional practice and health care outcomes. *Cochrane Database of Systematic Reviews, 3*, CD005470

Sholomskas, D. E, Syracuse-Siewert, G., Rounsaville, B. J., Ball, S. A., Nuro, K. F., & Carroll, K. M. (2005). We don't train in vain: A dissemination trial of three strategies of training clinicians in cognitive-behavioral therapy. *Journal of Consulting and Clinical Psychology, 73*, 106–115.

Sikkema, K. J., Kelly, J. A., Winett, R. A., Solomon, L. J., Cargill, V. A., Roffman, R. A., et al. (2000). Outcomes of a randomized community-level HIV prevention intervention for women living in 19 low-income housing developments. *American Journal of Public Health, 90*, 57–63.

Simmel, G. (1908). *Soziologie*. Leipzig: Duncker & Humblot.

Simpson, D. D., & Flynn, P. (2007). Moving innovations into treatment: A stage-based approach to program change. *Journal of Substance Abuse Treatment, 33*, 111–120.

Southam-Gerow, M. A., Austin, A. A., & Marder, A. M. (2008). Transportability and dissemination of psychological treatments: Research models and methods. In D. McKay (Ed.), *Handbook of research methods in abnormal and clinical psychology* (pp. 203–224). Newbury Park, CA: Sage.

Squires, D. D., Gumbley, S. J., & Storti, S. A. (2008). Training substance abuse treatment organizations to adopt evidence-based practices: The Addiction Technology Transfer Center of New England Science to Service Laboratory. *Journal of Substance Abuse Treatment, 34*, 293–301.

Stirman, S. W., Crits-Christoph, P., & DeRubeis, R. J. (2004). Achieving successful dissemination of empirically support psychotherapies: A synthesis of dissemination theory. *Clinical Psychology: Science and Practice, 11*, 343–359.

Tarde, G. (1903). *The laws of imitation*. New York: Henry Holt and Company.

Triandis, H. C. (1980). Values, attitudes and interpersonal behavior. In M. M. Page (Ed.), *Nebraska symposium on motivation beliefs, attitudes and values* (Vol. 1, pp. 195–259). Lincoln, NE: University of Nebraska Press.

Trist, E. (1985). Intervention strategies for interorganizational domains. In R. Tannenbaum, N. Margulies, & F. Massarik (Eds.), *Human systems development* (167–197). San Francisco: Jossey-Bass.

Valente, T. W., Hoffman, B. R., Ritt-Olson, A., Lichtman, K., & Johnson, C. A. (2003). Effects of a social-network method for group assignment strategies on peer-led tobacco prevention programs in schools. *American Journal of Public Health, 93,* 1837–1843.

Wolfe, R.A. (1994). Organizational innovation: Review, critique, and suggested research directions. *Organizational Dynamics, 4,* 3–21.

Zwarenstein, M., Hux, J. E., Kelsall, D., Paterson, M., Grimshaw, J., Davis, D., et al. (2007). The Ontario Printed Educational Message (OPEM) trial to narrow the evidence-practice gap with respect to prescribing practices of general and family physicians: A cluster randomized controlled trial, targeting the care of individuals with diabetes and hypertension in Ontario, Canada. *Implementation Science, 2,* 37. doi:10.1186/1748–5908-2–37

Training in Evidence-Based Psychological Interventions
R. Kathryn McHugh and David H. Barlow

Despite the emergence of information technology and other novel methods of psychological service delivery, the individual clinical provider continues to be the linchpin of mental health practice. Accordingly, training clinical providers in the application of evidence-based psychological interventions (EBPIs) is among the core elements of dissemination and implementation (D&I) efforts. EBPIs are complex and require both knowledge of the treatment model and its components and competence in the administration of these components flexibly based on the needs, preferences, and characteristics of individual patients. The complex and nuanced nature of these interventions, combined with barriers to the receipt of training (e.g., cost, negative perceptions of EBPIs), makes training one of the greatest challenges to successful implementation (McHugh & Barlow, 2010). Despite its importance, relatively little is known about the efficacy or effectiveness of training programs, or the necessary procedures for successful training. With increased attention to D&I in recent years, research on training has begun to proliferate and the science in this area is progressing rapidly. This chapter will provide an overview of the current status of clinician training including a description of training procedures, a brief review of the extant literature on the efficacy/effectiveness of training, and a discussion of novel approaches and future research directions in this area.

Training Procedures

Training procedures in EBPIs can be grouped into two broad categories corresponding to procedures to increase knowledge about an intervention (didactic training) and procedures to increase skill in the application of an intervention (competency training). The delivery of these procedures can be characterized by distinctions of time and place: synchronous/local, synchronous/distance, asynchronous/local, and asynchronous/distance (Weingardt, 2004). Specifically, the trainer and trainee can be engaging in procedures at the same (synchronous) or different times (asynchronous) from the same (local) or different (distance) locations.

For example, a clinician reading a treatment manual is an example of an asynchronous distance delivery method. A conference workshop is a synchronous local delivery method. Below, we describe didactic and competency training including a description of common procedures and delivery methods.

DIDACTIC TRAINING

Didactic training is analogous to the "hardware" training element of EBPIs and entails procedures aimed to increase knowledge about the intervention. Information provided in didactic training may include the procedural elements of the intervention, the timing and structure of the intervention, how to identify patients for whom the intervention would be relevant, and strategies for problem solving clinical complications and barriers to implementation. Another aim of didactic training can be to target myths and negative perceptions about EBPIs generally and the intervention specifically. Strategies for didactic training vary widely in their intensiveness, from the use of written materials to experiential exercises.

Low-intensity training mechanisms such as written manuals or texts describing EBPIs (e.g., Barlow, 2008; Nathan & Gorman, 2007; Roth & Fonagy, 2005) are easily accessible and can be readily distributed to large numbers of clinicians. In fact, many written resources can be accessed for free or low cost through organizations such as the Substance Abuse and Mental Health Services Administration in the United States. Higher intensity procedures, such as interactive, experiential trainings, increasingly have been used to facilitate knowledge acquisition and maintenance and enhance the engagement of trainees. This may include exercises such as small discussion groups and conducting role plays of important treatment components.

Traditionally, written materials and live workshops have made up the main delivery mechanisms for training. More recently, information technology (IT) has been utilized as a novel delivery method for synchronous and asynchronous distance learning. The application of IT can range from videos of expert clinicians administering or describing treatment elements to highly interactive computer-based programs. In web-based applications, video (either prerecorded or live), slides, interactive questions/polls, and other exercises can be utilized. Thus, such methods may combine some of the benefits of written materials (e.g., ability to reach large numbers of clinicians) with the benefits of live workshops (e.g., the use of interactive exercises).

COMPETENCY TRAINING

Competency training is analogous to the "software" training of EBPIs. This includes the procedural learning for the application of knowledge to a clinical encounter. Competency training has proven to be a greater challenge than didactic training and there remains a lack of consensus about its definition and measurement (e.g., Nelson et al., 2007; Roth & Pilling, 2007). However, despite such challenges, it is clear from both empirical studies of training outcomes (see below) and clinician report (Bennett-Levy, McManus, Westling, & Fennell, 2009) that competency training is necessary for skill acquisition. Competency training typically involves supervision by an advanced clinician, which incorporates feedback and guidance in treatment administration. This has long been thought to be a crucial element of training in psychological interventions, and is likely necessary for the successful training of EBPIs. The two main components of competency training are supervision/consultation in the administration of the intervention and monitoring with feedback.

Consistent with the development of any complex skill, practice is a necessary component of learning to administer an EBPI. Typically this involves administering a treatment to patients after completion of didactic training. Supervision of intervention administration is standard practice in graduate training programs and its importance in continuing education and D&I efforts is being increasingly emphasized. Guidance from an expert facilitates ongoing skill acquisition and aids in managing clinical complications. Such supervision either can be based on clinician self-report or can include varieties of "live" supervision, ranging from synchronous observation to review of video- or audiotaped sessions.

Miller and colleagues (Miller, Sorensen, Selzer, & Brigham, 2006) emphasize the importance of feedback to the early practice of administering a treatment, equating practice without feedback to trying to learn how to bowl in the dark. Such feedback may take many forms, such as quantitative feedback on performance in the form of ratings of adherence, competency, and patient outcomes (e.g., symptom improvement, satisfaction) or qualitative feedback from a supervisor/consultant on the administration of the intervention. This allows the learner to adjust the application of the intervention accordingly over time.

Delivery of competency training can occur in either individual or group structure in person or at a distance (e.g., phone or web-based conferencing). Given resource limitations, the major D&I efforts to date have typically focused on group distance competency training (e.g., weekly group consultation phone calls). The evaluation of the relative benefits of individual versus group and local versus distance approaches is still needed.

TRAINING MODELS

Procedures for training in EBPIs vary dramatically. Even in tightly controlled treatment efficacy trials—for which there have been calls to standardize the administration and reporting of training and treatment integrity procedures—there remains much inconsistency (e.g., Perepletchikova, Hilt, Chereji, & Kazdin, 2009; Perepletchikova, Treat, & Kazdin, 2007). In order to introduce greater standardization of procedures at this early stage, the development of models of training is much needed. In particular, such models should consider the complex interactions between trainees and contextual variables (e.g., organizational support) (Beidas & Kendall, 2010).

One early example is the ACCESS model. Stirman and colleagues (2010) developed the ACCESS model as an overarching model of training based on the available literature on training, experience with large implementation efforts, and research on adult learning. This model consists of six major components: assess and adapt, convey the basics, consult, evaluate work samples, study outcomes, and sustain. The first component (assess and adapt) involves evaluating the needs, values, and structure of the particular system and engaging providers and leaders in the process of training to maximize the fit of the intervention and the training program to the target setting. The second component (convey the basics) is the didactic training component: communicating information on the nature and application of the intervention to trainees. Stirman and colleagues emphasize the importance of small group and experiential exercises at this stage to maximize learning. The third (consult) and fourth (evaluate work samples) components are the competency training elements of the model. These elements include consultation and continued support as clinicians begin implementing the intervention in the setting with patients as well as evaluation of the competence and adherence with which the intervention is delivered. The fifth component (study the outcomes) includes the assessment of the effect of the training, including proximal outcomes (e.g., clinician attitudes, adherence) and distal outcomes (e.g., patient satisfaction and symptom outcomes). The final component (sustain) involves maintenance of the change and prevention of drift. The authors recommend both continued access to consultation and other opportunities to enhance learning and a plan for training new staff on an ongoing basis. Stirman and colleagues (Stirman, Buchhofer, McLaulin, Evans, & Beck, 2009) implemented the ACCESS model of training for providers in a large managed care organization in a state department of behavioral health. Although patient outcomes are not yet available, this program was successful in training more than 500 staff members in a brief time period (approximately 2 years) with more than 1,000 patients receiving treatment from trained clinicians during that time.

Empirical Evaluation of Training in Evidence-Based Psychological Interventions

Evaluation of continuing education in health care consistently indicates that didactic and workshop-based training alone is not effective for achieving desired clinical behavior change (David, Thomson, Oxman, & Haynes, 1995; Davis et al., 1999; Grimshaw et al., 2001; VandeCreek, Knapp, & Brace, 1990). Similar evidence has emerged from studies specific to psychological treatments (King et al., 2002; Sholomskas et al., 2005). However, the necessary elements for achieving and sustaining successful training outcomes is still in early stages of evaluation and much research has relied on nonexperimental paradigms and small sample sizes. Recently, comprehensive reviews have characterized this rapidly burgeoning research area (Beidas & Kendall, 2010; Herschell, Kolko, Bauman, & Davis, 2010; Rakovshik & McManus, 2010). Below, we briefly review the research base to date on training clinical providers.

NONEXPERIMENTAL, OPEN, AND NATURALISTIC STUDIES

A number of open studies have provided evidence for the success of training programs that include a competency component, typically expert supervision (e.g., Crits-Christoph et al., 1998; Lau, Dubord, & Parikh, 2004; Milne, Baker, Blackburn, James, & Reichelt, 1999; Morgenstern, Morgan, McCrady, Keller, & Carroll, 2001; Sobell, 1996). Likewise, didactic training alone seems to be ineffective for clinician behavior change using either written materials (Ducharme & Feldman, 1992; Rubel, Sobell, & Miller, 2000) or workshops (Lopez, Osterberg, Jensen-Doss, & Rae, in press; Saitz, Sullivan, & Samet, 2000). Studies comparing trainings including supervision to those without have found support for supervision in improving clinician competency (e.g., Sholomskas et al., 2005) and attenuation of treatment effects has been seen with the use of training models absent of ongoing consultation/supervision (Henggeler, Melton, Brondino, Scherer, & Hanley, 1997). Of supervisor variables that may impact outcomes, supervisor emphasis on treatment adherence in particular has been associated with both clinician adherence and patient outcomes (Schoenwald, Sheidow, & Chapman, 2009).

Studies of graded or stepwise training approaches—in which the dose of training is calibrated to each individual clinician—have suggested that different clinicians may require different intensities of training to achieve competency (e.g., Martino, Canning-Ball, Carroll, & Rounsaville, in press; Merrill, Tolbert, & Wade, 2003). Such approaches suggest that decision points can be used during training activities to determine which clinicians will require additional training. These adaptive training designs have the potential to maximize efficiency and minimize cost.

CONTROLLED TRIALS

One of the best systematic evaluations of training programs has been in the training of Motivational Interviewing (MI; Miller & Rollnick, 1991, 2002), a brief intervention originally developed for the treatment of substance use disorders. Early investigations demonstrated limited success of a standard workshop, particularly relative to maintenance of gains in competency (Baer et al., 2004) and the impact of skill gains on patient outcomes (Miller & Mount, 2001). A large randomized clinical trial compared (a) a workshop alone; (b) written manual and instructional tapes alone; and (c) a workshop plus feedback, coaching, or both (Miller, Yahne, Moyers, Martinez, & Pirritano, 2004). This study demonstrated that despite immediate gains in the workshop alone condition, these gains were not maintained over time, and that only clinicians receiving feedback, coaching, or their combination maintained gains over 12 months of follow-up. The manual/tapes-only condition was not successful in training clinicians. Two follow-up pilot studies of workshop plus ongoing supervision have replicated this success (Schoener, Madeja, Henderson, Ondersma, & Janisse, 2006; Smith et al., 2007). However, a subsequent study suggested that even with ongoing consultation, providers with lower baseline skills and less motivation to learn MI were unable to maintain gains in skill after initial training (Moyers et al., 2008).

Martino and colleagues (2011) randomized clinicians to one of three training conditions: self-study (receipt of written training materials alone), expert-led training (workshop led by an expert in MI plus follow-up supervision with feedback), and train-the-trainer training (same as expert-led but clinicians were trained to deliver the workshop and supervise at their own setting). Results indicated that both the expert training and train-the-trainer models yielded superior adherence and competence gains relative to self-study and that more clinicians met efficacy trial standards for competence (>50% in both groups, compared with 18% for the self-study group).

Lochman and colleagues (2009) randomized 57 public schools to receive one of three counselor training programs in Coping Power (Lochman & Wells, 2004), an evidence-based preventative intervention for aggressive behavior. Programs included a basic training, training plus feedback (which included individualized consultation and feedback), and a placebo comparison condition. Results indicated that the training plus feedback resulted in better outcomes (both reduction in externalizing behaviors and improvement in social and academic functioning) relative to both the basic and control conditions; the basic training did not evidence benefits over the control condition.

Sholomskas and colleagues (2005) assigned 78 clinicians to one of three training conditions in cognitive behavioral therapy (CBT) for substance abuse: manual only, manual plus web-based training, and manual plus workshop and supervision. Results indicated superior outcome in adherence and competency for the manual plus workshop and supervision conditions; the web-based training performed better than manual only but not as well as the supervision condition. Despite several limitations of this trial (including inability to randomize approximately 30% of the sample due to logistical considerations, and the lack of a web training plus supervision condition), this trial provided further support for the necessity of supervision to training outcomes.

COMPREHENSIVE REVIEWS AND SYNTHESES
OF THE LITERATURE

Qualitative reviews also support the finding that didactic training alone does not yield significant change in clinician behavior (Beidas & Kendall, 2010; Herschel et al., 2010). A large literature review concluded that training can increase therapist knowledge and change attitudes toward EBPIs but that clinician behavior change and patient symptom improvement were the most challenging outcomes to achieve (Beidas & Kendall, 2010).

In a comprehensive review of the literature on training in CBT, Rakovshik and McManus (2010) evaluated the elements of training relative to study outcomes to identify the training components that appeared to be associated with superior clinical outcomes. Results suggested that longer durations of training in general and longer duration of competency training in particular were associated with better clinical outcomes. Reviews consistently have called for greater consistency of research methods and measures to facilitate comparison and interpretation across studies.

Challenges and Future Directions in Training

Substantial advances have been made in the training of EBPIs. The expansion of research and improved methods for studying training hold promise for the rapid advancement of knowledge in this area. However, many questions remain unanswered, and continued development and study of training methods are of particular importance to the D&I agenda. Several of the major challenges and important directions for future study are discussed below.

WHEN, WHAT, AND WHO TO TRAIN?

Some of the most fundamental challenges of training are when to train, what interventions to provide training in, and who should serve as trainers. The foundational training in the mental health care field occurs at the graduate level; however, the sole utilization of graduate training is insufficient given both the urgent need for evidence-based services (prohibiting waiting for the next generation of trainees) and the constant improvement and development of EBPIs. Continuing education mechanisms, which are built into the licensure requirements in most professions for the majority of states in the United States as well as in other countries (e.g., continuing professional development requirements in Australia), provide an important complementary entry point for training efforts. However, current continuing education requirements are relatively minimal and continuing education activities are often not consistent with the level of involvement needed to achieve clinician behavior change. Given the evidence consistently suggesting that ongoing training and supervision is needed to achieve competency, the reconsideration of how continuing education can be used effectively is an important challenge for the field. Seeking out additional training is associated with significant time and financial cost that may not be possible for many clinical providers, especially those in service provision settings with a high workload burden and/or low funding.

The number of EBPIs for various psychological disorders continues to grow. The cost of training in multiple EBPIs is prohibitive if single-disorder interventions are trained individually. One potential solution to this problem is the evidence-based practice approach (e.g., Norcross, Hogan, & Koocher, 2008; see Chapter 1, this volume), which involves teaching providers to be consumers of the empirical literature and to incorporate this information into practice. Data from the use of this approach in medicine suggest that when it is integrated in practice settings (as opposed to a stand-alone training), it can yield change in clinician knowledge and behavior (Coomarasamy & Khan, 2004). An alternative solution to this training challenge is to distill the elements of EBPIs to more common elements through either the use of transdiagnostic interventions or trainings that focus on both general and disorder-specific competencies. Transdiagnostic interventions build on the commonalities among treatment approaches for different discrete disorders and the phenomenological overlap among disorders (Barlow et al., 2010; Fairburn et al., 2009; McHugh, Murray, & Barlow, 2009). Such interventions have several benefits relative to D&I such as providing greater coverage of disorders while requiring less training (McHugh et al., 2009). Other training approaches, such as those emphasized by the Improving Access to Psychological Therapies (IAPT) Program in the United Kingdom (see Chapter 4), train both in general competencies that are applicable across disorders and in disorder-specific strategies. The IAPT has taken an intensive approach to training clinicians to competently administer EBPIs and utilizing a year-long course consisting of modules in both general CBT skills (e.g., case conceptualization, decisional balance, behavioral experiments) and disorder-specific strategies (e.g., use of video feedback of performance in social phobia).

Trainings have historically been administered by experts in the intervention, typically treatment developers. Although this approach allows trainees to receive an expert perspective on the intervention, the feasibility of such a strategy in terms of both the number of clinical providers with access to training and the cost of trainings prevents wide-scale impact. Moreover, staff turnover is a particular issue in many mental health service provision settings, with estimates of mean annual staff turnover over 25% (Gallon, Gabriel, & Knudsen, 2003; Rollins, Salyers, Tsai, & Lydick, 2010). With an annual turnover rate of 25%, within 3 years following a training it is possible that less than half of trained staff will still be employed at the setting. One strategy is to have continued follow-up "booster" trainings to reinforce learning and refresh skills among those trained and to introduce the EBPI to new staff members. Another strategy is the train-the-trainer approach. Train-the-trainer strategies involve building a training workforce through teaching local clinicians/administrators how to train others in EBPIs. Thus, expert trainers can reach more clinicians through training trainers. Research on this model is ongoing and preliminary data are promising (Martino et al., 2011). See Chapter 5 of this volume for a description of an application of the train-the-trainer model.

DOSING AND TIMING

The necessary duration of supervision (e.g., 6 months, 12 months) and the need for "refresher" supervision or booster sessions is unclear from the extant literature.

Sustainability in D&I efforts rests largely on the maintenance of training effects over time (at least for face-to-face psychological interventions) and thus the appropriate dose of training and frequency and spacing of follow-up or booster trainings is crucial.

Some have proposed training approaches that dose training based on clinician characteristics, such as speed of acquisition of skill or level of pretraining experience (e.g., Martino et al., in press). Such graded training approaches use clinician experience or performance as markers of need for additional training. For example, competency may be assessed following stages of training (e.g., workshop, 3 months of supervision) and those meeting benchmarks may discontinue formal training while others continue with additional supervision/feedback. A particular benefit of this type of approach is the ability to provide more efficient—and presumably cost-effective—training by targeting the amount of training to the needs of the particular clinician. Such approaches have demonstrated preliminary success (see Rakovshik & McManus, 2010).

MECHANISMS

Much like the study of treatment efficacy, the active ingredients of training cannot be adequately established when training programs are tested as packages. The identification of the necessary and active ingredients of training (i.e., training mechanisms) will be of particular importance given the high cost of training efforts. By identifying the active ingredients, training programs can be refined to be as efficient as possible. Likewise, the identification of training mechanisms can inform decisions regarding training by suggesting the minimum necessary intervention to justify the cost of training. For example, investing limited resources in minimal strategies that are unlikely to yield desired outcomes can be avoided. Studies of mechanisms also can inform graded approaches by identifying the components that may be important for providers from varied backgrounds.

Given the consistency of findings indicating that supervision and feedback appear to be necessary for the achievement of competency, the identification of what specific elements of these efforts are active ingredients may help to streamline supervision. For example, this may inform whether group supervision is sufficient for skills gain and maintenance or whether individualized attention is necessary. For didactic training, mechanisms may include elements of training (e.g., specific types of exercises) and the delivery of those elements (e.g., video, lecture, written materials) that impact knowledge and attitude change. If, for example, the active elements of didactic training can be administered in a 1-day workshop as effectively as a 5-day workshop, significant cost savings can be achieved.

MEASUREMENT

There has been a large response to the need for systematic research on training in EBPIs in recent years. However, inconsistency in measurement strategies is a substantial limitation to these efforts. Both the development and testing of measures and establishment of the relevant outcomes for training efforts are needed at this time.

In a review of major D&I efforts, we (McHugh & Barlow, 2010) found that the outcomes evaluated varied widely even across state-of-the-art efforts. Across these efforts representing major programs at the national, state, and individual treatment levels, the outcomes evaluated included both patient outcomes (number of patients receiving services, pre/post symptoms, impairment/quality of life) and clinician training outcomes (assessment of competency by clinicians/supervisors/patients, feedback to clinicians, number of clinicians trained, clinician attrition, and percentage who achieve competency). We recommended that at this stage it is of particular importance to assess a wide range of variables including both proximal (e.g., clinician knowledge and skill change) and distal (e.g., patient satisfaction, symptom reduction) outcomes. The evaluation of too few outcomes and overreliance on therapist self-report are major limitations in both large-scale implementation efforts (McHugh & Barlow, 2010) and the training research literature (Herschell et al., 2010). The development and use of validated scales for evaluating relevant outcomes, such as fidelity and competency, are sorely needed.

Assessing competency outcomes has been particularly challenging. Outcomes may include both skill in administering the treatment and adherence to the treatment model. Skill in treatment administration can be difficult to operationalize and it is unclear what methods of evaluation (e.g., chart review; clinician, supervisor, or independent observer report) are valid and reliable markers of competency. The importance of the measurement of fidelity has been debated. For example, a meta-analytic review of the literature suggested that fidelity is not related to clinical outcomes (Webb, Derubeis, & Barber, 2010). However, this analysis was limited by examining only treatment efficacy trials, which typically are associated with intensive training, ongoing expert supervision, and quality standards, resulting in a ceiling effect precluding the ability to detect associations between outcomes and fidelity. Examination of effectiveness and D&I trials—characterized by a greater range of fidelity scores—indicates that stronger fidelity is associated with outcome (McHugh et al., 2009). This is further complicated by the finding that this association may not be linear and that moderate fidelity may be associated with the best patient outcomes (Barber et al., 2006; Hogue et al., 2008). This is consistent with the principle of "flexibility with fidelity" (Kendall, Gosch, Furr, & Sood, 2008), which emphasizes flexible application of EBPIs to the individual patient. Thus, at this time it appears that measurement of both competency/skill and adherence/fidelity may be of particular importance to understanding this complex relationship.

DISTANCE LEARNING, INFORMATION TECHNOLOGY, AND OTHER NOVEL APPROACHES

Future research on innovative approaches to training is important to the advancement of this research agenda. In particular, the use of IT has enormous potential for the advancement of training agendas. Some examples of IT applications in training are the use of web-based conferencing software for didactic training (e.g., slide presentations with discussion) and structured computer-based didactic applications. Computer-based software may include elements similar to workshop training and can include numerous features, such as testing/evaluation (e.g., multiple choice tests), videos of the intervention administration, and printable handouts and outlines. Such applications also vary widely and can include either "real-time" or self-paced (i.e., clinicians complete training on their own time) structures (Weingardt, 2004). IT trainings provide flexible, interactive tools that can be designed to facilitate engagement and learning and reduce complexity. There are numerous benefits to the use of technology, including providing increased access to providers who might have more difficulty accessing training due to financial and/or geographical barriers, providing standardization of training, and allowing for self-paced training. However, there are several unknown elements of this strategy, such as how to facilitate adherence in a distance learning format and whether there is a loss or mitigation of training efficacy when training is not conducted in person. The extension of IT to competency training is an interesting area for future research. Evaluation of such programs is in the very early stages and results thus far have been generally positive (Dimeff et al., 2009; Larsen et al., 2009; Weingardt, Cucciare, Bellotti, & Lai, 2009.). However, such studies are preliminary in nature, including having brief periods of assessment and focusing primarily on issues of feasibility (e.g., satisfaction), and thus future evaluation of such technologies is needed to determine their efficacy relative to traditional methods.

Innovation in the delivery of training is much needed. For example, social networking technology may be leveraged for maintenance of training, such as through consultation with peers. Peer consultation networks may facilitate both training/intervention administration as well as other challenges of D&I efforts (e.g., organizational behavior change). Other novel uses of IT, such as mobile phones (e.g., Ekberg et al., 2011) for support and delivery of EBPIs, are being explored.

Interdisciplinary approaches may also be needed to advance this area of practice and research. A recent report on continuing education published by the Institute of Medicine (2010) proposed the development of a national continuing education institute and the facilitation of greater integration of continuing education activities across the health care professions. Drawing from experience both from other health professions and from education (including adult learning theories) may aid in providing a comprehensive approach to training clinicians as well as maintaining knowledge and skill acquisition and facilitating ongoing learning as the field continues to advance with respect to EBPIs.

Conclusions and Summary

Training clinical providers in the administration of EBPIs is necessary to building workforce capacity to deliver interventions and improve access to effective care.

Recent years have seen a significant increase in interest in training along with the development of preliminary models for conceptualizing training and assessment. Moreover, there has been a call for both improved methodology in the study of training and the increasing use of information technology as a flexible and cost-effective method for delivery.

The literature to date suggests that didactic training alone—even that including active, experiential components—is insufficient to yield change in clinician behavior (i.e., administration of EBPIs). Ongoing consultation/supervision along with feedback may be necessary elements of training, at least for many providers. Of particular importance will be the determination of the "dose" of training that maximizes both impact and cost savings. Although the gold standard of training utilized in controlled treatment efficacy trials would likely achieve favorable outcomes, the cost associated with using this model broadly in mental health services is prohibitive. Thus, identification of the methods best suited to facilitate successful training is needed. In particular, the use of graded approaches that dose training based on clinician needs has the potential to increase efficiency and decrease cost.

Building an infrastructure for maintenance of training gains is similarly important. For example, the use of train-the-trainer models (see Chapter 5, this volume) has the potential to increase the capacity to continue training new staff and to provide continued learning opportunities for those already trained. The challenge of sustainability and provision of new training outside of formal graduate training will be a critical systems-level question.

REFERENCES

Baer, J. S., Rosengren, D. B., Dunn, C. W., Wells, E. A., Ogle, R. L., & Hartzler, B. (2004). An evaluation of workshop training in motivational interviewing for addiction and mental health clinicians. *Drug and Alcohol Dependence, 73,* 99–106.

Barber, J. P., Gallop, R., Crits-Christoph, P., Frank, A., Thase, M., Weiss, R. D., et al. (2006). The role of therapist adherence, therapist competence, and alliance in predicting outcome of individual drug counseling: Results from the National Institute on Drug Abuse Collaborative Cocaine Treatment Study. *Psychotherapy Research, 16,* 229–240.

Barlow, D. H. (Ed.). (2008). *Clinical handbook of psychological disorders* (4th ed.). New York: Guilford.

Barlow, D. H., Farchione, T. J., Fairholme, C. P., Ellard, K. K., Boisseau, C. L., Allen, L. B., et al. (2010). *Unified protocol for the transdiagnostic treatment of emotional disorders: Therapist guide.* New York: Oxford University Press.

Beidas, R. S., & Kendall, P. C. (2010). Training therapists in evidence-based practice: A critical review of studies from a systems-contextual perspective. *Clinical Psychology, 17,* 1–30.

Bennett-Levy, J., McManus, F., Westling, B. E., & Fennell, M. (2009). Acquiring and refining CBT skills and competencies: Which training methods are perceived to be most effective? *Behavioral and Cognitive Psychotherapy, 37,* 571–583.

Coomarasamy, A., & Khan, K. S. (2004). What is the evidence that postgraduate teaching in evidence based medicine changes anything? A systematic review. *British Medical Journal, 329*, 1017.

Crits-Christoph, R., Siqueland, L., Chittams, J., Barber, J. P., Beck, A. T., Frank, A., et al. (1998). Training in cognitive, supportive-expressive, and drug counseling therapies for cocaine dependence. *Journal of Consulting and Clinical Psychology, 66*, 484–492.

David, D. A., Thomson, M. A., Oxman, A. D., & Haynes, R. B. (1995). Changing physician performance: A systematic review of the effect of continuing medical education strategies. *Journal of the American Medical Association, 274*, 700–705.

Davis, D., O'Brien, M. A., Fremantle, N., Wolf, F. M., Mazmanian, P., & Taylor-Vaisey, A. (1999). The impact of formal continuing education: Do conference, workshops, rounds, and other traditional continuing education activities change physician behavior or health care outcomes? *Journal of the American Medical Association, 282*, 867–874.

Dimeff, L. A., Koerner, K., Woodcock, E. A., Beadnell, B., Brown, M. Z., Skutch, J., et al. (2009). Which training method works best? A randomized controlled trial comparing three methods of training clinicians in dialectical behavior therapy skills. *Behaviour Research and Therapy, 47*, 921–930.

Ducharme, J. M., & Feldman, M. A. (1992). Comparison of staff training strategies to promote generalized teaching skills. *Journal of Applied Behavior Analysis, 25*, 165–179.

Ekberg, J., Timpka, T., Bång, M., Fröberg, A., Halje, K., & Eriksson, H. (2011). Cell phone-supported cognitive behavioural therapy for anxiety disorders: A protocol for effectiveness studies in frontline settings. *BMC Medical Research Methodology, 11*, 3.

Fairburn, C. G., Cooper, Z., Doll, H. A., O'Connor, M. E., Bohn, K., Hawker, D. M., et al. (2009). Transdiagnostic cognitive-behavioral therapy for patients with eating disorders: A two-site trial with 60-week follow-up. *American Journal of Psychiatry, 166*, 311–319.

Gallon, S. L., Gabriel, R. M., & Knudsen, J. R. (2003). The toughest job you'll ever love: A Pacific Northwest Treatment Workforce Survey. *Journal of Substance Abuse Treatment, 24*, 183–196.

Grimshaw, J. M., Shirran, L., Thomas, R., Mowatt, G., Fraser, C., Bero, L., et al. (2001). Changing provider behavior: An overview of systematic reviews of interventions. *Medical Care, 39*, 8(Suppl. 2), 2–45.

Henggeler, S. W., Melton, G. B., Brondino, M. J., Scherer, D. G., & Hanley, J. H. (1997). Multisystemic Therapy with violent and chronic juvenile offenders and their families: The role of treatment fidelity in successful dissemination. *Journal of Consulting and Clinical Psychology, 65*, 821–833.

Herschell, A. D., Kolko, D. J., Baumann, B. L., & David, A. C. (2010). The role of therapist training in the implementation of psychosocial treatments: A review and critique with recommendations. *Clinical Psychology Review, 30*, 448–466.

Hogue, A., Henderson, C. E., Dauber, S., Barajas, P. C., Fried, A., & Liddle, H. A. (2008). Treatment adherence, competence, and outcome in individual and family therapy for adolescent behavior problems. *Journal of Consulting and Clinical Psychology, 76*, 544–555.

Institute of Medicine (2010). *Redesigning continuing education in the health professions.* Washington, DC: The National Academies Press.

Kendall, P. C., Gosch, E., Furr, J. M., & Sood, E. (2008). Flexibility with fidelity. *Journal of the American Academy of Child and Adolescent Psychiatry, 47*, 987–993.

King, M., Davidson, O., Taylor, F., Haines, A., Sharp, D., & Turner, R. (2002). Effectiveness of teaching general practitioners skills in brief cognitive behavior therapy to treat patients with depression: Randomised controlled trial. *British Medical Journal, 324,* 947–953.

Larson, M. J., Amodeo, M., Storti, S. A., Steketee, G., Blitzman, G., & Smith, L. (2009). A novel CBT web course for the substance abuse workforce: Community counselors' perceptions. *Substance Abuse, 30,* 26–39.

Lau, M. A., Dubord, G., & Parikh, S. (2004). Effective cognitive therapy education: A pilot study using a longitudinal interactive format. *Canadian Journal of Psychiatry, 49,* 696–700.

Lochman, J. E., Boxmeyer, C., Powell, N., Qu, L., Wells, K., & Windle, M. (2009). Dissemination of the Coping Power Program: Importance of intensity of counselor training. *Journal of Consulting and Clinical Psychology, 77,* 397–409.

Lochman, J. E., & Wells, K. C. (2004). The Coping Power Program for preadolescent aggressive boys and their parents: Outcome effects at the 1-year follow-up. *Journal of Consulting and Clinical Psychology, 72,* 571–578.

Lopez, M. A., Osterberg, L. A., Jensen-Doss, A., & Rae, W. A. (2011). Effects of workshop training for providers under mandated use of evidence-based practice. *Administration and Policy in Mental Health and Mental Health Services Research, 38,* 301–312.

Martino, S., Ball, S. A., Nich, C., Canning-Ball, M., Rounsaville, B. J., & Carroll, K. M. (2011). Teaching community program clinicians motivational interviewing using expert and train-the-trainer strategies. *Addiction, 106,* 428–441.

Martino, S., Canning-Ball, M., Carroll, K. M., & Rounsaville, B. J. (2011). A criterion-based stepwise approach for training counselors in motivational interviewing. *Journal of Substance Abuse Treatment, 40,* 357–365.

McHugh, R. K., & Barlow, D. H. (2010). Dissemination and implementation of evidence-based psychological interventions: A review of current efforts. *American Psychologist, 65,* 73–84.

McHugh, R. K., Murray, H. W., & Barlow, D. H. (2009). Balancing fidelity and adaptation in the dissemination of empirically-supported treatments: The promise of transdiagnostic interventions. *Behaviour Research and Therapy, 47,* 946–953.

Merrill, K. A., Tolbert, V. E., & Wade, W. A. (2003). Effectiveness of cognitive therapy for depression in a community mental health center: A benchmarking study. *Journal of Consulting and Clinical Psychology, 71,* 404–409.

Miller, W. R., & Mount, K. A. (2001). A small study of training in Motivational Interviewing: Does one workshop change clinician and client behavior? *Behavioural and Cognitive Psychotherapy, 29,* 457–471.

Miller, W. R., & Rollnick, S. (1991) *Motivational Interviewing: Preparing people to change addictive behaviour.* New York: Guilford Press.

Miller, W. R., & Rollnick, S. (2002). *Motivational Interviewing: Preparing people for change.* New York: Guilford Press.

Miller, W. R., Sorensen, J. L., Selzer, J. A., & Brigham, G. S. (2006). Disseminating evidence-based practices in substance abuse treatment: A review with suggestions. *Journal of Substance Abuse Treatment, 31,* 25–39.

Miller, W. R., Yahne, C. E., Moyers, T. B., Martinez, J., & Pirritano, M. (2004). A randomized trial of methods to help clinicians learn motivation interviewing. *Journal of Consulting and Clinical Psychology, 72,* 1050–1062.

Milne, D. L., Baker, C., Blackburn, I. M., James, I., & Reichelt, K. (1999). Effectiveness of cognitive therapy training. *Journal of Behavior Therapy and Experimental Psychiatry, 30*, 81–92.

Morgenstern, J., Morgan, T. J., McCrady, B. S., Keller, D. S., & Carroll, K. M. (2001). Manual-guided cognitive behavioral therapy training: A promising method for disseminating empirically supported substance abuse treatments to the practice community. *Psychology of Addictive Behaviors, 15*, 83–88.

Moyers, T. B., Manuel, J. K., Wilson, P. G., Henrickson, S. M. L., Talcott, W., & Durand, P. (2008). A randomized trial investigating training in motivational interviewing for behavioral health providers. *Behavioural and Cognitive Psychotherapy, 36*, 149–162.

Nathan, P. E., & Gorman, J. M. (Eds.). (2007). *A guide to treatments that work* (3rd ed.). New York: Oxford University Press.

Nelson, T. S., Chenail, R. J., Alexander, J. F., Crane, D. R., Johnson, S. M., & Schwallie, L. (2007). The development of core competencies for the practice of marriage and family therapy. *Journal of Marital and Family Therapy, 33*, 417–438.

Norcross, J. C., Hogan, T. P., & Koocher, G. P. (2008). *Clinician's guide to evidence-based practices: Mental health and the addictions.* New York: Oxford University Press.

Perepletchikova, F., Hilt, L. M., Chereji, E., & Kazdin, A. E. (2009). Barriers to implementing treatment integrity procedures: Survey of treatment outcome researchers. *Journal of Consulting and Clinical Psychology, 77*, 212–218.

Perepletchikova, F., Treat, T. A., & Kazdin, A. E. (2007). Treatment integrity in psychotherapy research: Analysis of the studies and examination of the associated factors. *Journal of Consulting and Clinical Psychology, 75*, 829–841.

Rakovshik, S. G., & McManus, F. (2010). Establishing evidence-based training in cognitive behavioral therapy: A review of current empirical findings and theoretical guidance. *Clinical Psychology Review, 30*, 496–516.

Rollins, A. L., Salyers, M. P., Tsai, J., & Lydick, J. M. (2010). Staff turnover in statewide implementation of ACT: Relationship with ACT fidelity and other team characteristics. *Administration and Policy in Mental Health and Mental Health Services Research, 37*, 417–426.

Roth, A., & Fonagy, P. (2005). *What works for whom? A critical review of psychotherapy research.* New York: Guilford Press.

Roth, A. D., & Pilling, S. (2007). *The competences required to deliver effective cognitive and behavioural therapy for people with depression and with anxiety disorders.* Retrieved May 7, 2008, from http://www.dh.gov.uk/en/Publicationsandstatistics/Publications/PublicationsPolicyAndGuidance/DH_078537

Rubel, E. C., Sobell, L. C., & Miller, W. R. (2000). Do continuing education workshops improve participants' skills? Effects of a motivational interviewing workshop on substance-abuse counselors' skills and knowledge. *Behavior Therapist, 23*(4), 73–77.

Saitz, R., Sullivan, L. M., & Samet, J. H. (2000). Training community-based clinicians in screening and brief intervention for substance abuse problems: Translating evidence into practice. *Substance Abuse, 21*, 21–31.

Schoener, E. P., Madeja, C. L., Henderson, M. J., Ondersma, S. J., & Janisse, J. J. (2006). Effects of motivational interviewing training on mental health therapist behavior. *Drug and Alcohol Dependence, 82*, 269–275.

Schoenwald, S. K., Sheidow, A. J., & Chapman, J. E. (2009). Clinical supervision in treatment transport: Effects on adherence and outcomes. *Journal of Consulting and Clinical Psychology, 77*, 410–421.

Sholomskas, D. E., Syracuse-Siewert, G., Rounsaville, B. J., Ball, S. A., Nuro, K. F., & Carroll, K. M. (2005). We don't train in vain: A dissemination trial of three strategies of training clinicians in cognitive-behavioral therapy. *Journal of Consulting and Clinical Psychology, 73*, 106–115.

Smith, J. L., Amrhein, P. C., Brooks, A. C., Carpenter, K. M., Levin, D., Schreiber, E. A., et al. (2007). Providing live supervision via teleconferencing improves acquisition of motivational interviewing skills after workshop attendance. *American Journal of Drug and Alcohol Abuse, 33*, 163–168.

Sobell, L. C. (1996). Bridging the gap between scientists and practitioners: The challenge before us. *Behavior Therapy, 27*, 297–320.

Stirman, S. W., Bhar, S. S., Spokas, M., Brown, G. K., Creed, T. A., Farabaugh, D. T., et al. (2010). Training and consultation in evidence-based psychosocial treatments in public mental health settings: The ACCESS model. *Professional Psychology: Research and Practice, 41*, 48–56.

Stirman, S. W., Buchhofer, R., McLaulin, J. B., Evans, A. C., & Beck, A. T. (2009). The Beck Initiative: A partnership to implement cognitive therapy in a community behavioral health system. *Psychiatric Services, 60*, 1302–1304.

VandeCreek, L., Knapp, S., & Brace, K. (1990). Mandatory continuing education for licensed psychologists: Its rationale and current implications. *Professional Psychology: Research and Practice, 21*, 135–140.

Webb, C. A., Derubeis, R. J., & Barber, J. P. (2010). Therapist adherence/competence and treatment outcome: A meta-analytic review. *Journal of Consulting and Clinical Psychology, 78*, 200–211.

Weingardt, K. R. (2004). The role of instructional design and technology in the dissemination of empirically supported, manual-based therapies. *Clinical Psychology: Science and Practice, 11*, 331–341.

Weingardt, K. R., Cucciare, M. A., Bellotti, C., & Lai, W. P. (2009). A randomized trial comparing two models of web-based training in cognitive-behavioral therapy for substance abuse counselors. *Journal of Substance Abuse Treatment, 37*, 219–227.

PART II

Dissemination and Implementation Programs

The English Improving Access to Psychological Therapies (IAPT) Program

HISTORY AND PROGRESS

David M. Clark

On World Mental Health Day in October 2007, the UK government announced a large-scale initiative for Improving Access to Psychological Therapies (IAPT) for depression and anxiety disorders within the English National Health Service (NHS). Between 2008 and 2011, at least 3,600 new psychological therapists will have been trained and employed in new IAPT clinical services offering the evidence-based psychological therapies that are recommended by the National Institute for Clinical Excellence (NICE). A further cohort of around 2,400 new psychological therapists should be trained between 2011 and 2014, so that the services will have sufficient therapist capacity to offer treatment to at least 15% of people in the community with depression and/or anxiety disorders. The training follows national curricula and initially particularly focused on cognitive behavioral therapy (CBT), as this was where the manpower shortage was considered greatest. As the program matures, training in other NICE-recommended treatments for depression is also being made available. The clinical and other outcomes of patients who access the services are carefully monitored. This article describes the background to the program, provides an overview of the training initiative and clinical service model, presents a summary of progress to date (early 2011), and anticipates future developments.

Motivating Circumstances

The IAPT program had its roots in a wide range of clinical and policy developments. However, two developments deserve particular mention. First, starting in 2004, NICE systematically reviewed the evidence for the effectiveness of a variety of interventions for depression and anxiety disorders. These reviews led to the publication of a series of clinical guidelines (NICE, 2004a, 2004b, 2005a, 2005b, 2006, 2009a, 2009b, 2011) that strongly support the use of certain psychological therapies. CBT is recommended for depression and all the anxiety disorders. Some other therapies (interpersonal psychotherapy, behavioral couples therapy, counseling, brief dynamic therapy) are also recommended (with varying indications) for depression, but not for anxiety disorders. In light of the evidence that some individuals respond well to "low-intensity" interventions (such as guided self-help and computerized CBT), NICE also advocates a stepped-care approach to the delivery of psychological therapies in mild to moderate depression and some anxiety disorders. In moderate to severe depression and in some other anxiety disorders (such as posttraumatic stress disorder [PTSD]), low-intensity interventions are not recommended and instead it is suggested that patients should be offered immediate "high-intensity" face-to-face psychological therapy. Table 4.1 summarizes the current NICE recommendations.

In the second development, economists and clinical researchers combined resources to argue that an increase in access to psychological therapies would largely pay for itself by reducing other depression- and anxiety-related public costs (welfare benefits and medical costs) and increasing revenues (taxes from return to work, increased productivity, etc.). This argument was advanced in academic articles (e.g., Layard, Clark, Knapp, & Mayraz, 2007), but also in the more populist pamphlets such as the *Depression Report* (Layard et al., 2006) and *We Need to Talk* (a report sponsored by numerous mental health and other charities). The latter were widely distributed to the public and to policymakers. For example, the *Depression Report* was included in every copy of a national newspaper (the *Observer*) on Sunday, June 18, 2006.

The UK government was receptive to the recommendations of NICE and to the broader arguments advanced in the *Depression Report* and elsewhere. A general political commitment to increase the availability of evidence-based psychological treatments was secured in 2005. However, before any decisions about the scale and form of the increase could be established, the government wisely decided to fund two pilot projects that would test whether the outcomes that one would expect from implementing NICE guidelines could be achieved in practice if a local area was given increased funding to recruit and deploy additional psychological therapists.

Doncaster and Newham Demonstration Sites

In 2006 the NHS in England consisted of 154 primary care trusts (PCTs), each of which had responsibility for the health care of its local population. Two PCTs (Doncaster and Newham) were chosen as pilot sites (termed "demonstration sites" by the Department of Health). Full details of the clinical services that were developed in the two demonstration sites and the outcomes they obtained in their first year can be found in Clark and colleagues (2009) and Richards and Suckling (2009).

Briefly, each demonstration site received substantial funds to recruit and deploy an expanded workforce of CBT-focused psychological therapists. Doncaster had

TABLE 4.1 Summary of NICE's Recommendations for the Psychological Treatment of Depression and Anxiety Disorders

Place in Stepped-Care Service	Disorder	Recommended Intervention
Step 3: High-intensity service (*Primarily weekly, face-to-face, one-on-one sessions with a suitably trained therapist. In some disorders, such as depression, CBT can also be delivered effectively to small groups of patients. Behavioral couples therapy naturally involves the therapist, the depressed client, and his or her partner*)	Depression: moderate to severe	CBT or IPT,[a] each with medication
	Depression: mild to moderate	CBT or IPT[a] Behavioral activation (BA)[a,b] Behavioral couples therapy (*if the patient has a partner, the relationship is considered to be contributing to the maintenance of the depression, and both parties wish to work together in therapy*) Counseling[a] or short-term psychodynamic therapy[a] (*consider if patient has declined CBT, IPT, BA, or behavioral couples therapy*)
	Panic disorder	CBT
	GAD	CBT
	Social phobia	CBT
	PTSD	CBT, EMDR
	OCD	CBT
Step 2: Low-intensity service (*Less intensive clinician input than the high-intensity service. Patients are typically encouraged to work through some form of self-help program with frequent, brief guidance and encouragement from a Psychological Well-Being Practitioner [PWP] who acts as a coach*)	Depression	Guided self-help based on CBT, computerized CBT, behavioral activation, structured physical activity
	Panic disorder	Self-help based on CBT, computerized CBT
	GAD	Self-help based on CBT, psychoeducational groups, computerized CBT
	PTSD	n/a[c]
	Social phobia	n/a
	OCD	Guided self-help based on CBT
Step 1: Primary care	Recognition of problem	Assessment/referral/active monitoring
	Moderate to severe Depression with a chronic physical health problem	Collaborative care (*consider if depression has not responded to initial course of high-intensity intervention and/or medication*)

Notes. CBT = cognitive behavioral therapy; IPT = interpersonal therapy; EMDR = eye movement desensitization reprocessing therapy (considered by many to be a form of CBT). Behavioral activation is a variant of CBT. Active monitoring includes careful monitoring of symptoms, psychoeducation about the disorder, and sleep hygiene advice.

[a]NICE's recent (*2009a, 2009*b) updates on the treatment of depression come in two parts: recommendations for the treatment of "depression" and recommendations for the treatment of "depression in people with a chronic physical health problem." The two guidelines are very similar. However, it should be noted that the "depression with a physical health problem" guideline does *not* recommend IPT, behavioral activation, counseling, or brief dynamic therapy as high-intensity interventions.

TABLE 4.1 Summary of NICE's Recommendations for the Psychological Treatment of Depression and Anxiety Disorders

[b]Although the recent update of the NICE Guidance for Depression (NICE, *2009a*) recommends behavioral activation for the treatment of mild to moderate depression, it notes that the evidence base is not as strong as for CBT or IPT.

[c]NICE does not recommend any low-intensity interventions for PTSD and recommends that you do NOT offer psychological debriefing.

NICE has not yet issued guidance on the treatment of social phobia. However, there is a substantial body of evidence supporting the effectiveness of high-intensity CBT. Low-intensity versions of CBT are being developed by several groups around the world and it seems likely that they will play a useful role in the future.

been pioneering the use of low-intensity therapies (especially guided self-help) and chose to particularly expand the workforce that delivered these treatments, although some additional capacity to deliver high-intensity interventions (face-to-face CBT) was also developed. Many of the guided self-help sessions were delivered over the telephone. As low-intensity interventions and stepped care are not recommended by NICE for PTSD, the Doncaster site excluded this anxiety disorder but encouraged referrals for other anxiety disorders, as well as depression. Newham initially placed greater emphasis on high-intensity CBT, although it also operated a stepped-care model when appropriate, using a newly recruited workforce of low-intensity therapists (subsequently called Psychological Well-being Practitioners or PWPs). The low-intensity therapies included computerized CBT (cCBT), guided self-help, and psychoeducation groups.

In order to determine whether the demonstration sites were able to achieve the outcomes one might expect from the randomized controlled trials that led to NICE's recommendations for the use of psychological treatments in depression and anxiety disorders, both demonstration sites agreed to adopt a session-by-session outcome-monitoring system that had demonstrated its worth in achieving high levels of pre/post treatment data completeness in community samples (Gillespie, Duffy, Hackmann, & Clark, 2002). At every clinical contact patients were asked to complete simple measures of depression (PHQ-9: Kroenke, Spitzer, & Williams, 2001) and anxious affect (GAD-7: Spitzer, Kroenke, Williams, & Lowe, 2006). If specific anxiety disorders (agoraphobia, social phobia, obsessive-compulsive disorder [OCD], PTSD, etc.) were being treated, patients were also encouraged to complete a validated measure of that disorder (e.g., the Revised Impact of Events Scale in PTSD: Weiss & Marmar, 1997). This is because the GAD-7 does not cover key features of specific anxiety disorders, such as phobic avoidance, compulsive behavior, and intrusive thoughts, images, or impulses.

Since the creation of the NHS in 1948, most patients who received specialist psychological therapy had to be referred by their general practitioner (GP), partly to help constrain NHS costs. However, there was some concern that requiring patients to be referred by a GP might be seen as an impediment to access for some members of the community. For this reason, the demonstration sites were allowed to also accept self-referrals as an experiment to see whether it identified people with mental health problems who would not otherwise have access to services.

The main findings from the first year of operation of the two demonstration sites were as follows:

Clinical problems: The two sites saw somewhat different populations. Although Doncaster did not use formal diagnoses, GP referral letters mentioned depression as the main problem in 95% of cases. In the remaining 5% anxiety was mentioned as the main problem, mainly generalized anxiety disorder (GAD) (3.9%). Newham established International Classification of Diseases, 10th edition (ICD-10) diagnoses. The main problems were depression (46% of patients), anxiety disorders (43%), and other problems (11%).

Numbers seen: Taken together, the two sites saw an impressively large number of people (over 3,500) in the first year, with the use of low-intensity therapies and stepped care being the key ingredients for managing large numbers. For this reason, as the year progressed the Newham site increased the size of its PWP workforce.

Data completeness: The session-by-session outcome-monitoring system ensured that almost all (over 99% in Doncaster and 88% in Newham) patients who received at least two sessions had pre- *and* posttreatment PHQ-9 and GAD-7 scores. For patients who discontinued therapy earlier than expected, the scores from the last available session were used as posttreatment scores. As well as the new session-by-session outcome-monitoring scheme, the sites also obtained outcome data on the CORE-OM (Barkham et al., 2001) using a more conventional pretreatment- and posttreatment-only data collection protocol. As is usual in community samples, this protocol produced a much lower data completeness rate (6% in Doncaster, 54% in Newham), mainly due to missing posttreatment scores. Figure 4.1 shows the mean improvements in depression (assessed by the PHQ-9) and anxiety (assessed by the GAD-7) in patients treated in Newham who did, and did not, provide posttreatment data on the conventional (CORE-OM–based) outcome-monitoring protocol. Patients who failed to provide posttreatment data on the conventional system showed less than half of the improvement of those who did provide posttreatment data. This finding led the IAPT national team to conclude that services that have substantial missing data rates are likely to overestimate their effectiveness. For this reason, session-by-session outcome monitoring was adopted in the subsequent national roll-out of IAPT (see below).

Self-referral versus GP referral: Newham, which has a mixed ethnic community, made extensive use of self-referral. Comparisons of self-referred and GP-referred patients indicated that the self-referrers had similarly high PHQ-9 and GAD-7 scores as the GP referrals but tended (nonsignificantly) to have had their problem longer. Importantly, self-referrals more accurately tracked the ethic mix of the community (minorities were underrepresented among GP referrals) and had higher rates of PTSD and social phobia, both conditions that traditionally tend to be

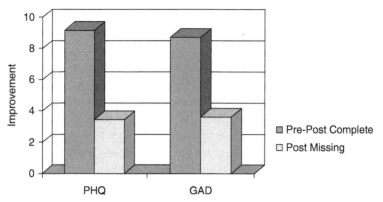

FIGURE 4.1 *Improvement in PHQ-9 and GAD-7 scores between initial assessment (pre-) and last available session (post-) in people who either completed both the pre- and posttreatment CORE-OM or who failed to complete the CORE-OM at posttreatment. Data from the Newham demonstration site. Figure derived from Clark and colleagues (2009).*

underrecognized. These findings led the government to include self-referral in the subsequent national roll-out.

Outcomes: The high level of data completeness on the PHQ-9 and GAD-7 made it possible to accurately assess any clinical improvements that patients achieved while being treated in the demonstration sites. All patients who received at least two sessions (including assessment) were included in the analysis, irrespective of whether they were coded as completers or dropouts by their therapist. As a group, patients treated in both sites showed large improvements (pre- and posttreatment uncontrolled effect sizes of 0.98 to 1.26). Individuals were considered clinically recovered if they scored above the clinical cut-off on the PHQ and/or the GAD at pretreatment and below the clinical cut-off on *both* at posttreatment. Using this criterion, 55% (Newham) and 56% (Doncaster) of patients recovered. Self-referrers and patients from ethnic minorities were no less likely to recover than GP referrals and Caucasians, respectively.

The economic argument for IAPT (Layard et al., 2007) was based on the assumption that clinical improvement would be sustained and that treatment would improve people's employment status as well as symptoms. To assess whether clinical improvements were sustained, patients in both sites were asked to recomplete the outcome measures 9 months (on average) after discharge. Unfortunately, data completeness at follow-up (36% in Newham and 51% in Doncaster) was much lower than at posttreatment (88% and 99%, respectively). However, among those people who did provide data, the gains that were achieved in therapy were largely maintained. To assess employment changes, pretreatment and posttreatment employment status was compared. It had been assumed that IAPT services would achieve an overall improvement in employment status in 4% of the total treated cohort (Layard et al., 2007). The observed rate was 5%.

Although the outcomes observed in the demonstration sites were broadly in line with expectations, it is important to realize that the sites were not set up as randomized controlled trials and it is likely that some of the observed improvement would have happened anyway (e.g., natural recovery). Various studies suggest that natural recovery rates over a period of time that is similar to the duration of IAPT treatment are high among recent-onset (<6 months) cases of depression and anxiety disorders but are substantially lower among more chronic cases. Building on this observation, Clark and colleagues (2009) separately computed the recovery rates among recent-onset and chronic cases. Most cases (83% in Newham, 66% in Doncaster) had been depressed or anxious for over 6 months and it seemed safe to conclude that treatment had provided added benefit to this group as the recovery rates (52% at each site) comfortably exceeded the 5% to 20% one might expect from natural recovery or minimal intervention. However, among the minority of cases with a recent onset, it was not possible to exclude the possibility that much of the improvement may have been due to natural recovery (see Clark et al., 2009, p. 919).

Description of the National Program

INITIAL FUNDING, GOALS, AND TARGETS

Following the success of the Newham and Doncaster demonstration sites and the submission of a detailed business case, which included reviews of controlled evaluations of CBT in depression and anxiety disorders, the UK government announced that it intended to greatly increase the availability of evidence-based psychological therapies for depression and anxiety disorders throughout England through a phased roll-out that would last several years. Funding for the first 3 years was announced: year 1: £33 million; year 2: an additional £70 million on top of the year 1 sum (which had become recurrent); year 3: an additional £70 million on top of the years 1 and 2 sums. The total over 3 years was £309 million.

The funding was allocated to train up to 3,600 new psychological therapists (60% high-intensity CBT therapists, 40% PWPs) and to deploy them, along with existing experienced clinicians, in new psychological treatment services for depression and anxiety disorders that operate on stepped-care principles. The training program initially focused on CBT as (a) it is recommended by NICE for both depression and anxiety disorders and (b) it is the therapy where the manpower shortage was considered to be greatest.

Targets were set for the number of patients that would be seen by the services in the first 3 years and there was an expectation that 50% would "move to recovery" in terms of their symptomatology. In addition, it was expected that 25,000 fewer people would be on sick pay or receiving state benefits. At least 20 of England's 154 PCTs were expected to establish new IAPT services during the first year (2008–2009), with more PCTs joining in future years.

In order to realize these goals, the Department of Health established a series of expert groups that helped devise the necessary training program and specified key features of the IAPT clinical services. A large number of documents providing guidance to courses and PCTs were produced, most of which can be viewed on the IAPT website (http://www.iapt.nhs.uk). Table 4.2 lists the key documents, including the *National Implementation Plan* (Department of Health, 2008).

During the first 2 years, all funds were held centrally by the Department of Health and distributed through England's 10 Strategic Health Authorities (SHAs), who commissioned appropriate regional training courses and selected the PCTs that would receive the new trainees and other resources needed to set up a new IAPT service. Rather than place a few trainees to each PCT, it was decided to initially allocate a substantial number of trainees to a few PCTs (early adopters), who would then have the resources to create a service with sufficient capacity to ensure patients are seen promptly. During the third year, the principle for distributing funds changed and much of the money for IAPT went into the general bundle of funds that PCTs receive to finance all of their health care work.

TRAINING

In order to guide the training of the new workforce, the Department of Health commissioned and distributed separate national curricula for the training of high-intensity CBT therapists and PWPs. As the main aim of the IAPT program is to increase the availability of treatments recommended by NICE, the high-intensity CBT curriculum is closely aligned to the particular CBT programs that had been shown to be effective in the randomized controlled trials that contributed to NICE's recommendations. A wide range of general CBT assessment and intervention

TABLE 4.2 Key IAPT Reference Documents with Publication Dates in Parentheses, When Relevant

---

IAPT Implementation Plan: National Guidelines for Regional Delivery *(February 2008)*
IAPT Implementation Plan: Curriculum for High-Intensity Workers
IAPT Implementation Plan: Curriculum for Low-Intensity Workers
IAPT Impact Assessment *(February 2008)*
IAPT Equality Impact Assessment *(February 2008)*
IAPT Supervision Guidance
IAPT Commissioning Toolkit *(April 2008)*
Realising the Benefits: IAPT at Full Roll-Out *(February 2010)*
The Operating Framework for the NHS in England 2011/12
No Health without Mental Health *(February 2010)*
Talking Therapies: A Four Year Plan *(February 2010)*
Which Talking Therapy for Depression
Commissioning Talking Therapies for 2011/12 *(March 2011)*
IAPT Data Handbook 2

---

strategies are included in the curriculum. In addition, trainees are required to be taught at least two evidence-based treatments for depression (cognitive therapy and behavioral activation) and at least one specific, evidence-based treatment for each anxiety disorder. In panic disorder, examples include Barlow and colleagues' CBT program (Craske & Barlow, 2007) and Clark and colleagues' cognitive therapy program (Clark et al., 1999). In PTSD, examples include Foa's imaginal reliving therapy (Foa, Hembree, & Rothbaum, 2007), Ehlers and Clark's cognitive therapy (Ehlers, Clark, Hackmann, McManus, & Fennell, 2005), and Resick's Cognitive Processing Therapy (Resick & Schnicke, 1996). Roth and Pilling (2008) developed a competency framework for many of the leading empirically-supported CBT treatments for depression and anxiety disorders and the high-intensity curriculum aims to ensure that these are covered in IAPT training programs. In addition to specifying the skills that trainees should acquire, the curriculum also specifies how these skills should be assessed (through a mixture of ratings of actual therapy sessions using the revised version of the Cognitive Therapy Rating Scale [CTS-R: Blackburn et al., 2001] and written assignments in the form of case reports and essays).

A separate curriculum was issued for PWP training. The four sections of the curriculum cover (a) engagement and assessment; (b) evidence-based low-intensity treatments; (c) values, policy, culture, and diversity; and (d) working within an employment, social, and health care context. As low-intensity working is relatively new, there are few published therapist manuals. To redress this shortfall, a substantial set of teaching aids developed by David Richards (one of the pioneers of low-intensity work) and his colleagues were produced to supplement the curriculum. As with the high-intensity curriculum, assessment procedures are also specified, with particular emphasis being placed on structured role plays covering a wide range of different skills.

Both the high-intensity CBT and the PWP training programs are conceived as joint university and in-service trainings. Over a period of approximately 1 year, high-intensity trainees attend a university-based course for lectures, workshops, and case supervision 2 days a week, while PWPs attend university for 1 day per week. For the rest of their time, both sets of trainees work in an IAPT service where they receive further regular supervision. The services are also encouraged to provide the trainees with the opportunity to directly observe therapy sessions conducted by experienced staff that work in the service.

IMPROVING ACCESS TO PSYCHOLOGICAL THERAPIES (IAPT) SERVICE MODEL

A general framework for IAPT services was outlined in the *National Implementation Plan* (Department of Health, 2008). The framework specifies several key principles for the operation of the services while leaving considerable scope for local determination. The key principles include:

- Access to the service through self-referral as well as referral by a general practitioner.

- A person-centered assessment that identifies the key problems that require treatment and their social and personal context. Goals for therapy are identified and a treatment plan is jointly agreed upon.
- Stepped care in which many people with mild to moderate depression or anxiety disorders are offered treatment with a PWP initially. Many people recover with such treatment. Individuals who do not should be offered a further course of high-intensity treatment. For people with more severe depression or anxiety and for everyone with PTSD, immediate high-intensity treatment is recommended. All treatments that are offered should be in line with NICE recommendations.
- Access to an employment advisor if employment (lack of, or danger of losing) is an issue. Services are encouraged to involve employment advisors in treatment plans from the very beginning as making progress with employment issues can greatly facilitate psychological recovery and vice versa.
- Use of the IAPT minimum dataset (see *IAPT Data Handbook 2* [Department of Health, 2011d] for full details). This includes giving the PHQ-9 and GAD-7 every session along with some other patient self-report measures that focus on specific anxiety disorders, when these are relevant. All data are entered into an electronic database that enables therapists and their supervisors to monitor patients' progress and adjust treatment plans, if required.
- All therapists should receive weekly, outcome-informed supervision, which ensures that all cases are discussed at regular intervals and decisions about step-up/step-down are made in a timely fashion (see *IAPT Supervision Guidance*).
- Because of the importance of obtaining outcome data on almost all patients who receive treatment, the services are asked to ensure that at least 90% of patients who are seen at least twice in a service have a pretreatment and posttreatment (or last available session) score on the main outcome measures. For patients who exceed the clinical cut-off for depression and/or anxiety at pretreatment, "recovery" is operationalized as moving to below the clinical cut-off for *both* depression and anxiety at posttreatment.

PROGRESS TO DATE

At the time of writing (Spring 2011), the IAPT program is midway through its third year. Progress to date includes:

- IAPT services have been established in 95% of PCTs. However, there is wide variation in the number of therapists employed in the services, and, as a consequence, they vary substantially in the number of patients that they are able to see. It is therefore calculated that only around 60% of the population has access to an IAPT service. For this reason, there is a need to further expand the services in the coming years (see later section on future developments).

- Over 3,660 new high-intensity therapists and PWPs have been appointed and will have completed their training by the end of the year.
- The IAPT services are currently seeing around 310,000 patients per annum and aim to see around 900,000 per annum by 2015 when the roll-out of the program should be complete.
- National data collected at the end of the second year of the program showed that it is on target in terms of the number of people seen (399, 460 compared to a target of 400,000) and the number of people who have moved off sick pay and/or state benefits (13,962 compared to a target of 11,100), and has recovery rates that are approaching expectation (an average of 40% compared to a target of 50%).

LESSONS FROM THE FIRST PHASE OF THE IMPLEMENTATION

In addition to the broad performance figures given above, the Department of Health has released two reports that provide more detailed analysis of the national IAPT program during its first year of operation (October 1, 2008, to September 39, 2009). During this period 35 PCTs established an IAPT service, 32 of which provided data for analysis.

The first report (Glover, Webb, & Evison, 2010) particularly focused on issues to do with equity of access, descriptions of the treatments offered, and overall outcome. With respect to equity of access, both genders were fairly represented in the year 1 IAPT services. The most recent Adult Psychiatric Morbidity Survey (McManus, Meltzer, Brugha, Bebbington, & Jenkins, 2009) shows that 61% of people in the community with a common mental disorder are female, which was very similar to the rate in IAPT services (66% female). However, people older than 65 years and people from the black and minority ethnic (BME) groups were somewhat underrepresented. Part of the reason for the latter finding may have been the slow development of a self-referral route into the services. Clark and colleagues (2009) found that self-referral produces a more equitable pattern of access for different ethnic groups, but only 10% of patients came through self-referral (compared to 21% in the Newham demonstration site). Looking at clinical conditions, it was difficult to assess equity of access accurately because for 39% of patients, an ICD diagnosis was not recorded. However, among the 61% for whom diagnoses were recorded, there was an overrepresentation of patients with depression or mixed anxiety and depressive disorder (MADD), compared to prevalence rates found in epidemiological studies. There was also underrepresentation of patients with persistent anxiety disorders, such as PTSD, OCD, panic disorder, social phobia, and agoraphobia, as less than 10% of patients had these diagnoses, whereas around a third of patients should have these disorders if access was equitable (see McManus et al., 2009).

The first report also found that the majority of patients received NICE-compliant treatment. The NICE-recommended low-intensity interventions that were provided included guided self-help, psychoeducation groups, behavioral activation, computerized CBT, and structured exercise. NICE recommends CBT as a high-intensity psychological therapy for depression and for all the anxiety disorders that are currently covered by guidelines. In line with this recommendation, almost everyone with a recorded diagnosis of social phobia, specific phobia, agoraphobia, or OCD received CBT. For patients with a recorded diagnosis of GAD or PTSD, CBT was also the most commonly provided treatment. However, a significant number of patients received counseling, which is not recommended by NICE for these conditions. For patients with a recorded diagnosis of depression, CBT and counseling were equally likely to be offered and both are recommended by NICE, although counseling has a more restricted recommendation in terms of the range of cases for which it is considered relevant (see Table 4.1). Turning to clinical outcomes, a recovery rate of 42% was observed among suitable patients who were likely to have received at least some treatment (defined as having at least two sessions on the assumption that the first session was always assessment). However, there was considerable between-site variability in recovery rates.

The second report (Gyani, Shafran, Layard, & Clark, 2011) explored the observed variability in recovery rates in further detail in order to identify site and other characteristics that were associated with higher recovery rates. The analyses focused on patients who were clinical cases on entry into the service, had received a least two sessions, and had completed their involvement with the services. Pre- to posttreatment data completeness for these patients was good (>90%). The findings, which are briefly summarized below, generally support the IAPT clinical model and highlight the value of following NICE guidelines.

Patients had a higher chance of meeting recovery criteria if they were treated at sites that had the following characteristics:

- Higher step-up rates from low-intensity to high-intensity therapy among those who had failed to respond adequately to the former (i.e., the services were making good use of stepped care)
- Higher average numbers of therapy sessions at low intensity and at high intensity (highlighting the importance of providing an adequate dose of treatment)

Although most patients received NICE-recommended treatments, for some clinical conditions a significant minority of patients received a treatment not recommended by NICE. This created a natural experiment in which it was possible to assess whether deviation from NICE recommendations was associated with a reduction in recovery rates. One of the natural experiments concerned the contrast between CBT and counseling. For depression, NICE recommends both treatments for mild to moderate cases. Consistent with this recommendation, there was no difference in the recovery rates associated with CBT and counseling among patients with a diagnosis of depression. In contrast to the recommendations for depression, NICE does not recommend counseling for the treatment of GAD. Consistent with this position, CBT was associated with a higher recovery rate than counseling among patients with a diagnosis of GAD. A further natural experiment concerned the contrast between guided self-help and pure (nonguided) self-help. NICE only recommends guided self-help for depression. Consistent with this position, guided self-help was associated with a higher recovery rate than pure self-help among patients with a diagnosis of depression. Taken together, these findings would appear to support the value of aligning clinical interventions with NICE guidance. However, this conclusion needs to be treated with caution as these "natural experiments" are not randomized clinical trials.

A final variable considered in the second report was initial severity. Patients with higher initial depression or anxiety scores were less likely to meet recovery criteria (dropping below the clinical/nonclinical threshold) at the end of treatment, but their overall amount of symptomatic improvement was at least as large as that observed in milder cases. This suggests that the IAPT services are beneficial for individuals with a wide range of symptom severity.

Future Development of the Program

Following the success of the first 3 years of the IAPT program, the government announced in February 2011 a further NHS investment of £400 million to complete and extend the program over the period 2011–2015. Full details of the next phase can be found in the mental health policy entitled *No Health without Mental Health* (Department of Health, 2011b) and in the accompanying document entitled *Talking Therapies: Four Year Plan of Action* (Department of Health, 2011c).

Briefly, a major component of the next phase is completion of the roll-out of IAPT services for adults. This will require the training of a further 2,400 new high-intensity and PWP therapists. At the same time, continuing profession development (CPD) short courses will be used to further enhance and update existing clinicians' skills in non-CBT therapies that are recommended by NICE for the treatment of mild to moderate depression, in order to widen patient choice for evidence-based treatments within IAPT services. The CPD courses are aligned to national curricula and published competencies (available at www.iapt.nhs.uk) and cover interpersonal psychotherapy, couples therapy, a form of brief psychodynamic therapy (dynamic interpersonal therapy), and counseling.

A challenge for the completion of the program is a change in the way funding for the training and new posts will be managed. In the first 2 years of the program, all funds were centrally held and ring fenced. It was therefore possible to ensure that they were exclusively spent on the IAPT workforce. In year 3 (2010–2011), a significant proportion of the funds were allocated within general NHS budgets (technically termed "PCT baseline funding"), as are the funds for most mainstream NHS activities. Unfortunately, there is evidence that some of this money was not spent on IAPT, although the numbers of new trainees in that year remained on target. In the next phase, almost all funds will be allocated within general NHS training and PCT budgets and there is a risk that some geographical areas will invest less in IAPT than expected. To mitigate this risk, the Department of Health has specifically highlighted the importance of IAPT by including it for the first time in the *Operating Framework for the NHS* (Department of Health, 2010). To assist local commissioners in their decision making, a guidance document that highlights the value of extending IAPT has been issued. *Commissioning Talking Therapies for 2011/12* (Department of Health, 2011a) outlines the major savings in other costs to the NHS and to society that can be realized by increasing the availability of evidence-based psychological treatments for depression and anxiety disorders. One of the NHS savings relates to the medical treatment of chronic physical health problems, such as coronary heart disease, obstructive pulmonary disease, and diabetes, all of which are more costly to medically manage when a person is also depressed.

A further challenge concerns the relationship between IAPT and other NHS mental health services. The decision to deploy the IAPT workforce in new services was important to ensure consistency of the training experience and clinical supervision, compliance to NICE guidance, and high levels of data completeness. However, it is also important that the new services are well integrated with other NHS provisions for mental health problems. For this to happen, local areas need to develop coherent care pathways that provide clarity about who should be seen, by which service, and at which point in their care. Transition between services should be facilitated, whenever it is appropriate. It is essential that commissioners understand what their local IAPT service can and cannot offer when considering any reorganization of other services so they do not inadvertently reduce provision for individuals with some conditions or complexities whose care is best provided elsewhere.

Reporting on the performance of IAPT services will also be enhanced in the next phase to provide clinicians with valuable information they can use to further develop the accessibility and effectiveness of their IAPT services, as well as increasing transparency for commissioners and the public.

A new feature of the next phase will be the creation of a version of the IAPT program for children and young people. Many of the anxiety disorders that are seen in adult services start in adolescence or earlier and can severely interfere with social and educational development. For this reason, it is important to make effective psychological treatments for these conditions, as well as other mental health problems, available in childhood and adolescence. The underrepresentation of people older than 65 years and people from BME communities that was evident in some

IAPT services in the first phase of the program will also be addressed by initiatives that focus on these individuals.

Conclusions

England is midway through the development of a large-scale program that aims to greatly increase the availability in the NHS of NICE-recommended psychological therapies for depression and anxiety disorders. Following successful pilot work in Doncaster and Newham, a phased national roll-out was planned and is processing broadly in line with expectations. Training of the new workforce has been closely aligned to the skills and competencies required for the specific treatments recommended by NICE and a session-by-session outcome-monitoring system has ensured unprecedentedly high levels of pre- to posttreatment data completeness for key outcome measures. Large numbers of people who would not previously have had the option of a psychological treatment have accessed the services. Average recovery rates are approaching, but are not yet at, those expected from the randomized controlled trials that generated the NICE recommendations. As expected, gains in terms of employment and reductions in state benefits have also been observed. Lessons from the early phases of the program suggest ways in which less-well-performing services may evolve to achieve the outcomes shown by the best services (which are in line with, or exceed, expectations). In the meantime, the extremely high levels of data completeness achieved by IAPT has brought greater transparency to mental health services and helped clinicians and commissioners to identify both areas of excellence and areas that require further attention as the NHS strives to further improve the care it offers people with depression and anxiety disorders.

Acknowledgements

The views expressed by the author are personal and are not necessarily the same as those of the Department of Health. DMC acknowledges the support of the Wellcome Trust (Grant 069777) and the NIHR Biomedical Research Centre at the South London & Maudsley NHS Foundation Trust and Kings College London, UK.

REFERENCES

Barkham, M., Margison, F., Leach, C., Lucock, M., Mellor-Clark, J., Evans, C., et al. (2001). Service profiling and outcomes benchmarking using the CORE-OM: Towards practice-based evidence in the psychological therapies. *Journal of Consulting and Clinical Psychology, 69*, 184–196.

Blackburn, I. M., James, I. A., Milne, D. L., Baker, C., Standart, S., Garland, A., et al. (2001). The revised cognitive therapy scale (CTS-R): Psychometric properties. *Behavioural and Cognitive Psychotherapy, 29*, 431–446.

Clark, D. M., Layard, R., Smithies, R., Richards, D. A., Suckling, R., & Wright, B. (2009) Improving access to psychological therapy: Initial evaluation of two UK demonstration sites. *Behaviour Research and Therapy, 47*, 910–920.

Clark, D. M., Salkovskis, P. M., Hackmann, A., Wells, A., Ludgate, J., & Gelder, M. (1999). Brief cognitive therapy for panic disorder: A randomized controlled trial. *Journal of Consulting and Clinical Psychology, 67*, 583–589.

Craske, M. G., & Barlow, D. H. (2007). *Mastery of your anxiety and panic: Therapist guide* (4th ed.) New York: Oxford University Press.

Department of Health. (2008). *IAPT implementation plan: National guidelines for regional delivery*. London, UK: Author. Retrieved from www.iapt.nhs.uk

Department of Health. (2010). *The operating framework for the NHS in England 2011/12*. London, UK: Author. Retrieved from www.iapt.nhs.uk

Department of Health. (2011a). *Commissioning talking therapies for 2011/12*. London, UK: Author. Retrieved from www.iapt.nhs.uk

Department of Health. (2011b). *No health without mental health*. London, UK: Author. Retrieved from www.iapt.nhs.uk

Department of Health. (2011c). *Talking therapies: A four year plan*. London, UK: Author. Retrieved from www.iapt.nhs.uk

Department of Health (2011d). *The IAPT data handbook* (version 2.0.1). London, UK: Author. Retrieved from www.iapt.nhs.uk

Ehlers, A., Clark, D. M., Hackmann, A., McManus, F., & Fennell, M. (2005). Cognitive therapy for PTSD: Development and evaluation. *Behaviour Research and Therapy, 43*, 413–431.

Foa, E. B., Hembree, E. A., & Rothbaum, B. O. (2007). *Prolonged exposure therapy for PTSD: Therapist guide*. New York: Oxford.

Gillespie, K., Duffy, M., Hackmann, A., & Clark, D. M. (2002). Community based cognitive therapy in the treatment of posttraumatic stress disorder following the Omagh bomb. *Behaviour Research and Therapy, 40*, 345–357.

Glover, G., Webb, M., & Evison, F. (2010). *Improving access to psychological therapies: A review of progress made by sites in the first roll-out year*. North East Public Health Observatory. Retrieved from www.iapt.nhs.uk

Gyani, A., Shafran, R., Layard, R., & Clark, D. M. (2011). *Enhancing recovery rates in IAPT services: Lessons from analysis of the year one data*. Retrieved from www.iapt.nhs.uk

Kroenke, K., Spitzer, R. L., & Williams, J. B. (2001). The PHQ-9: Validity of a brief depression severity measure. *Journal of General and Internal Medicine, 16*, 606–613.

Layard, R., Bell, S., Clark, D. M., Knapp, M., Meacher, M., Priebe, S., et al. (2006). *The Depression Report: A new deal for depression and anxiety disorders* (Centre for Economic Performance Report). London: London School of Economics. Retrieved from http// cep.lse.ac.uk

Layard, R., Clark, D. M., Knapp, M., & Mayraz, G. (2007). Cost-benefit analysis of psychological therapy. *National Institute Economic Review, 202*, 90–98.

McManus, S., Meltzer, H., Brugha, T., Bebbington, P., & Jenkins, R. (2009). *Adult psychiatric morbidity in England 2007: Results of a household survey*. London, UK: The Health and Social Care Information Centre.

National Institute for Clinical Excellence. (2004a). *Anxiety: Management of anxiety (panic disorder, with and without agoraphobia, and generalised anxiety disorder) in adults in primary, secondary and community care* (Clinical Guidance 22). London, UK: National Institute for Clinical Excellence. Retrieved from www.nice.org.uk

National Institute for Clinical Excellence. (2004b). *Depression: Management of depression in primary and secondary care* (Clinical Guide 23). London, UK: National Institute for Clinical Excellence. Retrieved from www.nice.org.uk

National Institute for Clinical Excellence. (2005a). *Obsessive-compulsive disorder: Core interventions in the treatment of obsessive-compulsive disorder and body dysmorphic disorder* (Clinical Guideline 31). London, UK: National Institute for Clinical Excellence. Retrieved from www.nice.org.uk

National Institute for Clinical Excellence. (2005b). *Post-traumatic stress disorder (PTSD): The management of PTSD in adults and children in primary and secondary care* (Clinical Guideline 26). London, UK: National Institute for Clinical Excellence. Retrieved from www.nice.org.uk

National Institute for Clinical Excellence. (2006). *Computerized cognitive behaviour therapy for depression and anxiety* (Technology Appraisal 97). London, UK: National Institute for Clinical Excellence. Retrieved from www.nice.org.uk

National Institute for Clinical Excellence. (2009a). *Depression: Treatment and management of depression in adults* (Clinical Guideline 90). London, UK: National Institute for Clinical Excellence. Retrieved from www.nice.org.uk

National Institute for Clinical Excellence. (2009b). *Depression in adults with a chronic physical health problem: Treatment and management* (Clinical Guideline 91). London, UK: National Institute for Clinical Excellence. Retrieved from www.nice.org.uk

National Institute for Clinical Excellence. (2011). *Common mental health disorders: Identification and pathways to care* (Clinical Guideline 123). London, UK: National Institute for Clinical Excellence. Retrieved from www.nice.org.uk

Resick, P. A., & Schnicke, M. K. (1996). *Cognitive processing therapy for rape victims.* London: Sage Publications.

Richards, D. A., & Suckling, R. (2009). Improving access to psychological therapies: Phase IV prospective cohort study. *British Journal of Clinical Psychology, 48,* 377–396.

Roth, A. D., & Pilling, S. (2008). Using an evidence-based methodology to identify the competencies required to deliver effective cognitive and behavioural therapy for depression and anxiety disorders. *Behavioural and Cognitive Psychotherapy, 36,* 129–147.

Spitzer, R. L., Kroenke, R., Williams, J. B., & Lowe, B. (2006). A brief measure for assessing generalized anxiety disorder: The GAD-7. *Archives of Internal Medicine, 166,* 1092–1097.

Weiss, D. S., & Marmar, C. R. (1997). The Impact of Event Scale Revised. In J. P. Wilson & T. M. Keane (Eds.), *Assessing psychological trauma and PTSD* (pp. 399–411). New York: Guilford Press.

Implementation of Evidence-Based Psychological Treatments in the Veterans Health Administration

Josef I. Ruzek, Bradley E. Karlin, and Antonette Zeiss

The U.S. Department of Veterans Affairs (VA) operates the nation's largest integrated health care system. Administered by the Veterans Health Administration (VHA), the VA health care system addressed the comprehensive health care needs of approximately 5.5 million veterans in fiscal year 2009 (October 1, 2008, through September 30, 2009), of a total of 8 million enrolled veterans. Care is provided to veterans at more than 150 hospitals, more than 900 community-based outpatient clinics, 134 nursing homes (now called "community living centers"), and 271 Readjustment Counseling Centers (or "Vet Centers"). VHA provides a full spectrum of mental health services in inpatient, residential, and outpatient mental health settings at its medical centers and clinics. Mental health services are provided for a diverse range of problems, including posttraumatic stress disorder (PTSD), other anxiety disorders, depression, substance use disorders (SUDs), and psychotic disorders.

Since 2005, VA has been working to transform its mental health care delivery system (Edwards, 2008). As part of this transformation process, VHA has expanded and restructured its mental health operations, increasing the number of VA mental health care staff by over 6,000 to a total of more than 20,000 full-time-equivalent mental health workers. A major focus of this re-engineering of the service system has been on nationally promoting the delivery of evidence-based and recovery-oriented mental health services, including evidence-based practices (EBPs). To promote the delivery of EBPs, VA has developed national initiatives to disseminate evidence-based psychotherapies throughout the VA mental health care system. Since 2007, VA has been working to disseminate Prolonged Exposure Therapy (PE; Foa, Hembree, & Rothbaum, 2007) and Cognitive Processing Therapy (CPT; Resick, Monson, & Chard, 2007) for PTSD, cognitive behavioral therapy (CBT; Beck, Rush, Shaw, & Emery, 1979; Wenzel, Brown, & Karlin, 2010) and Acceptance and Commitment Therapy (ACT; Hayes & Smith, 2005; Walser & Chartier, 2010) for depression, and social skills training (SST) for serious mental illness (SMI; Bellack, Muesser, Gingerich, & Agresta, 2004). These interventions have been established as standards of care within the VA health care system through the development of large-scale training programs and complementary systems interventions designed to support delivery of these EBPs.

Motivating Circumstances

In April 2002, President George Bush's New Freedom Commission on Mental Health conducted a comprehensive study of the U.S. mental health care delivery system and made recommendations for improving the service system, effectively calling for a transformation in the nation's mental health care delivery system to improve service access and quality. The report envisioned a transformed mental health treatment system in which "consistent use of evidence-based, state-of-the-art medications and psychotherapies will be standard practice." In July 2003, the Under Secretary for Health of the Veterans Health Administration charged a workgroup to review the New Freedom Commission's final report to determine the relevance of the commission's goals and recommendations to veterans' mental health programs and to develop an action plan tailored to the special needs of the veteran population. This effort led to the development of a VHA action agenda, "Achieving the Promise: Transforming Mental Health Care in VA," and to the establishment of a mental health task force charged with operationalizing the goals and recommendations outlined in the action agenda. This culminated in the development of a comprehensive VHA Mental Health Strategic Plan (MHSP). One of the overarching goals of the MHSP for achieving transformation in mental health care in VHA was promoting the availability of evidence-based approaches to mental health treatment.

Underlying this process has been a recognition that mental health providers deliver evidence-based psychological treatments at low rates in most delivery settings (Goisman, Warshaw, & Keller, 1999; Jameson, Chambless, & Blank, 2009; Stewart & Chambless, 2007; van Minnen, Hendriks, & Olff, 2010), including VHA (Rosen et al., 2004). VHA saw an opportunity to realize the potential of EBPs and bridge the gap between research and practice so that veterans have access to highly effective treatments for PTSD and other mental health conditions. Further, the wars in Iraq and Afghanistan have given added impetus to efforts to ensure that VA is readily providing the most efficacious and scientifically established mental health services to returning veterans (Ruzek, Vasterling, Schnurr, & Friedman, 2011), as well as to veterans of previous conflicts.

Description of Programs

FUNDING

To help accomplish implementation of EBPs in VHA, significant funding has been allocated to support the hiring of additional mental health staff, the development and implementation of national EBP training programs, and the implementation of other systems changes described below. From October 2007 through September 2010, VA budgeted over $20 million for its national competency-based EBP training programs in CPT and PE for PTSD, CBT and ACT for depression, and SST for serious mental illness. This funding covered all direct costs associated with the development and administration of the training programs, training workshop delivery, staff travel, and ongoing consultation/supervision. As of the end of September 2010, VA has provided training in these EBPs to over 3,800 VA staff members, with some of these staff receiving training in more than one therapy. In addition, VA has provided training to over 800 Department of Defense personnel.

GOALS, TARGETS, AND STANDARDS OF CARE

The VA goal is to ensure that all veterans with mental health problems that include PTSD, depression, and serious mental illness have access to EBPs for these conditions. Following the development and implementation of the VHA Mental Health Strategic Plan, VA established national requirements for the range of evidence-based and recovery-oriented mental health services that must be available to all veterans through the VA care system. These requirements are delineated in VHA Handbook 1160.01, *Uniform Mental Health Services in VA Medical Centers and Clinics* (VHA, 2008). Included in the handbook are specific requirements that veterans have full access to evidence-based psychotherapies. Specifically, the handbook requires that all veterans with PTSD have access to CPT or PE; that all veterans with depression have access to CBT, ACT, or interpersonal therapy (IPT); and that all veterans with serious mental illness have access to SST. The handbook further requires that medical centers and large clinics have full staff capacity to provide these treatments. Additional therapies may be available to veterans, though the *Uniform Mental Health Services* handbook is designed to ensure that the above therapies are available, at a minimum, and offered to all veterans who can benefit from them. Of course, the selection of a particular treatment for a specific patient is made by the patient, in collaboration with his or her therapist. These recommendations are consistent with the Clinical Practice Guidelines jointly developed by VA and the Department of Defense (DoD). Based on review of research evidence and informed by expert consensus, VA/DoD Clinical Practice Guidelines related to mental disorders include guidelines for management of PTSD, major depressive disorder, substance use disorder, and bipolar disorder in adults.

Needs Assessment/Fit to System Needs

VA's efforts to nationally disseminate and implement EBPs began with initiatives to disseminate EBPs for PTSD. PTSD is among the most highly prevalent mental health problems experienced by veterans returning from Iraq and Afghanistan and, indeed, by veterans of Vietnam and other conflicts (Seal et al., 2009). PTSD is a problem for which veterans from Operation Iraqi Freedom and Operation Enduring Freedom (the conflicts in Iraq and Afghanistan, respectively) have been increasingly seeking treatment, and it is a disorder for which there are effective treatments (e.g., Foa, Keane, Friedman, & Cohen, 2008). As in other public and private sectors, depression is also among the most common presenting mental health conditions in VHA. Further, VA saw an opportunity to develop training in and adapted VA protocols for CBT and ACT for depression that focus on enhancing clinician competencies in the core components of these therapies. Utilizing a core competency approach to training in this way can provide opportunities to subsequently adapt competencies to other conditions and achieve greater training yield. Further, CBT and ACT core competencies include key psychotherapy skills that are in many ways transdiagnostic.

VHA also has a major investment in treating veterans with serious mental illness. SST is a treatment procedure that has been developed to directly address social problem-solving skills deficits in the SMI population, with the goal of enhancing social functioning. SST interventions are tailored to meet the real-life, current-day difficulties that affect the social experiences of each veteran, via a highly structured educational procedure that employs didactic instruction, breaking skills down into discrete steps, modeling, behavioral rehearsal (role playing), and social reinforcement.

Given the limited research on and experience with large-scale dissemination of EBPs, VA's dissemination initiatives are regarded as learning opportunities that can inform future systems changes. Each of the initiatives has included interactive training workshops and posttraining consultation, program evaluation components, and mechanisms for assessing and addressing barriers to implementation. Lessons learned are shared among the initiatives. Experience and expertise in training and system change is increasing so that future efforts will be based on a better understanding of the requirements of effective dissemination and implementation.

Training Model

CLINICIAN TRAINING PROCESS

While the specifics of training processes vary slightly among the initiatives, all adhere to a basic empirically informed training model. Training begins with an intensive workshop that includes demonstration of skills components and practice in treatment delivery. Participants then begin treating patients at their home facilities while receiving telephone or face-to-face consultation that generally lasts for a 6-month period. Each initiative has defined criteria for completion of training that include completion of both the workshop and consultation elements. Research suggests that these elements of training—interactive skills training, active trainee participation, and posttraining supervision—are key components of effective training in mental health interventions (Crits-Christoph et al., 1998; Fixsen, Naoom, Blase, Friedman, & Wallace, 2005; Grol & Grimshaw, 2003; Miller, Yahne, Moyers, Martinez, & Pirritano, 2004; Rakovshik & McManus, 2010; Sholomskas et al., 2005).

As an example, the 4-day PE clinician training workshops begin with an explanation of the foundational theory and evidence base for the intervention. This is followed by a discussion of assessment of PTSD to reinforce that patients receiving PE should be diagnosed with PTSD and deemed to be a good fit for the treatment. Training then focuses on the treatment rationale, implementation of in vivo and imaginal exposure, and the making of procedural modifications when needed. Training explores issues specific to veteran patients and lessons learned about implementation in VHA settings. Since focus groups and early experience indicated that many clinicians employed narrow selection criteria in determining that PE was appropriate for their patients, training illustrates delivery of PE to a range of veteran patients, including Vietnam veterans with chronic PTSD, recent returnees from Iraq and Afghanistan, sexual assault survivors, angry patients, and highly emotional patients. Key topics include motivation of the veteran to participate in the treatment and establishment of a strong therapeutic alliance, both of which are obstacles to engagement in treatment with many veterans. Training uses a standardized workshop structure that includes a set of slide presentations and 7 hours of videotaped materials showing delivery of the core elements of PE. After the workshop, trainees receive weekly telephone or face-to-face consultation in small groups of three or four training participants. These are supplemented by brief individual consultation sessions as needed. Training participants send tapes of their sessions to the consultant, who listens to selected portions of the session and provides detailed feedback on performance.

Postworkshop consultation processes are operationalized in consultant manuals. For example, the VA CBT for depression consultant training manual (Brown, Peterson, Cunning, Taylor, & Karlin, 2010) describes the policies, guidelines, procedures, and required forms associated with the training initiative, including the application process, the training workshop, the 6-month follow-up training consultation process, and criteria for completion of the training program.

Research also suggests that to be effective, EBPs must be delivered with fidelity to the treatment models (McHugh, Murray, & Barlow, 2009). The various training programs work to promote treatment fidelity and adherence to the EBP protocols while recognizing challenges associated with large-scale dissemination. In several of the VA EBP training programs, training participants' therapy tapes are regularly reviewed by training consultants and rated using therapy rating scales, and feedback is discussed with training participants. For example, in the CBT for depression training program, sessions are rated using the Cognitive Therapy Rating Scale (Young & Beck, 1980), a gold-standard CBT rating measure, and feedback is provided during weekly telephone consultation sessions.

DEVELOPMENT OF TRAINERS AND CONSULTANTS

Demonstrations of the capacity of evidence-based interventions for PTSD to effect behavior change in efficacy or effectiveness trials do not establish that these interventions can be successfully implemented on larger scales. The intensive training followed by ongoing consultation/supervision necessary to effect change in therapist behavior is difficult to take to scale, due in part to limited availability of experts to offer training and extended supervision. Often, training and/or supervision is provided by the experts who develop an intervention. To address this obstacle, Cahill, Foa, Hembree, Marshall, and Nacash (2006) have suggested a train-the-trainer model designed to create a larger pool of experts who can provide training and ongoing supervision of therapists. Such a model has been employed in the VA EBP training programs. Each initiative has engaged in selection and training of both "trainers" (workshop leaders) and "training consultants" (individuals who provide telephone or face-to-face case supervision during the training process). For example, the VA SST training program plans to train at least 21 master trainers (minimum of one per VHA region) to serve as expert trainers and consultants.

In all of the VA EBP training programs, trainers and training consultants identify and nominate very strong training participants as potential future training consultants, considering both demonstration of mastery of the full protocol and excellent interpersonal skills. In the PE training program, for example, approximately 25% to 30% of participants are selected and approached about possibly becoming training consultants. Those who are interested participate in a 5-day consultant training program that reinforces understanding of the PE intervention and explores issues related to the consultation process. All training consultants are routinely evaluated by their consultees through surveys, which allows for identifying and addressing any difficulties with consultant performance.

Strategies to Target Barriers to Adoption

Theoretical models of implementation science (e.g., Durlak & DuPre, 2008; Fixsen et al., 2005; Greenhalgh, Robert, MacFarlane, Bate, & Kyriakidou, 2004; Wandersman et al., 2008) include a range of variables that may affect likelihood of effective implementation. Delivery of training, even when evidence-based training methods are used, is unlikely to be sufficient to ensure successful adoption of EBPs. Across the VHA initiatives, a variety of barriers to widespread implementation have been identified and potential solutions are being explored. Key barriers include practitioner availability, trainer/consultant availability, practitioner skills deficits and attitudes, patient attitudes, and barriers related to time (time for clinicians to participate in training and time for consultants to offer telephone consultation). In addition to these systems solutions, the individual dissemination initiatives undertake to identify intervention-specific barriers as part of the planning process.

This is accomplished via literature reviews; focus groups targeted at clinicians, patients, and/or managers; and online surveys of participating clinicians.

PRACTITIONER AVAILABILITY

The ability to deliver EBPs to significant numbers of veterans depends first and foremost on a workforce adequate in size to match the need for these treatments. With the influx of veterans seeking services in VHA, VA has worked to significantly increase the size of the mental health workforce. Since 2005, VA has hired over 6,000 new mental health staff. VA has also significantly expanded the number of VA psychology internship and postdoctoral fellowship positions. These positions provide a strong pipeline of highly qualified psychologists to VA, including many with a strong training background in EBP; approximately 70% of VA psychologists have received training in VA. Further, many medical centers and clinics have restructured services and clinics to increase provider capacity to deliver EBPs. The availability of clinician capacity to deliver EBPs to all veterans, of the 8 million enrolled in VHA, who can benefit from these treatments is an ongoing area of focus.

TRAINER/CONSULTANT AVAILABILITY

In order for training to be delivered across the system of care, trainers and consultants must be available in sufficient numbers to support training participants. For several of the EBPs, VHA had experts already working within the health care system who took on the initial roles of trainer (e.g., Dr. Patricia Resick for CPT, Dr. Robyn Walser for ACT, Dr. Alan Bellack for SST). For others, external trainers were used at first, and then VHA personnel were prepared to become trainers. In the PE training program, Drs. Edna Foa and Elizabeth Hembree of the University of Pennsylvania conducted the 4-day training workshops during the first 2 years of implementation; thereafter, 16 VA PE trainers delivered the workshops. As the initiatives are maturing, additional trainers are being selected and trained for all of the EBPs.

As noted above, consultation is a significant component of VA's EBP training programs and has shown to be vital for promoting skill mastery and self-efficacy as practitioners undertake to apply their newly learned skills (Karlin et al., 2010). While trainers must be available only for a relatively brief training event, the consultation process is time-consuming in that it occurs on a weekly basis for a period of at least 6 months. When large numbers of clinicians are being trained, a very large cadre of consultants must be available. The VA EBP dissemination initiatives have included sufficient funding to mobilize such a consultant group. Some have relied on funded external consultants to meet the need initially; others have primarily used training consultants internal to VHA. Increasingly, efforts are being made across the programs to focus on identification and training of additional consultants. For example, the PE dissemination initiative currently has 79 trained consultants internal to VHA.

PRACTITIONER SKILLS DEFICITS

Skills deficits among mental health practitioners represent perhaps the greatest obstacle in achieving widespread implementation of EBPs, and training is especially important because psychological treatments require mastery of complex skill sets (Karlin et al., 2010; McHugh & Barlow, 2010). Unfortunately, presentation of didactic information alone or participation in a training workshop is unlikely to effect change in practitioner behavior. Workshop impact increases when demonstration of skills and opportunities for behavior rehearsal (Fixsen et al., 2005) and interactive participation via discussion, peer performance feedback, and group planning (Grol & Grimshaw, 2003) are included. Such training processes can be effective in changing practice (Crits-Christoph et al., 1998; Miller et al., 2004). Recent studies have shown the effectiveness of combination workshop training and ongoing supervision in training community service providers in PE (Cahill et al., 2006; Foa et al., 2005). Initial program evaluation results available from VA's EBP training programs indicate that intensive workshop training followed by ongoing expert consultation can significantly increase clinician competencies and that without ongoing consultation, clinician competency and adoption of newly learned therapies are often significantly lower (Karlin, 2009; Karlin et al., 2010).

STAFF ATTITUDINAL BARRIERS

Training is designed to develop skills but also to address the provider attitudinal barriers that can also impede practitioner adoption and implementation. These barriers differ among EBPs so that trainings tackle these barriers in individualized ways. For PE, studies suggest that clinicians are concerned about the safety of exposure therapy (e.g., Becker, Zayfert, & Anderson, 2004), despite the absence of evidence that more patients drop out of PE or that PE causes symptom worsening relative to other treatments (Riggs, Cahill, & Foa, 2006).

In addition, for some of the interventions, materials designed to promote attitude change and address misperceptions have been produced. For example, slide sets have been developed and distributed for use by PE and CPT training consultants to support presentations at local facilities. Videos and brochures targeted at "marketing" EBPs to clinicians, other health care staff, and hospital administrators have been produced and distributed.

PATIENT ATTITUDINAL BARRIERS

For the EBPs to be effectively implemented, patients must be interested in participating in a course of such treatment. Even better, patients should request to receive these treatments. Efforts to educate VHA patients about the EBPs being disseminated in VHA include the creation of patient brochures and patient education videos. To date, a variety of patient education brochures related to the EBPs being nationally disseminated in VHA have been developed. Patient education videos are under development and have a potentially important role in increasing motivation to participate in these EBPs. These videos are designed to be shown to individuals entering mental health treatment as part of a general clinic orientation (e.g., embedded in PTSD education classes) and/or when the patient and provider are considering whether these treatments will be part of treatment. In these videos, patients who have benefited from the specific interventions describe their treatment experiences.

Generally, efforts have been made to ensure that veteran perspectives inform the dissemination effort. Their feedback about the experience of participating in the EBPs is gathered, and the impact on their symptoms is measured. Veterans have volunteered to be involved in the making of the patient and clinician videos and have provided testimonials used to market the programs.

Perceptions of psychological treatments are likely to become increasingly positive when patients learn that others like themselves are benefiting from the treatments (e.g., Devilly & Huther, 2008). As the VA EBP dissemination initiatives gather increasing amounts of outcome data, providers are being encouraged to share treatment results with veterans who may benefit from the therapy. Further, as more patients benefit from the interventions, it is anticipated that they will share their experiences with their peers and help to "market" the services.

Pretherapy processes have been implemented in many VA medical centers and clinics, whereby clinicians inform veterans about EBPs that are available. This process may occur individually or in groups and involves promoting awareness of the treatment and its availability, providing brief education about the treatment and what it involves, and providing information about the efficacy and effectiveness of the intervention, as well as its clinical utility. The process of reviewing one or more treatments and their potential value for a particular patient is designed to promote informed choice among veterans and can help to motivate patients to engage in EBPs.

TIME TO LEARN

Insufficient time to attend training activities and to learn and practice intervention methods is routinely identified as a fundamental barrier to effective dissemination (e.g., Gray, Elhai, & Schmidt, 2007). In the present initiatives, too, time constraints have, in some instances, presented obstacles to implementation of the treatments. Busy VHA practitioners often experience difficulties in protecting time each week needed to participate in the consultation phase of training, which involves preparing for sessions, participating in consultation sessions, recording and sending tapes of their sessions to consultants, and completing other administrative tasks related to outcomes monitoring and program evaluation. Beyond the individual practitioner, clinic managers are tasked with establishing productive work environments and may sometimes experience the training activities as interfering with direct patient care responsibilities.

In the present initiatives, several steps have been taken to address these barriers. First, requirements for and expectations of training are carefully explained to clinicians, managers, and regional mental health leadership prior to recruitment of trainees. It is made clear that individuals will not be considered to have completed training unless they complete both the workshop and consultation phases of training. Attendees are required to sign a training agreement, which details expectations regarding participation; their direct supervisors also sign the agreement. Nomination of attendees is coordinated by regional mental health leaders. In this way, regional and local leadership are brought into the planning process and approve participation in the training programs.

A significant challenge has been to ensure that workshop trainees follow through and complete the consultation process. Difficulties with nonparticipation were encountered early in the dissemination process, and the steps noted above have improved participation and completion rates. The PE training initiative, despite its scale, has achieved a very high rate of participation in weekly consultation calls. At the time of this writing, 534 (53%) of workshop-trained participants have completed the minimum of two cases under weekly telephone consultation, 338 (33%) are actively participating in the consultation process, and 143 (14%) have dropped out of the consultation process.

The centrality of consultation is now emphasized in every communication with training participants. In addition to clarification of expectations and signing of agreements, training participants are asked to identify suitable intervention cases before they attend the clinical training workshops, so consultation can commence immediately following the workshop training. Training participants are also asked to initiate treatment with more than one case, to ensure continuity of consultation in the event of treatment dropout, and they are given a specific 6-month timeline in which to complete consultation. Furthermore, training participants remain with the same training consultant throughout the collaborative consultation process, and their direct experience makes clear the usefulness of consultation in mastering new therapy skills.

TIME TO TRAIN

As with clinicians who receive training, those who deliver telephone consultation and workshop training are busy clinicians. Consultation is an additional duty for most. Clinical programs face conflicting expectations regarding clinic workload, and consultants who are involved with the training process see fewer patients as a result of their consultation commitment to the national EBP training programs. This has led some clinic managers to restrict permission for their clinicians to serve as consultants within the initiatives. To help address this challenge, VHA's Office of Mental Health Services (OMHS) has provided funding to reimburse VHA facilities for the time that consultants devote to the training that can be used by the local facilities to augment their therapist capacity.

ADDITIONAL SYSTEMS CHALLENGES

Leadership "buy-in." OMHS has also taken steps to modify systems factors that may affect rates of clinician participation in training as well as rates of eventual delivery of these treatments. First, steps have been taken to secure leadership "buy-in." As noted above, regional mental health managers are brought into the process of selection of trainees to ensure that their viewpoints and needs are addressed. Letters signed by the chief of mental health in VHA have been sent to region and hospital directors explaining the initiatives and requesting leadership support. OMHS leaders frequently make visits to local facilities and discuss the EBP dissemination initiatives with key regional decision makers.

Clinic redesign. The VA EBP training programs and the systems changes described above have mobilized efforts to integrate EBPs into workflow processes. Mental health service managers have begun to re-engineer their clinics to accommodate EBPs. Local clinical infrastructure changes have also been made, including changing scheduling practices to accommodate 90-minute PE sessions, for example, and coordinating combined delivery of individual and group CPT. In-person site consultation and written materials have been provided to a number of facilities to help identify effective ways to integrate EBPs into local programs and services.

Internet support and communities of practice. The Internet is a key potential tool that can be used to support delivery of EBPs (Ruzek, 2010). Within VHA, a national OMHS website has been established for each of the EBPs being disseminated in VHA that allows for information sharing and access to EBP materials across the initiatives. For example, the CPT training program supplements its extensive set of materials with video teleconferences in which Dr. Resick and other training program staff members conduct advanced lectures on a variety of topics, including group adaptations of the protocol, working with patients with comorbid PTSD and substance abuse, and managing challenging cases. Lectures are also audiotaped and posted on the intranet site, as are video therapy vignettes. These sites assist with development of communities of practice organized around the several implementation initiatives. Training participants and other staff interact with one another and with consultants and trainers on planned telephone calls and Internet discussion forums. Therapists undergoing training and those who have completed training collaborate to give presentations at conferences, discuss relevant research findings, and discuss challenging cases.

Measurement of EBP implementation. EBP documentation "templates" located within VHA's computerized patient record system have been created and are being piloted at a number of VA medical centers. Once implemented, clinicians will use these templates for documenting therapy notes following EBP sessions. With such a record system in place, it will be possible to track delivery and fidelity of EBPs. Furthermore, the inclusion of the core components of the therapies in the templates will allow the templates to serve as heuristic tools for clinicians new to or still learning a therapy.

Evaluation

Each of the EBP dissemination initiatives has established systems of evaluation of training and implementation of therapy to examine training effectiveness, implementation of therapy, protocol adherence, and patient outcomes. Earlier in the dissemination process (February 2009), a national survey assessing CPT and PE treatment availability and capacity was sent to VA medical centers. Results indicated that 96% of facilities were providing CPT or PE, and 72% were providing both therapies. Most of the sites that had not yet implemented CPT or PE were working on specific plans for doing so. A follow-up survey was administered in July 2010; results of this survey revealed that all VA medical centers are now providing CPT or PE, with 98% of medical centers providing both therapies.

Effectiveness of training is also continuously evaluated. For example, in the PE training program, clinicians complete online surveys before and after the 4-day training workshops and again on completion of the consultation phase. The surveys assess a number of domains, including self-efficacy related to delivery of the treatment, perceived benefits of PE, and perceived drawbacks of PE. Results to date have indicated significant increases in reported self-efficacy to deliver PE from pre-training to postworkshop and also pre- and postconsultation (Karlin et al., 2010).

This evaluation process has enabled a comparison of quality of clinician training in PE during delivery of training by external expert trainers (Drs. Foa and Hembree) versus VHA staff trainers. Results indicated no difference in the degree of change in self-efficacy to deliver PE reported under the two training conditions. Also, there was no difference between training participants trained by Drs. Foa and Hembree and by VA trainers in the degree to which presenters were reported to have met specific training objectives, including enhancement of knowledge of empirically supported cognitive-behavioral treatments for PTSD and their comparative efficacy; learning how to implement treatment components of PE; or learning how to modify procedures of PE to manage emotional responses and promote effective emotional engagement (Karlin et al., 2010).

As noted above, VHA is also establishing a system for measuring the delivery of EBPs and the fidelity of implementation through the development of documentation templates for the EBPs. These therapy templates will yield data on session-by-session delivery of each of the therapies that will assist with local and national planning efforts. Moreover, the VA EBP documentation templates have been developed with specific health factors that will allow data from each specific session template to be extracted and aggregated across sessions and patients.

Perhaps most important, program evaluation associated with VA EBP dissemination initiatives is closely tracking outcomes of patients receiving these therapies. Preliminary results based on available treatment completer data provided by training participants as part of the initial implementation of program evaluation efforts suggest significant positive effects for CPT and PE. Initial program evaluation data reveal an overall average decline of close to 30% (or 20 points) in PTSD Checklist (PCL) scores among PE completers treated by clinician training participants, with similar outcomes for CPT (28.4%; $N = 93$) and PE (33.2%; $N = 381$) (Karlin et al., 2010). It is noteworthy that many veterans with PTSD receiving CPT or PE (as well as other EBPs) have complex symptoms and histories, often with multiple health and/or mental health comorbidities. Moreover, these outcomes are from therapists still learning these therapies. Program evaluation data from the CBT and ACT training programs reveal very similar patient gains typically by about the 10th therapy session and substantial increases in therapist competencies as a result of the training (Karlin, 2009).

As a direct result of the VA SST dissemination initiative, at least 152 SST groups have been implemented throughout VHA. These 152 groups have provided care to at least 1,200 veterans, who have expressed an overwhelmingly positive response to treatment. Of 424 veterans who responded to a survey about their experiences receiving SST, 93% agreed or strongly agreed that they were satisfied with the social skills training.

VHA is in the process of implementing broader outcomes measurement that, when fully implemented, will supplement these early findings and enable more systematic review of the effects of EBP (and other mental health service) delivery. However, these early findings provide for significant optimism and establish a model for mental health services outcomes monitoring in the largest integrated health care system in the United States.

Toward Sustained Implementation

It is recognized within VHA that successful initial implementation itself will not guarantee sustained delivery of these services. Several strategies are being used to work toward sustained implementation of EBPs. First, the centralized training model in which training activities and implementation activities more generally were managed by EBP-specific core leadership teams is transitioning to a decentralized model. Decentralization entails establishing training and consultation capacity within each of VHA's 21 Veterans Integrated Service Networks or regions from which planning, oversight, and coordination of care is directed within that geographical area. The decentralized training capacity will enable regions to expand EBP training to include a broader range of qualified mental health providers (e.g., those that spend a smaller amount of time treating patients with PTSD or other mental health conditions than have been the primary focus of the centralized trainings), provide training opportunities for mental health trainees (e.g., interns), and provide ongoing training to new staff members entering the system. Increasingly, Internet-based training resources can supplement face-to-face training. For example, online training in CPT has been created by the Medical University of South Carolina and Navy Medicine (available at http://cpt.musc.edu/index), and online training in PE and CBT is under development. Technologies are also being explored in terms of their capacity to support delivery of EBPs. VHA's MyHealtheVet national patient web portal will include tools to facilitate construction of in vivo exposure hierarchies, and cell phone applications are being created to support delivery of EBPs, such as PE and CPT.

Sustainability will also be enhanced by efforts to coordinate training in some of the EBPs (e.g., CPT, PE, CBT for depression) between VA and DoD. Such coordination will signal that commitment to EBPs is enduring and will facilitate sharing of training resources and strategies, establish common outcome measures and standards for documentation, and stimulate communication and mutual support via online "chat rooms" for VA and DoD mental health clinicians delivering EBPs.

VHA also now has in place several "human infrastructures" designed to support delivery of EBPs. Perhaps most significantly, Local Evidence-Based Psychotherapy Coordinators have been established at all VA medical centers to support VA's EBP dissemination and implementation efforts. The overall responsibility of individuals in this part-time (16 hours per week) role is to support the local facility, both clinically and administratively, in the implementation and sustainability of evidence-based psychotherapies. Local EBP Coordinators have received training in one or more of the EBPs and have experience in providing EBP services. It is intended that the coordinators can function as facilitators of systems change (Sullivan, Blevins, & Kauth, 2008) and thereby improve success of implementation efforts. For example, they have worked with facility-based informatics staff to incorporate 90-minute sessions into scheduling procedures.

A second infrastructure is provided by the various VHA mental health centers of excellence (COEs) whose mission is to research mental health services and facilitate integration of research findings, training and education, and clinical care. Several of these centers have helped serve as field coordinating sites for managing the day-to-day administration of the EBP training programs, working closely with the National Mental Health Director for Psychotherapy and Psychogeriatrics and OMHS. For example, two divisions of the National Center for PTSD have served as field coordinating sites for the CPT and PE training programs; the Sierra-Pacific Mental Illness Research, Education, and Clinical Center has served as the coordinating site for the CBT and ACT for depression training programs; and the Mental Illness Research, Education, and Clinical Centers in VHA regions 5 and 22 have served as the coordinating sites for the SST training program. These centers sometimes develop additional capabilities important to the EBP dissemination initiatives. The VA National PTSD Mentoring Program has as one of its objectives to support delivery of EBPs for PTSD. This program is designed to engage PTSD clinic managers in the EBP implementation process. Each region has identified two PTSD management mentors who participate in monthly phone calls and other methods of communication with one another and with program leadership. These mentors then hold monthly regional calls. The Mentoring Program intranet website enables sharing of valuable materials and discussion about issues related to EBP delivery within the context of clinics and serves as an exchange in which ways of re-engineering design of clinics can support EBP delivery.

The Future of Veterans Health Administration Evidence-Based Practice Implementation

Treatment improvement is an ongoing process, so implementation and training needs will continuously present themselves. New priorities for treatment delivery will be identified based on gap analyses and emerging research findings both internal and external to VHA. Beyond the EBP dissemination programs discussed herein, VHA is developing national initiatives to disseminate additional EBPs for marital distress, insomnia, substance use disorders, motivation and adherence, and other mental health conditions and behavioral health issues that will be largely based on, and will hopefully benefit from, the experiences and success of VA's existing EBP dissemination initiatives.

Just as practitioners need to see themselves as "lifelong learners," it is important that VHA support ongoing learning by mental health personnel so that implementation of evidence-based treatments can be sustained and available services remain consonant with evolving practice guidelines, new research findings, and emerging best practices. To accomplish this, ongoing dissemination infrastructures (Ruzek & Rosen, 2009) will be needed to facilitate dissemination and implementation of an ongoing stream of innovations across time. Key components of this organizational dissemination infrastructure might include systems/procedures for identification of dissemination priorities; marketing of practices; organization or site preparation; training and supervision; systems-level intervention; measurement of practitioner behaviors and monitoring of implementation and adherence; evaluation of dissemination effectiveness; and dialogue with system practitioners and patients. Processes of dissemination and implementation themselves must be researched and become evidence-based. To facilitate such developments, VHA is increasingly developing and utilizing expertise in research, training, and implementation science. Its extensive network of Centers of Excellence and Mental Illness Research, Education, and Clinical Centers are researching implementation processes and sharing information on best practices. Quality Enhancement Research Initiative Centers have amassed significant experience in managing and researching system change (e.g., Hagedorn et al., 2006), for example, related to the integration of mental health services delivery in primary care (Rubenstein et al., 2010).

To evaluate future dissemination initiatives, it will be necessary to establish means of outcomes monitoring in mental health services. Only when such outcome data are routinely and continuously available will the ultimate success of implementation initiatives—improvement in patient symptoms, functioning, and quality of life and improvement of well-being of family members—be capable of being established. VHA is committed to increasing utilization of outcomes data to drive decision making at the individual, program, and systems levels. Significant steps have already been taken to establish such monitoring systems. For example, VHA has recently implemented systematic, ongoing monitoring of outcomes for veterans with PTSD, using well-validated measurement instruments. VHA also conducts universal screening for PTSD, depression, substance abuse, military sexual trauma, and traumatic brain injury. National implementation of measurement systems will drive the spread of evidence-based clinical decision making at multiple levels of analysis.

Conclusion

The initiatives described in this chapter are resulting in large numbers of VA mental health clinicians being trained in delivery of specific EBPs. In the process, VHA is accumulating experience with large-scale implementation initiatives that can be used to sustain and expand the achievements of these projects. Human and technology infrastructures are being created that will facilitate more effective implementation. The many activities described here should enable improved performance in future implementation efforts, and thus improve VHA's ability to achieve its mission of delivering state-of-the-art mental health treatment for veterans that will effectively reduce their mental health symptoms and improve their ability to function in their families, work environments, and communities.

REFERENCES

Beck, A. T., Rush, A. J., Shaw, B. F., & Emery, G. (1979). *Cognitive therapy of depression.* New York: Guilford.

Becker, C. B., Zayfert, C., & Anderson, E. (2004). A survey of psychologists' attitudes towards and utilization of exposure therapy for PTSD. *Behaviour Research and Therapy, 42*, 277–292.

Bellack, A. S., Mueser, K. T., Gingerich, S., & Agresta, J. (2004). *Social skills training for schizophrenia: A step-by-step guide* (2nd ed.). New York: Guilford Press.

Brown, G. K., Peterson, L., Cunning, D., Taylor, C. B., & Karlin, B. (2010). *Training consultant manual: VA cognitive behavioral therapy for depression initiative.* Washington, DC: VA Central Office.

Cahill, S. P., Foa, E. B., Hembree, E. A., Marshall, R. D., & Nacash, N. (2006). Dissemination of exposure therapy in the treatment of posttraumatic stress disorder. *Journal of Traumatic Stress, 19*, 597–610.

Crits-Christoph, R., Siqueland, L., Chittams, J., Barber, J. P., Beck, A. T., Frank, A., et al. (1998). Training in cognitive, supportive-expressive, and drug counseling therapies for cocaine dependence. *Journal of Consulting and Clinical Psychology, 66,* 484–492.

Devilly, G. J., & Huther, A. (2008). Perceived distress and endorsement for cognitive- or exposure-based treatments following trauma. *Australian Psychologist, 43*, 7–14.

Durlak, J. A., & DuPre, E. P. (2008). Implementation matters: A review of research on the influence of implementation on program outcomes and the factors affecting implementation. *American Journal of Community Psychology, 41*, 327–350.

Edwards, D. J. (2008). Transforming the VA: The New Freedom Commission's report guides changes at the VA. *Behavioral Healthcare, 28*, 14–17.

Fixsen, D. L., Naoom, S. F., Blase, K. A., Friedman, R. M., & Wallace, F. (2005). *Implementation research: A synthesis of the literature* (FMHI Publication #231). Tampa, FL: University of South Florida, Louis de la Parte Florida Mental Health Institute, The National Implementation Research Network.

Foa, E. B., Hembree, E. A., Cahill, S. P., Rauch, S. A., Riggs, D. S., Feeny, N. C., & Yadin, E. (2005). Randomized trial of prolonged exposure for PTSD with and without cognitive restructuring: Outcome at academic and community clinics. *Journal of Consulting and Clinical Psychology, 73*, 955–964.

Foa, E. B., Hembree, E. A., & Rothbaum, B. O. (2007). *Prolonged Exposure therapy for PTSD: Emotional processing of traumatic experiences.* New York: Oxford University Press.

Foa, E., Keane, T., Friedman, M., & Cohen, J. (Eds.). (2008). *Effective treatments for PTSD. Practice guidelines from the International Society for Traumatic Stress Studies* (2nd ed.). New York: Guilford Press.

Goisman, R. M., Warshaw, M. G., & Keller, M. B. (1999). Psychosocial treatment prescriptions for generalized anxiety disorder, panic disorder, and social phobia, 1991–1996. *American Journal of Psychiatry, 156*, 1819–1821.

Gray, M. J., Elhai, J. D., & Schmidt, L. O. (2007). Trauma professionals' attitudes toward and utilization of evidence-based practices. *Behavior Modification, 31*, 732–748.

Greenhalgh, T., Robert, G., MacFarlane, F., Bate, P., & Kyriakidou, O. (2004). Diffusion of innovations in service organizations: Systematic review and recommendations. *The Milbank Quarterly, 82*, 581–629.

Grol, R., & Grimshaw, J. (2003). From best evidence to best practice: Effective implementation of change in patients' care. *Lancet, 362*, 1225–1230.

Hagedorn, H., Hogan, M., Smith, J., Bowman, C., Curran, G., Espadas, D., et al. (2006). Lessons learned about implementing research evidence into clinical practice: Experiences from VA QUERI. *Journal of General Internal Medicine, 21*(Suppl. 2), S21–S24.

Hayes, S. C., & Smith, S. (2005). *Get out of your mind and into your life: The new Acceptance and Commitment Therapy.* Oakland, CA: New Harbinger.

Jameson, J. P., Chambless, D. L., & Blank, M. B. (2009). Utilization of empirically supported treatments in rural community mental health centers: Necessity is the mother of innovation. *Community Mental Health Journal, 65,* 723–735.

Karlin, B. E. (July, 2009). *Dissemination of evidence-based psychotherapy in a health care system: National strategy and initial evaluation outcomes.* Plenary presentation at the Department of Veterans Affairs National Mental Health Conference, Baltimore, MD.

Karlin, B. E., Ruzek, J. I., Chard, K. M., Eftekhari, A., Monson, C. M., Hembree, E. A., et al. (2010). Dissemination of evidence-based psychological treatments for post-traumatic stress disorder in the Veterans Health Administration. *Journal of Traumatic Stress, 23,* 663–673.

McHugh, R. K., & Barlow, D. H. (2010). The dissemination and implementation of evidence-based psychological treatments: A review of current efforts. *American Psychologist, 65*, 73–84.

McHugh, R. K., Murray, H. W., & Barlow, D. H. (2009). Balancing fidelity and adaptation in the dissemination of empirically supported treatments: The promise of transdiagnostic interventions. *Behaviour Research and Therapy, 47*, 946–953.

Miller, W. R., Yahne, C. E., Moyers, T. B., Martinez, J., & Pirritano, M. (2004). A randomized controlled trial of methods to help clinicians learn motivational interviewing. *Journal of Consulting and Clinical Psychology, 72*, 1050–1062.

Rakovshik, S. G., & McManus, F. (2010). Establishing evidence-based training in cognitive behavioral therapy: A review of current empirical findings and theoretical guidance. *Clinical Psychology Review, 30*, 496–516.

Resick, P. A., Monson, C. M., & Chard, K. M. (2007). *Cognitive processing therapy: Veteran/ military version*. Washington, DC: Department of Veterans Affairs.

Riggs, D. S., Cahill, S. P., & Foa, E. B. (2006). Prolonged exposure treatment of posttraumatic stress disorder. In V. M. Follette & J. I. Ruzek (Eds.), *Cognitive-behavioral therapies for trauma* (2nd ed., pp. 65–95). New York: Guilford Press.

Rosen, C. S., Chow, H. C., Finney, J. F., Greenbaum, M. A., Moos, R. H., Sheikh, J. I., et al. (2004). VA practice patterns and practice guidelines for treating posttraumatic stress disorder. *Journal of Traumatic Stress, 17*, 213–222.

Rubenstein, L., Chaney, E., Ober, S., Felker, B., Sherman, S., Lanto, A., et al. (2010). Using evidence-based quality improvement methods for translating depression collaborative care research into practice. *Families, Systems, & Health, 28*, 91–113.

Ruzek, J. I. (2010). Disseminating best practices and information in post-trauma care: Towards online training and support for providers serving trauma survivors. In A. Brunet, R. A. Ashbaugh, & F. C. Herbert (Eds.), *Internet use in the aftermath of trauma* (pp. 179–191). Amsterdam, Netherlands: IOS Press.

Ruzek, J. I., & Rosen, R. C. (2009). Disseminating evidence-based treatments for PTSD in organizational settings: A high priority focus area. *Behaviour Research and Therapy, 47*, 980–989.

Ruzek, J. I., Vasterling, J. J., Schnurr, P. P., & Friedman, M. J. (Eds.). (2011). *Caring for veterans with deployment-related stress disorders: Iraq, Afghanistan, and beyond*. Washington, DC: American Psychological Association Press.

Seal, K. H., Metzler, T. J., Gima, K. S., Bertenthal, D., Maguen, S., & Marmar, C. R. (2009). Trends and risk factors for mental health diagnoses among Iraq and Afghanistan veterans using Department of Veterans Affairs health care, 2002–2008. *American Journal of Public Health, 99*, 1651–1658.

Sholomskas, D. E., Syracuse-Siewert, G., Rounsaville, B. J., Ball, S. A., Nuro, K. F., & Carroll, K. M. (2005). We don't train in vain: A dissemination trial of three strategies of training clinicians in cognitive-behavioral therapy. *Journal of Consulting and Clinical Psychology, 73*, 106–115.

Stewart, R. E., & Chambless, D. L. (2007). Does psychotherapy research inform treatment decisions in private practice? *Journal of Clinical Psychology, 63*, 267–281.

Sullivan, G., Blevins, D., & Kauth, M. R. (2008). Translating clinical training into practice in complex mental health systems: Toward opening the "black box" of implementation. *Implementation Science, 3*, 33.

van Minnen, A., Hendriks, L., & Olff, M. (2010). When do trauma experts choose exposure therapy for PTSD patients? A controlled study of therapist and patient factors. *Behaviour Research and Therapy, 48*, 312–320.

Veterans Health Administration. (2008). *Uniform mental health services in VA medical centers and clinics* (VHA Handbook 1160.01). Washington, DC: Government Printing Office.

Walser, R. D., & Chartier, M. (2010). Laying out in anxiety: Acceptance and Commitment Therapy for values-based living. In G. Burns (Ed.), *Happiness, healing, enhancement* (pp. 176–189) Hoboken, NJ: John Wiley & Sons, Inc.

Wandersman, A., Duffy, J., Flaspohler, P., Noonan, R., Lubell, K., Stillman, L., et al. (2008). Bridging the gap between prevention research and practice: The interactive systems framework for dissemination and implementation. *American Journal of Community Psychology, 41*, 171–181.

Wenzel, A., Brown, G. K., & Karlin, B. E. (2010). *Cognitive behavioral therapy for depressed veterans and military service members.* Washington, DC: U.S. Department of Veterans Affairs.

Young, J. E., & Beck, A. T. (1980). *Cognitive therapy rating scale manual.* Philadelphia: University of Pennsylvania.

6

Development and Application of the NCCTS Learning Collaborative Model for the Implementation of Evidence-Based Child Trauma Treatment

Lori Ebert, Lisa Amaya-Jackson, Jan Markiewicz, and John A. Fairbank

Among the estimated 15 million children with a mental disorder in the United States, only 20% to 30% receive specialized mental health care in a given year (American Psychological Association [APA] Task Force on Evidence-Based Practice for Children and Adolescents, 2008). Fewer still receive appropriate treatment grounded in scientific evidence (APA Task Force on Evidence-Based Practice for Children and Adolescents, 2008; Glisson, 2002; Weisz, Jensen, & McLeod, 2005). It follows that despite recent progress in the development of efficacious treatments for posttraumatic stress reactions in children (e.g., Cohen, Mannarino, & Deblinger, 2006; Kolko & Swensen, 2002; Lieberman, Gosh Ippen, & Van Horn, 2006), use of these evidence-based treatments (EBTs) in the community settings that serve most traumatized youth remains limited (Chadwick Center for Children and Families, 2004). Exposure to trauma among children is a major public health concern increasing risk for a range of mental health problems, including posttraumatic stress disorder (PTSD), substance abuse, and depression (Fairbank, Putnam, & Harris, 2007). In this chapter, we describe the National Center for Child Traumatic Stress Learning Collaborative Model, an approach to implementing evidence-based psychotherapeutic interventions intended to support the skillful delivery and sustained use of effective child trauma treatments in community practice settings.

Efforts to adopt empirically supported psychotherapies are often initiated under the assumption that these interventions can be transferred to community settings without modification and that clinical training is sufficient to change clinical practice (Fixsen, Naoom, Blase, Friedman, & Wallace, 2005; Gotham, 2006; Stirman, Crits-Christoph, & DeRubeis, 2004). But, as numerous investigators have noted (e.g., Hoagwood, Burns, & Weisz, 2002; Southam-Gerow, Chorpita, Miller, & Gleacher, 2008), there are many differences between the contexts and conditions under which EBTs are developed and those in which most psychological services are delivered. A recent report by the APA's Task Force on Evidence-Based Practice for Children and Adolescents (2008) identified several factors that can hamper implementation of EBTs in children's mental health services. These include the challenge of integrating evidence-based practice into fragmented child-serving systems, costs associated with training and supervision and their impact on productivity, assessment and measurement issues, difficulties engaging caregivers struggling with multiple social and family problems, and concerns about the effectiveness of manualized treatments for the severe, complex cases often seen in community clinics.

Only a handful of publications have addressed factors affecting implementation of EBTs designed to address posttraumatic reactions in children. The training process, including practitioners' perception that trainers had little experience delivering the intervention in everyday practice settings, was one barrier identified in research with community practitioners serving maltreated children; limited access to or lack of effective model-based supervision was another (Aarons & Palinkas, 2007; Baumann, Kolko, Collins, & Herschell, 2006). The belief that the intervention was not well suited to the needs of some of the families served was an additional barrier along with concerns that aspects of the intervention (e.g., requirements for increased documentation) would decrease providers' efficiency (Aarons & Palinkas, 2007).

The Kauffman Best Practices Project "Closing the Quality Chasm in Child Abuse Treatment" (Chadwick Center for Children and Families, 2004) identified several putative barriers to broad implementation of EBTs for abused children and their families. First, funding levels for most community programs that serve maltreated youth do not allow for the costs typically incurred in adopting and adapting a new intervention, including costs associated with lost productivity during training, consultation from trainers, regular model-based supervision, and monitoring of fidelity. In addition, supervisors trained in child trauma EBTs are in short supply and high staff turnover rates can make it difficult to sustain these practices due to the burden of constantly needing to train new staff in a complex intervention (Woltmann et al., 2008). Organizational characteristics are considered an important factor in EBT implementation (Fixsen et al., 2005; Gotham, 2006; Stirman et al., 2004). Historically underfunded, many child abuse service settings lack the attributes of "learning organizations" including strong and stable leadership, a reliable resource base to support continuous improvement, and mechanisms for identifying and disseminating best practices from emerging research (Chadwick Center for Children and Families, 2004). Even organizations that are well informed about efficacious treatments for child trauma may face financial disincentives to adopting these since reimbursement is still often determined by the quantity not the quality of services delivered.

Information dissemination (e.g., publication of research, distribution of practice guidelines) and training remain two of the most widely used strategies for attempting to spread new practices (Fixsen et al., 2005). However, there is growing consensus that these methods are insufficient for ensuring the broad and sustained use of mental health EBTs; longer-term multilevel implementation strategies are necessary (Fixsen et al., 2005; Proctor et al., 2009; Stirman et al., 2004). Quality collaboratives are one methodology that has been used to support change across multiple levels of a hospital or other health care system in order to implement innovations in medicine and improve quality of care (Kilo, 1999; Ovretveit et al., 2002; Schouten, Hulscher, van Everdingen, Huijsman, & Grol, 2008; Wilson, Berwick, & Cleary, 2003). In 1995, the Institute for Healthcare Improvement (IHI) introduced the Breakthrough Series Collaborative (BSC), a quality collaborative model that brings together multidisciplinary teams from different organizations to work in a structured way with each other and recognized experts to accelerate the spread of a best practice (Institute for Healthcare Improvement, 2003). Teams learn quality improvement techniques, which they apply in their local setting to make the organizational and system changes necessary to implement innovative health care practices. To hasten progress, successful changes are shared across the collaborative along with lessons learned. Despite extensive use in medicine (e.g., Asch et al., 2005; Benedetti, Flock, Pedersen, & Ahern, 2004, Schonlau et al., 2005; Vargas et al., 2007) and recent applications in child welfare (Casey Family Programs, 2005; Miller & Ward, 2008) the BSC methodology has not been widely used in mental health service settings. We were only able to identify one published study describing use of the BSC model in child mental health (Cavaleri et al., 2006). In that project, a BSC was conducted to increase engagement of urban youth and families in mental health services (i.e., to improve attendance at clinic appointments). No prior applications of the BSC to support broad implementation of a child trauma EBT or any other evidence-based psychotherapy were found.

In 2000, the U.S. Congress established the National Child Traumatic Stress Network (NCTSN), a collaboration of academic and community-based service centers funded by the Substance Abuse and Mental Health Services Administration (SAMHSA) to enhance services and access to care for traumatized children and their families (Pynoos et al., 2008).[1] Network activities are coordinated by the National Center for Child Traumatic Stress (NCCTS), which is co-located at the University of California, Los Angeles, and Duke University Medical Center. Over the past 6 years, the NCCTS and its network partners have worked together to adapt the BSC methodology, melding high-quality training with improvement science, to support broad and skillful implementation of evidence-based psychotherapies for children affected by trauma through learning collaboratives (LCs). Below we describe the development of the NCCTS Learning Collaborative Model along with essential components of the model as currently conceived. Selected evaluation data are also provided.

---

[1] For more information about network centers, products, and resources please see the NCTSN website (www.nctsn.org).

Model Development

Development of the NCCTS Learning Collaborative Model has been an iterative process informed by both implementation science and repeated application in community service settings. Along with the research literature on implementation of EBTs, the development process has benefited from extensive consultation with experts in implementation science and quality improvement including the Institute for Healthcare Improvement, National Initiative for Children's Healthcare Quality, Casey Family Programs, and the University of North Carolina/Cincinnati Children's Hospital's Center for Healthcare Improvement. Collaboration with professionals from other NCTSN centers, staff at community agencies with countless years of experience serving traumatized youth working alongside intervention developers, contributed vast expertise in the area of child trauma treatment. The current model (detailed in a later section) reflects multiple iterations informed by lessons learned from conducting more than 25 collaboratives—information gleaned through both formal evaluation and informal feedback from collaborative faculty and participants. As illustrated in Table 6.1, the development process was informed by state, regional, and national collaboratives focused on the implementation of multiple treatment models. Below we offer an overview of that process.

EARLY EFFORTS AT COLLABORATIVE LEARNING: REGIONAL LEARNING COMMUNITIES

The NCCTS conducted its first version of an LC in 2004, bringing together clinicians from multiple agencies to learn a new child trauma treatment. The Southern Regional Learning Collaborative was composed of four agencies in the southeast

TABLE 6.1 Overview of Collaboratives Conducted Using Key Components of the NCCTS Learning Collaborative Model and Contributing to Its Development

Intervention	Scope	Number
Child-Parent Psychotherapy (CPP)	National	2
Cognitive Behavioral Intervention for Trauma in Schools (CBITS)	National	1
Life Skills, Life Story	Regional	1
Structured Psychotherapy for Adolescents Responding to Chronic Stress (SPARCS)	National	2
Trauma Adaptive Group Education and Therapy (TARGET)	Regional	1
Trauma-Focused Cognitive Behavioral Therapy (TF-CBT)	State, regional, national	18
Trauma Systems Therapy (TST)	Regional	1
Wraparound	State	1
Total		27

that were interested in adopting Trauma-Focused Cognitive Behavioral Therapy (TF-CBT; Cohen et al., 2006). Shortly thereafter, the NCCTS coordinated three collaboratives on three different group treatments for traumatized adolescents— TARGET (Trauma Adaptive Recovery Group Education and Therapy; Ford & Russo, 2006), Life Skills/Life Story (Cloitre, Koenen, & Cohen, 2006), and SPARCS (Structured Psychotherapy for Adolescents Responding to Chronic Stress; DeRosa & Pelcovitz, 2009). During this same period, the NCTSN sponsored a small LC on Child-Parent Psychotherapy (CPP; Lieberman, Van Horn, & Gosh-Ippen, 2005), an intensive, dyadic, attachment-based treatment for young children exposed to interpersonal violence. These early efforts drew on aspects of the BSC model that provide a structure for collaborative learning. However, the primary focus was on promoting clinical competence through intensive training rather than on address-ing barriers to implementing and sustaining the practice at an organizational level. Quality improvement techniques were introduced in these collaboratives but were limited in scope and not broadly applied. Instead, the emphasis was on integrating adult learning principles into the training process and fostering collaboration to improve practice (e.g., participants were encouraged to share clinical resources with practitioners at other agencies).

Theory and research on the dissemination of innovations suggests that "early adopters" can play an important role in accelerating the diffusion of an innovation (Berwick, 2003; Rogers, 1995). One early lesson was that applying this principle in LCs, by highlighting the successes of clinicians who eagerly and skillfully imple-mented the new treatment, motivated others to try it out. Elevating early adopters also encouraged them to serve as supportive role models and to "spread the word" regarding the feasibility and benefits of the EBT in their agencies and communities. In a field where trainers and experienced supervisors are in short supply, staff from agencies that participated in early collaboratives have played an important role in helping to disseminate trauma-focused treatment by serving as faculty in subse-quent LCs, including in state initiatives outside the NCTSN. Evaluation data sug-gest that LCs can also support the diffusion of an intervention within a community. For example, in the 1-year follow-up evaluation of the NCTSN BSC (see below), more than half of the participating organizations reported having facilitated the spread of TF-CBT to partner or affiliate organizations in their community.

NCTSN BREAKTHROUGH SERIES COLLABORATIVE

In 2005, the NCCTS launched its first national BSC with the overarching goal of supporting the full and sustained implementation of TF-CBT in a diverse, national sample of community agencies. The NCCTS chose to focus on implementation of TF-CBT because it has a strong evidence base (Chadwick Center for Children and Families, 2004; Cohen et al., 2006) and because there was a high level of interest in TF-CBT among NCTSN centers (Agosti et al., 2007). TF-CBT is a time-limited, outpatient psychotherapy designed to treat posttraumatic stress and related emotional and behavior problems in children ages 3 to 18 (Cohen et al., 2006). Caregiver participation in treatment is an integral component of the model.

Consistent with the BSC's emphasis on organizational change and engagement, after topic selection, the NCCTS collaborative leadership group convened an expert panel to draft a collaborative change framework, or *change package*, designed to offer a vision of what an organization needs to do to fully implement TF-CBT. The expert panel consisted of individuals in a range of roles considered integral to successful implementation, including clinicians, supervisors, and administrators from community agencies that were implementing TF-CBT; family members of children who had received trauma treatment ("family consumers"); the developers of TF-CBT; and other child trauma experts. The composition of the BSC faculty mirrored that of the expert panel. The faculty and leadership group selected 12 sites to participate through a competitive application process. Because the BSC is intended as a model for adaptation and spread—a step beyond training—participating agencies were expected to have clinical staff who had received basic training in TF-CBT. Due to funding constraints, only NCTSN grantees were eligible to participate. Each agency team included at least one high-level administrator, clinicians, and supervisors; participation of family consumers and community partners representing key stakeholders for trauma-focused treatment was also encouraged.

Over a 9-month period, collaborative participants came together for three 2-day "learning sessions" during which they met intensively with faculty, other teams, and members of their own team. Learning sessions emphasized interactive training in best practices for implementing TF-CBT (e.g., approaches to quality supervision of TF-CBT) and the use of Plan-Do-Study-Act (PDSA) cycles to overcome implementation challenges and adapt practices to local settings. The PDSA cycle, considered one of the cornerstones of BSC, is a structured method for rapidly testing improvement strategies on a small scale. In the action periods between learning sessions, teams test and refine changes to address barriers and improve practice. Effective strategies are then shared and spread across the collaborative to accelerate progress. Monthly cross-site conference calls are used to maintain momentum during the action periods, providing teams an opportunity to share successes and lessons learned from the changes they have tested. A collaborative intranet, an interactive password-protected website, was developed to share information and foster collaboration during the action periods. Teams were also expected to develop simple measures or *metrics* to track their progress on a monthly basis and post these to the intranet.

Findings from the formative evaluation of the NCTSN BSC suggested that, overall, participating agencies made substantial progress toward the overarching goal of broad and skillful implementation of TF-CBT (Agosti et al., 2007). Sixty-eight clinicians representing 10 teams[2] delivered TF-CBT

---

[2] One site, which was unable to institute a program to serve traumatized youth, did not participate in the collaborative evaluation. Due to staff attrition, 2 of the remaining 11 sites were

to 463[3] youth during the collaborative. Over 40% of these clinicians ($n = 27$, 43%) had not delivered TF-CBT prior to the NCTSN, representing a 75% increase in the number of TF-CBT providers over the 9-month collaborative. The change package for the NCTSN BSC identified best practices in five domains considered essential to skillful implementation of TF-CBT: (a) organizational readiness to implement EBTs, (b) organizational readiness to monitor and evaluate clinical processes and outcomes, (c) clinical competence in delivering TF-CBT, (d) quality training and supervisory skills, and (e) effective child and family engagement. Teams tested changes in all five domains and the collaborative evaluation pointed toward related practice improvements. For example, the number of sites that offered weekly or biweekly supervision in TF-CBT increased from four to nine, with over 80% of participating staff reporting that their agency had made "a lot" of progress in building capacity to offer quality supervision in TF-CBT over the course of the collaborative.

FURTHER DEVELOPMENT OF THE LEARNING COLLABORATIVE MODEL

The BSC is intended as a model for adaptation and spread. Unless a critical mass of practitioners in an organization have already received the intensive training necessary to build competency in delivering an EBT, the BSC model cannot be fully effective. Because clinicians at many community agencies have not had training in evidence-based child trauma treatments, subsequent iterations of the LC model have sought to meld effective training in a child trauma EBT with training in quality improvement methods designed to help organizations fully implement and sustain effective practices. Clinical training in LCs emphasizes the application of evidence-based teaching processes and adult learning principles to foster clinically competent delivery of the intervention with fidelity. Drawing on lessons learned in the NCTSN BSC and more than a dozen subsequent collaboratives, the NCCTS has worked diligently to tailor the BSC methodology, which was designed to support process improvements in health care (e.g., to improve access in primary care, reduce adverse drug events), to implementation of an evidence-based mental health treatment. Below we provide an overview of that development process.

One significant development was a major revision of the change package, the document that specifies the collaborative aims and recommended change strategies. The change package developed for the NCTSN BSC drew heavily on the work of Casey Family Programs, which has adapted the IHI BSC to improve child welfare practices. The evaluation of the NCTSN BSC suggested that the content of the change package was sound, but the format could be improved. The BSC change

---

not providing TF-CBT at the time of the first learning session and one did not resume provision until after the collaborative ended.

[3] This number excludes clients who dropped out of treatment prior to the end of the collaborative.

package emphasized broad aspirational goals and included numerous objectives embedded in a lengthy narrative. Conversely, the collaborative change framework now used to guide the work of LCs specifies a small number of measureable goals and includes an organizational assessment that emphasizes behavioral indicators of implementation rather than aspirations and attitudes toward evidence-based practice. The metrics used to measure progress toward the collaborative goals have also changed. In the BSC, teams were tasked with developing and calculating their own metrics, which proved impractical. The collaborative leadership group now develops an initial set of metrics, including measures of treatment fidelity, which the NCCTS implements and provides to teams and faculty each month.

Other adaptations have been made to tailor the BSC model to the needs of agencies implementing a complex psychotherapeutic intervention. For example, it has become increasingly evident that a well-constructed launch phase is essential in a collaborative focused on evidence-based treatment. Without intensive preparatory work prior to the first learning session many agencies are unable to quickly implement the treatment and, in turn, cannot take full advantage of the resources available through the collaborative. Launch activities are now designed not only to introduce participants to the practice but also to help agencies identify appropriate referral sources, implement a screening protocol, and develop the skills and infrastructure necessary to use clinical assessments in treatment planning. We have also modified the format used for calls during the action periods. Conference calls in a BSC typically included the full collaborative membership; however, evaluation data suggested that this approach was not well suited to the needs of clinical staff learning a new intervention. Therefore, calls focused on clinical skill building are now conducted in a small group format with three to four teams who convene regularly with one of the faculty. This format also affords faculty greater familiarity with particular teams and, in turn, allows the collaborative leadership to better support teams that encounter significant challenges. It also makes it easier to recognize and draw on teams' strengths.

A growing recognition of the critical role agency leadership plays in implementing and sustaining an evidence-based mental health treatment has resulted in a greater emphasis on "senior leader" involvement in recent collaboratives. Consistent with reports from quality collaboratives in health care (e.g., Nolan, 2007; Reinertsen, Bisognano, & Pugh, 2008), without a substantial commitment from agency leadership it can be difficult to address significant barriers to implementing a mental health EBT, which often require organizational or system change. Learning collaboratives initiated subsequent to the NCTSN BSC have all required agency teams to include a senior leader. However, the level of senior leader involvement has progressed from participation in bimonthly conference calls, to also expecting senior leaders to attend the second learning session, to having a dedicated senior leader track at each learning session along with regular conference calls. Moreover, feedback from recent collaboratives (see below) has prompted efforts to foster leadership team connections between agency senior leaders and clinical supervisors to address cross-cutting organizational issues (e.g., balancing productivity demands with the need for model-based supervision).

Included in our later efforts have been partnerships with organizations leading initiatives to roll out EBTs across the states of Connecticut (Connecticut Center for Effective Practice), Mississippi (Catholic Charities), North Carolina (N.C. Child Treatment Program—University of North Carolina-Duke University), South Carolina (Project BEST—Dee Norton Lowcountry Children's Center), and Tennessee (University of Tennessee Center for Excellence for Children in State Custody). These initiatives have contributed to the development of the LC model through application outside the NCTSN and by providing an opportunity to work in partnership to adapt the model to fit a particular state's needs. For example, the North Carolina Child Treatment Program has adapted the LC model for private practitioners and Project BEST has adapted the model to have more of a community focus rather than an organizational one.

FUNDING FOR LEARNING COLLABORATIVES

Funding to develop the LC methodology and to conduct all LCs within the NCTSN has come from grants that participating NCTSN centers received through the SAMSHA National Child Traumatic Stress Initiative. Funded network centers covered costs associated with staff time and travel via their grants. An effort was made to curtail cost by having sites host the learning sessions on a rotating basis. Costs for the intranet and conference calls were funded by the NCCTS. It is worth noting that all NCTSN collaboratives, except the BSC, have included teams from "nonnetwork" sites; nonnetwork teams paid for their own travel but participated at no cost. The state initiatives described above have received support from a variety of sources, including direct funding from their respective states as well as grants from foundations and other institutions. Several of these initiatives have benefitted from a funded evaluation component in addition to development efforts in prior collaboratives.

The NCCTS Learning Collaborative Model

The NCCTS Learning Collaborative Model is an adaptation of the BSC intended to support implementation of evidence-based child trauma treatments in diverse community practice settings by fostering the clinical competence necessary to skillfully execute such treatments and the "implementation competence" necessary to adapt, deliver, and sustain them. In keeping with the NCTSN vision, collaborative learning across disciplines, roles, and organizations is at the heart of this model (Pynoos et al., 2008). Collaboration among faculty and teams is essential to achieving the balance between flexibility and fidelity necessary to implement the treatment in a manner that is developmentally appropriate, culturally competent, and effective (Fixsen et al., 2005; Stirman et al., 2004). Because implementation of an evidence-based mental health treatment requires not only practice change on the part of direct service providers but also changes in organizational practices, policies, and procedures, collaboration among individuals in different roles at participating organizations is also critical (Aarons & Palinkas, 2007; Fixsen et al., 2005; Gotham, 2006; Stirman et al., 2004). Finally collaboration across teams supports rapid implementation (Institute for Healthcare Improvement, 2003). There is no reason for each organization to start from scratch in solving every problem it encounters; each has strengths on which others can draw. Learning collaboratives accelerate progress by providing regular opportunities for teams to capitalize on the successes of other organizations and learn from their mistakes. Adult learning theories and methods permeate the teaching–learning process used in this model and are an essential ingredient to giving individuals and agencies the tools necessary to quickly implement a mental health EBT and sustain it. This includes fostering the development of interagency peer support networks that can help support and spread the practice after the collaborative ends.

Below we outline the core components of the NCCTS Learning Collaborative Model—an emerging methodology in which collaborative learning, improvement science, and high-quality training are used to foster broad and sustained use of evidence-based child trauma treatments.

THE MODEL FOR IMPROVEMENT

The Model for Improvement (Langley, Nolan, Nolan, Norman, & Provost, 1996), a framework designed to accelerate improvements that organizations must make to successfully adopt a best practice, is integral to both the Breakthrough Series and LC models. Key components include (a) setting aims, (b) establishing measures, and (c) selecting and systematically testing changes. A "collaborative change framework" (CCF) specifies the collaborative mission and goals and provides guidelines for achieving the mission and goals. The collaborative change framework, developed by the collaborative planning group and expert panel,[4] provides a "roadmap" for how to implement the practice with fidelity and sustain it. Figure 6.1 offers a sample statement of the mission and goals for an LC focused on implementation of TF-CBT. The CCF also includes an organizational assessment that teams complete at the start and end of the collaborative to evaluate their practices with respect to each of the goals and to identify potential improvements. For example, with respect to the first goal identified in Figure 6.1, does the agency have a standard screening protocol for the treatment (i.e., TF-CBT)? Is the protocol consistently administered

---

[4] See description of the NCTSN Breakthrough Series Collaborative for information about the expert panel.

Collaborative Mission

The mission of this learning collaborative is:

1. To improve access for children and their families across the United States to an evidence-based child trauma treatment, Trauma-Focused Cognitive Behavioral Therapy (TF-CBT), implemented with fidelity.

2. To build organizational capacity necessary for participating agencies to implement, sustain, and continue to improve the delivery of TF-CBT and other evidence-based treatments (EBTs).

Collaborative Goals

Clinical competence in delivering TF-CBT is a critical component of effective adoption. However, organizational support and capacity and family and youth engagement also are essential. To successfully adopt an EBT, an organization must have the capacity to implement the practice, have worked through implementation barriers in the organizational culture, and have an infrastructure in place to collect and use data. Additionally, implementation of TF-CBT requires an understanding of the effects of trauma on child development and family systems and a commitment to family and youth engagement.

This TF-CBT Learning Collaborative will provide training to effect improvements in three domains: (a) clinical competence in delivering TF-CBT, (b) effective family and youth engagement, and (c) organizational support and capacity for implementing EBTs. Improvements in these three domains are targeted for participating agencies to make progress toward five overarching goals:

1. Youth eligible for psychotherapy are screened for referral to TF-CBT using a standard protocol.
2. Therapists who provide TF-CBT receive ongoing consultation/supervision in the model through their agency.
3. Therapists who provide TF-CBT implement the model with skill and fidelity, balanced with appropriate flexibility.
4. The progress of clients receiving TF-CBT is evaluated using standardized assessments.
5. Procedures are established for obtaining TF-CBT training for additional staff and for preparing additional staff to supervise TF-CBT.

FIGURE 6.1. *Sample mission and goals for a TF-CBT Learning Collaborative.*

to all youth eligible for psychotherapy through the agency? Are findings from the screening regularly reviewed with the caregiver and youth?

In an LC, simple measures, or metrics, are used to track progress toward the mission and goals articulated in the CCF. Although these data can sometimes be used for other purposes (e.g., evaluation), monthly metrics should first and foremost serve as a tool to guide participating organizations' efforts to implement the intervention. Faculty also use the metrics toward that end, for instance, to help determine if certain teams need additional support or which skills to emphasize on conference calls. To be useful, metrics must be sensitive to change in the short term; to be practicable, they must be brief and easy to complete. Incorporating measures that assess participants' skill in implementing the core components of the treatment is strongly recommended. Metrics for an LC, with the goals articulated in Figure 6.1, might include the number of clients receiving TF-CBT (during the past month), the percentage of clinicians who received 2 hours or more of TF-CBT supervision, and mean skill ratings for providers' implementation of core components of the treatment (e.g., coping skills, trauma narrative). Each month participating teams receive a set of graphs that charts their progress on the metrics. Metrics data are also used to provide teams and faculty with bimonthly progress reports that summarize implementation efforts across the collaborative.

As in a BSC, organizations participating in an LC are trained to use Plan-Do-Study-Act (PDSA) cycles, to make organizational and practice changes necessary to implement the new treatment. Agencies often spend a significant amount of time planning changes, then move directly from planning to full-scale implementation. The PDSA method allows ideas to be tested in small increments, where the consequences are minimized before a change is rolled out to the organization. Because small changes are tested in rapid succession, less time is spent on abstract planning and more time is spent refining ideas based on real practice in context. PDSAs provide a structured approach for agency staff in a variety of roles to address barriers to EBT implementation by planning changes with clear objectives (e.g., developing materials to improve caregiver participation in treatment), testing those changes on a small scale (e.g., with one family), studying their impact, and then acting to adjust, expand, or discard the change based on what was learned. Metrics, in turn, serve as an important tool for evaluating whether the changes teams are testing result in measureable improvements.

COLLABORATIVE STRUCTURE

Figure 6.2 provides a schematic of the structure and flow of a typical LC. After the expert panel has met to develop the CCF, a collaborative leadership group is established to design and implement the collaborative. The leadership group includes teaching faculty and staff responsible for coordinating collaborative activities, from meeting logistics to metrics. The teaching faculty includes not only experts in the intervention but also an improvement advisor, clinicians who have delivered the intervention in community settings, and other individuals in key roles necessary to implement and sustain the practice, including an agency administrator and clinical supervisor. Interested organizations complete a written application developed by the leadership group that describes the collaborative and specifies expectations for participation. Systematic reviews have shown interprofessional collaboration to be an effective strategy leading to positive changes in care (Hammick, Freeth, Koppel, Reeves, & Barr, 2007; Zwarenstein, Goldman, & Reeves, 2009). Therefore, like the teaching faculty, agency teams are broadly representative of organizational roles and functions necessary to implement the intervention with fidelity and sustain it, including senior leadership in the organization, clinical supervisors, and clinicians. Applicants are encouraged to identify other key stakeholders, including consumers, to serve as adjunct team members. The leadership group reviews completed applications and selects 5 to 12 teams with a minimum of 25 participants to join the collaborative. In general, conducting a collaborative with fewer than five teams is not

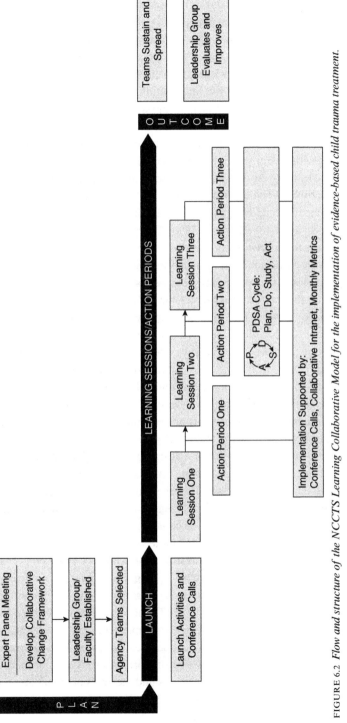

FIGURE 6.2 *Flow and structure of the NCCTS Learning Collaborative Model for the implementation of evidence-based child trauma treatment.*

cost-effective and limits opportunities for cross-team sharing (J. Agosti, personal communication, March 27, 2008). Initiatives with more than 12 teams may be feasible with experienced faculty and appropriate resources.

Three 2-day learning sessions (face-to-face meetings), each followed by an action period, provide a structure within which faculty and teams work together over a period of 9 to 12 months to learn, implement, and develop the organizational capacity necessary to sustain the intervention. Evidence-based teaching–learning processes and adult learning principles are a vital, supportive ingredient during learning sessions and action periods. Adult-styled learning is a purpose-driven and self-directed activity that is influenced by the learner's experience and readiness to learn, along with task or solution orientation toward that learning (Knowles, 1990). Through the learning process, adults seek to be able to apply knowledge and skill to immediate problems (Bain, 2004; Knowles, 1990). To facilitate learning, the teaching environment should be egalitarian, collaborative, and interactive and promote mutual respect and trust (Knowles, 1990; Savery & Duffy, 1996); therefore, LCs are designed such that participants' knowledge and experiences are highlighted from the start, with participants given increasing opportunities to provide content for learning sessions as the collaborative progresses.

It is within this context of a partnership with collaborative participants that LC faculty seek to optimize EBT uptake by applying best practices in the teaching–learning process. Research is identifying a growing set of adult learning methods and characteristics that have a positive effect on provider behavior in the care of their patients (Dunst & Trivette, 2009; Stuart, Tondora, & Hoge, 2004): interactive, participatory environments; reflection and self-assessment; audit and feedback; practice illustration; reminders (e.g., fidelity checklists); and mastery. The NCCTS Learning Collaborative Model incorporates training techniques with these characteristics, specifically sequencing them with an eye toward fostering fidelity and sustaining the practice. Before the first learning session, launch activities (e.g., a team-based organizational assessment, training in screening and assessment) are offered in an effort to ensure that all of the teams are prepared to begin delivering the intervention. The launch period begins the reflection and self-assessment process and introduces feedback via consultation. Learning sessions emphasize interactive, participatory learning techniques and processes through the use of experiential skill-building exercises (rather than lectures), energizers, small group discussion, role play, and team problem solving. Learning session one emphasizes clinical skill building in the EBT. Learning session two dives deeper into the skills necessary to maintain fidelity to the EBT, and also formally introduces quality improvement tools to address barriers to implementation and support spread. Planning to sustain the practice (e.g., documenting procedures for training new staff, use of data to monitor quality and support spread) is a major focus at learning session three, where team presentations and meetings predominate to promote mastery and reflection. Collection and discussions of metrics throughout the collaborative supports audit and feedback.

Another prominent consideration in the design of learning sessions is creating a structure that promotes collaboration within and across agency teams to accelerate progress in implementing the EBT. For example, at learning sessions, individuals in comparable roles at different organizations are given opportunities to meet to share information and address common challenges and most small group activities include staff from multiple sites. This supports the adult learning characteristic of self-direction, and task or solution orientation to learning. Agency teams often report that the day-to-day demands of work make it difficult for the full team to convene regularly; therefore, teams are also given time to meet together at learning sessions to clarify and address significant implementation challenges (e.g., to review metrics and develop PDSAs). Because support of organizational leaders is considered essential for successful implementation of evidence-based practices (Aarons & Palinkas, 2007; Fixsen et al., 2005 Vaughn et al., 2006), engagement of senior leaders is another priority. Whenever possible, a senior leader track, led by the agency administrator on faculty, is offered at each learning session. Team-based learning in multiple ways permits communities of practice to evolve where individuals learn from each other, which, in turn, supports ongoing learning at work. Structured and unstructured workplace learning assists in mastering organizational processes, negotiating the political, and dealing with the atypical (Boud & Middleton, 2003). Implementing a new EBT or improving the use of one inherently results in atypical and unseen situations, which teams can work together to solve.

In the action periods between learning sessions, collaborative participants return to their local communities to implement the treatment and receive periodic group coaching from faculty via conference calls. From an adult learning perspective, action periods are a time for individual and team reflection, audit and feedback, and practice illustration; thus, they support a learn, work, learn loop. Coaching also exposes individuals to role models and teachers who are positive about the use of an evidence-based practice (Hoge, Tondora, & Stuart, 2003). Monthly (or biweekly) conference calls for clinical staff focus on developing competence in the intervention. Clinical consultation emphasizes learning to deliver the core components of the treatment with fidelity while tailoring the components to the specific needs (e.g., culture, stage of development) of the client populations served. Barriers to successful implementation, such as difficulty engaging families with complex needs, are also addressed. Monthly conference calls for supervisors addressing supervisory practice (e.g., use of techniques that foster evidence-based skill development) are offered to enhance agency capacity to provide effective supervision in the EBT. Bimonthly conference calls for senior leaders emphasize the role of leadership in improving practice. Areas addressed include engaging key stakeholders in the community, facilitating effective team meetings, using metrics to guide and maintain EBT implementation, infrastructure and staff development, and sustainability planning. In addition to regularly scheduled calls, a collaborative intranet, an interactive password-protected website, is available to support asynchronous learning and serve as a central information store and communications center during the action periods. The intranet facilitates communication by enabling teams to access training materials, share resources, engage in online discussions, review their monthly metrics, and post PDSAs.

Evaluation of the NCCTS Learning Collaborative Model

As documented in this volume, a true science of mental health services implementation is just beginning to emerge (see also Proctor et al., 2009). Although a small number of systematic approaches to implementing mental health EBTs are being developed and tested, well-supported implementation strategies demonstrated effective across a range of psychotherapeutic interventions for children and families are lacking. In contrast to the extant implementation approaches, the majority of which have been developed through grant-supported research, the NCCTS Learning Collaborative Model grew out of a SAMHSA initiative focused on service delivery. Although the LC model has not yet been tested using a controlled design, LCs coordinated by the NCCTS have included an evaluation component and those evaluation data have informed development of the model. At the end of each collaborative, a process evaluation, consisting of a self-report questionnaire and focus group discussions, has been conducted to evaluate participants' use of key components of the LC model and their perceived utility. Data from metrics and organizational assessments have provided information about progress toward implementing the treatment made by each of the participating agencies. To evaluate the long-term impact of collaborative participation, 1-year follow-up evaluations were conducted with agencies that participated in two TF-CBT LCs conducted in 2007 as well as the NCTSN BSC.

Promoting clinical competence in the delivery of child trauma EBTs to a diverse group of consumers has been a priority in the design of LCs. At the same time, rigorous evaluation of treatment fidelity outside a research context has proved challenging. Treatment developers have worked with the NCCTS to create metrics to monitor providers' skill in delivering EBTs implemented through LCs. However, efforts to rigorously evaluate treatment fidelity have been hampered by the lack of validated fidelity measures suitable for use in community practice settings. Further, despite a strong emphasis on using clinical assessments to inform treatment, LC faculty have been unable to monitor client outcomes. Because of the funding structure of the NCTSN (e.g., only a relatively small percentage of grantees' funds could be allocated to evaluation), requiring sites to submit clinical assessments tailored to each of the interventions implemented through LCs has not been feasible. Some assessment data on youth receiving services from clinicians participating in LCs has been collected through an NCTSN core dataset that focuses on client-level data and outcomes. Analyses of that dataset are under way with relevant findings to be reported at a later date.

Below we offer some early findings from evaluations of LCs. We begin with a brief overview of implementation data from NCTSN LCs offered subsequent to the NCTSN BSC. We then demonstrate how evaluation data have informed and continue to inform the development of the LC model. Additionally, we provide some preliminary results from a 1-year follow-up evaluation of two NCTSN LCs, which point to the potential utility of LCs for supporting the sustained use of child trauma EBTs. Finally, we offer some initial results from the North Carolina Child Treatment Program, a state initiative that included a research component in the pilot program.

Table 6.2[5] provides an overview of the scope of efforts to support the implementation of evidence-based child trauma treatments through NCTSN LCs conducted between 2006 and 2009. As previously noted, training was offered in a variety of treatment modalities (i.e., individual, group, and dyadic) and provided in diverse settings serving youth from infancy through adolescence. Although most of the 57 agencies that participated in these collaboratives were current or former NCTSN grantees, 30% were nonnetwork sites. All but one of the participating agencies delivered the treatment in which they were being trained during the collaborative; one nonnetwork site in the SPARCS II collaborative began but was unable to complete a SPARCS group. Retention of youth in treatment appeared to be better than average. Research on client attrition suggests that over 45% of clients terminate psychotherapy prematurely (Wierzbicki & Pekarik, 1993). In NCTSN LCs overall treatment dropout rates were 7% for Cognitive Behavioral Intervention for Trauma in Schools (CBITS), 23% for TF-CBT, and 29% for CPP.[6] While the number of clients served by different agencies varied widely, from 3 to 188, during these seven collaboratives, a total of 1,078 youth received evidence-based child trauma treatment from 280 community-based providers.

Each of the LCs in Table 6.2 included an evaluation component. After the final action period, the feedback participants provided in the process evaluation was combined with data from the collaborative metrics and organizational assessments to evaluate the extent to which participating agencies made progress toward the collaborative mission and goals. Working within a framework in which data are used to improve practice, in reviewing these data careful consideration was given to how the LC process may have affected sites' implementation efforts with lessons learned applied to subsequent collaboratives. For example, the most recent ("National") NCTSN TF-CBT LC was the first to include regular calls for supervisors and a dedicated senior leader track at each learning session. With respect to supervisory practice, data from the collaborative evaluation indicated good progress in this area,

---

[5] The numbers in Table 6.2 exclude clients who dropped out of treatment prior to the end of a collaborative and clinicians who did not deliver the treatment (e.g., because they left the agency or were transferred to another program).

[6] Accurate information about treatment dropout rates for the 2006 SPARCS Learning Collaborative was not available at the time this manuscript was prepared.

TABLE 6.2 Implementation of Child Trauma Treatments through NCTSN Learning Collaboratives Subsequent to the NCTSN BSC

Collaborative	Description of Treatment & Settings Delivered	Sites Trained Total (Non-NCTSN)	Clinicians Providing	Clients Receiving
CPP I	Dyadic intervention for young children (ages 0–5) exposed to family violence and their caregivers	4 (1)	18	49
SPARCS II	Group treatment for adolescents delivered in schools, shelters, clinics, and residential treatment	8 (4)	39	105
Western TF-CBT	Individual treatment for youth (ages 3–18) and caregivers delivered in shelters, residential treatment, homes, and clinics	8 (3)	26	158
Eastern TF-CBT	Individual treatment for youth and caregivers delivered in residential treatment, homes, and clinics	10 (3)	52	141
National TF-CBT	Individual treatment for youth and caregivers delivered in residential treatment, foster care, homes, and clinics	11 (3)	54	207
National CPP	Dyadic intervention for young children exposed to family violence and their caregivers delivered in homes and clinics	11 (2)	46	118
National CBITS	Group treatment for youth (ages 10–15) delivered in schools	5 (1)	45	300

[a]Excludes clients who dropped out of treatment before the end of the collaborative.

[b]SPARCS is Structured Psychotherapy for Adolescents Responding to Chronic Stress.

[c]CPP is Child-Parent Psychotherapy.

[d]CBITS is Cognitive Behavioral Intervention for Trauma in Schools.

with 90% of participants reporting "some" (30%) or "a lot" (60%) of progress toward ensuring that staff received quality supervision in TF-CBT. Consistent with these perceptions, by the time of the final learning session, 9 of the 11 agencies in the collaborative (82%) were offering 2 hours or more of TF-CBT supervision each month, with the remaining 2 agencies regularly providing 1 to 2 hours of TF-CBT supervision. With respect to senior leader involvement, senior leaders all considered the opportunity to meet with other senior leaders at learning sessions to have been "very" important to their agencies' efforts to implement TF-CBT. Although it is difficult to gauge the specific impact of senior leader involvement, focus group data suggested that the LC model did change the way in which participating senior leaders viewed adopting a new practice: "This is a new way of thinking about a program that needs to be established, standardized, and sustained." "I didn't realize how free wheeling we used to do things; we weren't thinking about the future before the collaborative." At the same time, the focus groups pointed to a need for greater communication and coordination between supervisors and senior leaders during the implementation process. This lesson is being carried into subsequent collaboratives where testing and refining mechanisms for forging a stronger partnership between supervisors and senior leaders is a priority.

A defining characteristic of the LC model is its emphasis on sustainability planning. Therefore, early in 2009, the NCCTS conducted a 1-year follow-up evaluation of the 2007 NCTSN (Eastern and Western) TF-CBT LCs to assess the extent to which participating agencies had been able to sustain and spread the practice of TF-CBT. To minimize burden, each agency was asked to complete a single web-based survey, which broadly assessed delivery of TF-CBT through the agency, including current practices with respect to TF-CBT supervision and fidelity monitoring. All 18 agencies completed the survey; all but one were continuing to provide TF-CBT to youth in their community. One nonnetwork site serving youth in residential treatment did not have clinicians on staff who were available to provide TF-CBT at the time of the survey. The team's senior leader had left the agency and there was no longer support for the practice at an organizational level. The vast majority of the remaining sites ($n = 15$; 83%) reported having more clinicians on staff available to provide TF-CBT than at the end of the collaborative. All but two reported having at least the same number of clients currently receiving TF-CBT, with 12 (67%) reporting more TF-CBT cases. With respect to spread of the practice, 15 sites (83%) reported use of TF-CBT in additional agency programs or locations and 5 (28%) reported supporting spread to other agencies in the community. Providing regular supervision in an EBT and monitoring treatment fidelity are both important in ensuring that the practice is skillfully delivered and spread. Nearly all of the agencies currently delivering TF-CBT offered regular supervision focused specifically on TF-CBT skills and cases ($n = 15$; 88%). Most ($n = 14$; 82%) also reported regularly evaluating the skill and fidelity with which agency staff were implementing TF-CBT; however, supervisors observed or viewed recordings of TF-CBT sessions to monitor fidelity at only six of these agencies. Finally, seven agencies (39%) had received funding to provide or disseminate TF-CBT that they had not had prior to participating in the LC, suggesting that developing the capacity to deliver and sustain an EBT could have fiscal benefits.

The application of an adaptation of the NCCTS Learning Collaborative Model to individual practitioners in a pilot for a statewide dissemination of TF-CBT included the most rigorous evaluation of the model to date. Designed using public health principles, the North Carolina Child Treatment Program (http://ncctp.med.unc.edu) assessed client symptoms pre- and posttreatment (i.e., PTSD, depression, and behavior problems) and treatment fidelity. The fidelity assessment included a structured rating scale completed by TF-CBT trainers based on regular consultation and case review with each trainee. Clients who completed TF-CBT evidenced significant improvement on all symptom measures. Moreover, better adherence to the treatment model (i.e., higher fidelity scores) was associated with significantly greater improvements in PTSD symptoms (Amaya-Jackson, Hagele, & Socolar, 2009; Amaya-Jackson et al., 2011).

Summary and Conclusions

There is clear evidence that American youth suffer high rates of exposure to violence, abuse, and other traumatic stressors (Fairbank et al., 2007; Finkelhor, Turner, Ormrod, & Hamby, 2009); it is also clear that such experiences can adversely affect physical, psychological, and social functioning into adulthood (Fairbank et al., 2007; Fergusson, Boden, & Horwood, 2008). Although tremendous progress has been made in the development of EBTs for posttraumatic reactions in children and adolescents, the challenge of broadly implementing these treatments remains (Chadwick Center for Children and Families, 2004). Developed within a national network of academic and community service centers, the NCCTS Learning Collaborative Model is designed to address the challenge of making effective trauma treatments widely available in communities across the United States. Learning collaboratives are structured to foster clinically competent delivery of child trauma EBTs by applying best practices in training and consultation including the use of interactive, participatory educational techniques; intensive skill practice and feedback by faculty coaches; self-assessment and audit via monthly metrics; and mastery of core treatment components via a learn, work, learn loop. Partnering with intervention developers and experienced trainers ensures a thoughtful balance between flexibility and fidelity in adapting the treatment to the specific needs of the clients being served.

Learning collaboratives are structured to not only facilitate clinically competent delivery of an evidence-based child trauma treatment but to also help community agencies develop the implementation competence necessary to rapidly implement and sustain the treatment. Many of the barriers to implementing evidence-based practices in child mental health services pertain to organizational and system factors (APA Task Force on Evidence-Based Practice for Children and Adolescents, 2008; Hemmelgarn, Glisson, & James, 2006). Therefore, LCs seek to broadly engage an organization in the process of adopting a child trauma EBT, with teams composed of agency leadership, supervisors, and clinicians all working together to address barriers and improve agency practice. Teams receive training in quality improvement methods to help them test and refine strategies to addressing barriers and improving practice and learn to use measures to evaluate the effectiveness of those strategies. Effective strategies are then shared and spread across the collaborative to accelerate progress. Collaboration across teams is also encouraged to foster the development of interagency peer support networks that can help to sustain and spread the practice after the collaborative ends. In collaborative evaluations, the opportunity to meet and share resources with staff from other agencies is consistently evaluated as one of the most helpful aspects of the collaborative for supporting progress toward implementation. In order to enhance this capacity for cross-agency learning and collaboration, the NCCTS recently launched a TF-CBT implementers website. The site archives all of the materials, discussions, and clinical tools that were developed during previous TF-CBT LCs coordinated by the NCTSN. In addition, the site allows users to continue to share resources and engage in dialogue with each other and interested faculty through an active discussion board and an area to post clinical tools and improvement strategies.

The impact of the NCTSN Learning Collaborative Model goes well beyond the providers who use it and the children and families who receive improved services. The changes that could result from its widespread use have broad policy implications for mental health service delivery to children and families affected by trauma. Over the past decade, both public and private sectors (APA Task Force on Evidence-Based Practice for Children and Adolescents, 2008; Goodheart, Kazdin, & Sternberg, 2006; President's New Freedom Commission on Mental Health, 2003) have demonstrated increasing interest in transporting EBTs to everyday practice settings. Federal initiatives, such as the SAMHSA National Child Traumatic Stress Initiative, can provide funding that, coupled with state funding, can facilitate the use of LCs for state, regional, and national efforts to make EBTs increasingly available to traumatized children and families. The principle of collaboration that is an essential element of LCs means that this model has the capacity to bring together not only intervention developers and staff from specific agencies as they work to integrate EBTs into their local settings but also administrators and practitioners from multiple agencies within one state, or even across states. Leadership from multiple agencies can and have worked in partnership to influence reimbursement, legal, and regulatory policies that affect evidence-based practice. For example, in one state initiative, collaborating agency leaders used their experience with the LC model to successfully petition insurance companies to expand a service definition (that of allowing TF-CBT to be delivered in 90-minute sessions vs. the usual 60). Another LC brought together state mental health and state social services program staff to inform state legislators on the need and feasibility of spreading EBTs for traumatized youth. Additionally, the evaluation efforts that are built into LCs can provide evidence about positive change that is critically important for policymakers who have to make difficult budget decisions. At the federal level, the success of the LC model can also inform policymakers during the development and implementation of health care reform efforts. The ability of the LC to shape integrated care and to build accountability and continuous improvement of care into the treatment of traumatized children makes this a valuable tool for national health care change.

The NCCTS Learning Collaborative Model was developed through an iterative process informed by work with experts in both child trauma treatment and implementation methods, along with application and evaluation of the model in over 20 regional, state, and national initiatives. As is true of other successful programs for implementing EBTs for children and families (e.g., Chamberlain, 2003; Henggeler, Schoenwald, Letourneau, & Edwards, 2002), the LC model includes intensive clinical training, regular consultation with supervisors with advanced skills in the treatment (i.e., treatment developers and trainers), and mechanisms to engage and support agency leadership. Learning collaboratives attempt to combine the benefits of these programs, which provide intensive oversight to support implementation with a high degree of fidelity, with the strengths of the BSC and other quality collaboratives. Quality collaboratives seek to accelerate the pace of diffusion of best practices through the efficient use of experts to support effective implementation, through training in quality improvement methods to make organizational and practice improvements, and by fostering the exchange of ideas, expertise, and resources across organizations to hasten progress. Evaluation findings suggest that agency staff view LCs as a valuable and practicable approach for implementing child trauma EBTs in diverse community settings. Evaluation findings also indicate that LCs foster rapid implementation of child trauma EBTs and, for the vast majority of agencies, the organizational capacity necessary to sustain the practice. Although early findings from the North Carolina Child Treatment Program are promising, additional research is needed to determine whether child trauma EBTs implemented through LCs consistently improve outcomes for traumatized children and families. Research is also needed to determine whether the NCCTS Learning Collaborative Model is cost-effective and to determine which components of the model contribute to its effectiveness. The chasm between best practice and everyday practice noted by the Institute of Medicine in 2001 remains a challenge to health care delivery systems. The NCCTS Learning Collaborative Model, in conjunction with the broader efforts of the NCTSN to raise the standard of care for children and families affected by trauma, shows promise as one way to begin to close that chasm.

Acknowledgments

This paper was developed in part under grant number 2U79SM054284–08 from the Center for Mental Health Services (CMHS), Substance Abuse and Mental Health Services Administration (SAMHSA), U.S. Department of Health and Human Services (HHS). The views, policies, and opinions expressed are those of the authors and do not necessarily reflect those of SAMHSA or HHS. The authors gratefully acknowledge the UCLA-Duke NCCTS Training and Implementation Program team for their assistance in preparation of this chapter, and Dr. Ellen Gerrity for her generous editorial assistance.

REFERENCES

Aarons, G. A., & Palinkas, L. A. (2007). Implementation of evidence-based practice in child welfare: Service provider perspectives. *Administration and Policy in Mental Health and Mental Health Services Research, 34*, 411–419.

Agosti, J., Ebert, L., Amaya-Jackson, L., Kisiel, C., Markiewicz, J., & Maze, J. (2007). Improving the adoption of evidence-based practice in community agencies. *Using the breakthrough series collaborative methodology in child trauma: Final report.* Los Angeles, CA, and Durham, NC: National Center for Child Traumatic Stress.

Amaya-Jackson, L., Hagele, D., & Socolar, R. S. (2009, January). *Pilot to policy: Dissemination of Trauma-Focused CBT in North Carolina.* Presented at the annual San Diego International Conference on Child and Family Maltreatment, San Diego, CA.

Amaya-Jackson, L., Hagele, D., Socolar, R. S., Briggs-King, E., Potter, D., Keen, L., et al. (2011). *Statewide rostering and quality threshold for dissemination and implementation of trauma focused evidence-based treatment.* Manuscript in preparation.

American Psychological Association Task Force on Evidence-Based Practice for Children and Adolescents. (2008). *Disseminating evidence-based practice for children and adolescents: A systems approach to enhancing care.* Washington, DC: American Psychological Association.

Asch, S., Baker, D., Keesey, J., Broder, M., Schonlau, M., Rosen, M., et al. (2005). Does the collaborative model improve care for chronic heart failure? *Medical Care, 43*, 667–675.

Bain, K. (2004). *What the best college teachers do.* Boston: Harvard University Press.

Baumann, B. L., Kolko, D. J., Collins, K., & Herschell, A. D. (2006). Understanding practitioner's characteristics and perspectives prior to the dissemination of an evidence-based intervention. *Child Abuse and Neglect, 30*, 771–787.

Benedetti, R., Flock, B., Pedersen, S., & Ahern, M. (2004). Improved clinical outcomes for fee-for-service physician practices participating in a diabetes care collaborative. *Joint Commission Journal on Quality and Safety, 30*, 187–194.

Berwick, D. (2003). Disseminating innovations in health care. *Journal of the American Medical Association, 289*, 1969–1975.

Boud, D., & Middleton, H. (2003). Learning from others at work: Communities of practice and informal learning. *Journal of Workplace Learning, 15*, 194–202.

Casey Family Programs. (2005). Recruitment and retention of resource families: Promising practices and lessons learned. *Report on the Breakthrough Series Collaborative*, 001. Retrieved from http://www.casey.org/Resources/Publications/BreakthroughSeries_RecruitmentRetention.htm

Cavaleri, M., Gopalan, G., McKay, M., Appel, A., Bannon Jr., W., Bigley, M., et al. (2006). Impact of a learning collaborative to improve child mental health service use among low-income urban youth and families. *Best Practices in Mental Health: An International Journal, 2*, 67–79.

Chadwick Center for Children and Families. (2004). *Closing the quality chasm in child abuse treatment: Identifying and disseminating best practices.* San Diego, CA: Author.

Chamberlain, P. (2003). Some challenges of implementing science-based interventions in the "real-world." In *Treating chronic juvenile offenders: Advances made through the*

Oregon multidimensional treatment foster care model (pp. 141–149). Law and Public Policy. Washington, DC: American Psychological Association.

Cloitre, M., Koenen, K. C., & Cohen, L. R. (2006). *Treating survivors of childhood abuse: Psychotherapy for the interrupted life.* New York: Guilford Press.

Cohen, J. A., Mannarino, A. P., & Deblinger, E. (2006). *Treating trauma and traumatic grief in children and adolescents.* New York: Guilford Press.

DeRosa, R., & Pelcovitz, D. (2009). Igniting SPARCS of change: Structured psychotherapy for adolescents responding to chronic stress. In J. Ford, R. Pat-Horenczyk, & D. Brom (Eds.), *Treating traumatized children: Risk, resilience, and recovery* (pp. 225–239). New York: Routledge.

Dunst, C. J., & Trivette, C. M. (2009). Let's be PALS: An evidence-based approach to professional development. *Infants and Young Children, 22*(30), 164–176. doi:10.1097/IYC.0b013e3181abe169

Fairbank, J., Putnam, F., & Harris, W. (2007). The prevalence and impact of child traumatic stress. In M. Friedman, T. M. Keane, & P. A. Resick (Eds.), *Handbook of PTSD: Science and practice* (pp. 229–251). New York: Guilford Press.

Fergusson, D. M., Boden, J. M., & Horwood, L. J. (2008). Exposure to childhood sexual and physical abuse and adjustment in early adulthood. *Child Abuse and Neglect, 32*(6), 607–619. doi:10.1016/j.chiabu.2006.12.018

Finkelhor, D., Turner, H., Ormrod, R., & Hamby, S. L. (2009). Violence, abuse, and crime exposure in a national sample of children and youth. *Pediatrics, 124*(5), 1–14. doi:10.1542/peds.2009–0467

Fixsen, D. L., Naoom, S. F., Blasé, K. A., Friedman, R. M., & Wallace, F. (2005). *Implementation research: A synthesis of the literature.* Tampa, FL: National Implementation Research Network.

Ford, J. D., & Russo, E. (2006). Trauma-focused, present-centered, emotional self-regulation approach to integrated treatment for posttraumatic stress and addiction: Trauma Adaptive Recovery Group Education and Therapy (TARGET). *American Journal of Psychotherapy, 60,* 335–355.

Glisson, C. (2002). The organizational context of children's mental health services. *Clinical Child and Family Psychology Review, 5*(4), 233–253. doi:10.1023/A:1020972906177

Goodheart, C. D., Kazdin, A. E., & Sternberg, R. J. (Eds.). (2006). *Evidence-based psychotherapy: Where practice and research meet.* Washington, DC: American Psychological Association.

Gotham, H. (2006). Advancing the implementation of evidence-based practices into clinical practice: How do we get there from here? *Professional Psychology: Research and Practice, 37*(6), 606–613. doi:10.1037/0735-7028.37.6.606

Hammick, M., Freeth, D., Koppel, I., Reeves, S., & Barr, H. (2007). A best evidence systematic review of interprofessional education: BEME Guide no. 9. *Medical Teacher, 29*(8), 735–751. doi:10.1080/01421590701682576

Hemmelgarn, A. L., Glisson, C., & James, L. R. (2006). Organizational culture and climate: Implications for services and interventions research. *Clinical Psychology: Science and Practice, 13*(1), 73–89. doi:10.1111/j. 1468–2850.2006.00008.x

Henggeler, S. W., Schoenwald, S. K., Letourneau, J. G., & Edwards, D. L. (2002). Transporting efficacious treatments to field settings: The link between supervisory practices and therapist fidelity in MST programs. *Journal of Clinical Child & Adolescent Psychology, 31*(2), 155–167.

Hoagwood, K., Burns, B. J., & Weisz, J. R. (2002). A profitable conjunction: From science to service in children's mental health. In B. J. Burns & K. Hoagwood (Eds.), *Community treatment for youth: Evidence-based interventions for severe emotional and behavioral disorders* (pp. 327–338). New York: Oxford University Press.

Hoge, M., Tondora, J., & Stuart, G. (2003). Training in evidence-based practice. *Psychiatric Clinics of North America, 26,* 851–865. doi:10.1016/S0193–953X(03)00066–2

Institute for Healthcare Improvement. (2003). *The breakthrough series: IHI's collaborative model for achieving breakthrough improvement* (IHI Innovation Series white paper). Cambridge, MA: Author. Retrieved from http://www.ihi.org/IHI/Results/WhitePapers/

Institute of Medicine. (2001). *Crossing the quality chasm: A new health system for the twenty-first century.* Washington, DC: National Academy Press.

Kilo, C. M. (1999). Improving care through collaboration [Supplement]. *Pediatrics, 103*(1), 384–393.

Knowles, M. S. (1990). *The adult learner: A neglected species* (4th ed.). Houston, TX: Gulf.

Kolko, D. J., & Swenson, C. C. (2002). *Assessing and treating physically abused children and their families: A cognitive behavioral approach.* Thousand Oaks, CA: Sage.

Langley, G. J., Nolan, K. M., Nolan, T. W., Norman, C. L., & Provost, L. P. (1996). *The improvement guide: A practical approach to enhancing organizational performance.* San Francisco, CA: Jossey-Bass.

Lieberman, A. F., Ghosh Ippen, C., & Van Horn, P. (2006). Child-Parent Psychotherapy: 6-month follow-up of a randomized control trial. *Journal of the American Academy of Child and Adolescent Psychiatry, 45*(8), 913–918. doi: 10.1097/01.chi.0000222784.03735.92

Lieberman, A. F., Van Horn, P., & Ghosh Ippen, C. (2005). Toward evidence-based treatment: Child-Parent Psychotherapy with preschoolers exposed to marital violence. *Journal of the American Academy of Child and* Adolescent Psychiatry, *44*(12), 1241–1248. doi:10.1097/01.chi.0000181047.59702.58

Miller, O., & Ward, K. (2008). Emerging strategies for reducing racial disproportionality and disparate outcomes in child welfare: The results of a national breakthrough series collaborative. *Child Welfare, 87*(2), 211–240.

Nolan, T. W. (2007). *Execution of strategic improvement initiatives to produce system-level results* (IHI Innovation Series white paper). Cambridge, MA: Institute for Healthcare Improvement. Retrieved from http://www.ihi.org/IHI/Results/WhitePapers/

Ovretveit, J., Bate, P., Cleary, P., Cretin, S., Gustafson, D., McInnes, K., et al. (2002). Quality collaboratives: Lessons from research. *Quality and Safety in Health Care, 11,* 345–351. Retrieved from http://qshc.bmj.com

President's New Freedom Commission on Mental Health. (2003). *Achieving the promise: Transforming mental health in America* (Final report). Rockville, MD: DHHS. Retrieved from http://www.mentalhealthcommission.gov/reports/FinalReport/downloads/downloads.html

Proctor, E. K., Landsverk, J., Aarons, G., Chambers, D., Glisson, C., & Mittman, B. (2009). Implementation research in mental health services: An emerging science with conceptual, methodological, and training challenges. *Administration and Policy in Mental Health and Mental Health Services Research, 36,* 24–34. doi:10.1007/s10488–008-0197–4

Pynoos, R. S., Fairbank, J. A., Steinberg, A. M., Amaya-Jackson, L., Gerrity, E., Mount, M., et al. (2008). The National Child Traumatic Stress Network: Collaborating to improve the standard of care. *Professional Psychology: Research and Practice, 39*(4), 389–395. doi:10.1037/a0012551

Reinertsen, J. L., Bisognano, M., & Pugh, M. D. (2008). *Seven leadership leverage points for organization-level improvement in health care* (2nd ed.) (IHI Innovation Series white paper). Cambridge, MA: Institute for Healthcare Improvement. Retrieved from http://www.ihi.org/IHI/Results/WhitePapers/

Rogers, E. M. (1995). *Diffusion of innovations* (4th ed.). New York: Free Press.

Savery, J., & Duffy, T. (1996). Problem based learning: An instructional model and its constructivist framework. In B. G. Wilson (Ed.), *Constructivist learning environments: Case studies in instructional design* (pp. 135–150). Englewood Cliffs, NJ: Educational Technology.

Schonlau, M., Mangione-Smith, R., Chan, K., Keesey, J., Rosen, M., Louis, T., et al. (2005). Evaluation of a quality improvement collaborative in asthma care: Does it improve processes and outcomes of care? *Annals of Family Medicine, 3*(3), 200–208. doi:10.1370/afm.269

Schouten, L. M., Hulscher, M. E., Van Everdingen, J. J., Huijsman, R., & Grol, R. P. (2008). Evidence for the impact of quality improvement collaboratives: Systematic review. *British Medical Journal, 336*(7659), 1491–1494. doi:10.1136/bmj.39570.749884.BE

Southam-Gerow, M. A., Chorpita, B. F., Miller, L. M., & Gleacher, A. A. (2008). Are children with anxiety disorders privately referred to a university clinic like those referred from the public mental health system? *Administration and Policy in Mental Health, 35*(3), 168–180. doi:10.1007/s10488–007-0154–7

Stirman, S. W., Crits-Christoph, P., DeRubeis, R. J. (2004). Achieving successful dissemination of empirically supported psychotherapies: A synthesis of dissemination theory. *Clinical Psychology: Science and Practice, 11*(4), 343–359. doi:10.1093/clipsy/bph091

Stuart, G., Tondora, J., & Hoge, M. (2004). Evidence-based teaching practice: Implications for behavioral health. *Administration and Policy in Mental Health, 32*(2), 107–130. doi:10.1023/B:APIH.0000042743.11286.bc

Vargas, R., Mangione, C., Asch, S., Keesey, J., Rosen, M., Schonlau, M., et al. (2007). Can a chronic care model collaborative reduce heart disease risk in patients with diabetes? *Society of General Internal Medicine, 22*, 215–222. doi:10.1007/s11606–006-0072–5

Vaughn, T., Koepke, M., Kroch, E., Lehrman, W., Sinha, S., & Levey, S. (2006). Engagement of leadership in quality improvement initiatives: Executive quality improvement survey results. *Journal of Patient Safety, 2*(1), 2–9.

Weisz, J., Jensen, A., & McLeod, B. (2005). Development and dissemination of child and adolescent psychotherapies: Milestones, methods, and a new deployment-focused model. In E. D. Hibbs & P. S. Jensen (Eds.), *Psychosocial treatments for child and adolescent disorders: Empirically based strategies for clinical practice* (2nd ed., pp. 9–39). Washington, DC: American Psychological Association.

Wierzbicki, M., & Pekarik, G. (1993). A meta-analysis of psychotherapy dropout. *Professional Psychology: Research and Practice, 24*, 190–195. doi:10.1037/0735–7028.24.2.190

Wilson, T., Berwick, D. M., & Cleary, P. D. (2003). Performance improvement: What do collaborative improvement projects do? Experience from seven countries. *Joint Commission Journal on Quality and Safety, 29*(2), 85–93.

Woltmann, E. M., Whitley, R., McHugo, G. J., Brunette, M., Torrey, W. C., Coots, L., et al. (2008). The role of staff turnover in the implementation of evidence-based practices in mental health care. *Psychiatric Services, 59*(7), 732–737. doi:10.1176/appi.ps.59.7.732

Zwarenstein, M., Goldman, J., & Reeves, S. (2009). Interprofessional collaboration: Effects of practice-based interventions on professional practice and healthcare outcomes. *Cochrane Database of Systematic Reviews, 3.* doi:10.1002/14651858.CD000072.pub2

7

Evidence-Based Practice and Autism

BUILDING SYSTEMIC CAPACITY BASED ON THE NATIONAL STANDARDS PROJECT

Susan M. Wilczynski, Dennis C. Russo, and Walter P. Christian

Internationally, we are faced with a growing number of children and adolescents receiving a diagnosis of an autism spectrum disorder (ASD). While reeling in response to this devastating news, parents need to make a number of important decisions. At the same time, allied health professionals and educational staff are confronted with the rising demand for appropriate services for individuals on the autism spectrum. Parents and professionals are challenged to select from among a dizzying array of treatment options, many of which have limited or no evidence of effectiveness.

Imagine your child being diagnosed with a serious, chronic disease and learning there are hundreds of treatment options for this devastating medical condition. You search the web, meet with a variety of professionals, and poll families whose children have the disease without arriving at consensus. You would feel compelled to take timely action and to select wisely in order to obtain the best care for your child. But the task is overwhelming and you cannot find any single source of credible information on what works for the particular challenges that your child faces. This scenario is very much the case today with respect to treating ASD.

The National Autism Center was created in 2005 in response to the growing need for reliable information about autism treatments. The National Autism Center is a not-for-profit organization dedicated to serving children and adolescents with ASD by providing reliable information, promoting best practices, and offering comprehensive resources for families, practitioners, and communities. The first goal of the National Autism Center has been, with the support and guidance of an expert panel composed of nationally recognized scholars, researchers, and other leaders representing diverse fields of study, to undertake a rigorous multiyear project to provide the most comprehensive analysis available to date about treatment effectiveness for ASD. The goal was to apply rigorous methodology to the autism treatment literature and to develop a mechanism for disseminating this information broadly to parents, professionals, and other stakeholders. The purpose of this dissemination process was the delivery of information across large numbers of people who have a need for such information across great distances.

The National Standards Project, a primary initiative of the National Autism Center, serves to support parents and professionals as they make critical treatment decisions for the children and adolescents with ASD who share their lives. The National Standards Project addresses the need for evidence-based practice guidelines. This project culminated in the *National Standards Report* (National Autism Center [NAC], 2009b), which identified the strength of evidence supporting a broad range of treatments that target the core and associated symptoms of these neurological disorders. The report also outlines the extent to which favorable outcomes have been reported in the literature—this information is available based on age, diagnostic population, and treatment targets—and describes the future direction of ASD treatment research that must be conducted to better arm families and service providers in all settings with the answers they need to make informed decisions.

In addition to the presentation of findings from the comprehensive systematic review of the ASD treatment literature, the *National Standards Report* (NAC, 2009b) strongly advocates for decision makers to adopt the process of evidence-based practice. Evidence-based practice is defined here as the integration of research findings with (a) professional judgment and data-based clinical decision making; (b) the values and preferences of families, including the individual on the spectrum; and (c) the capacity to implement an intervention with sufficient treatment fidelity.

One of the primary reasons for providing detailed analysis of the literature is to improve the likelihood that individuals on the autism spectrum will get access to treatments that are shown to be effective and will help them reach their full potential. For the purposes of this chapter, we focus predominantly on the systemic efforts required to accurately implement empirically-supported treatments on a large scale. These complex treatment selection decisions will need to occur in a variety of settings (e.g., hospitals, homes, schools, and community-based health centers). However, given that most children and adolescents with ASD will be served in treatment centers or schools, the present chapter uses the results of the National Standards Project to serve as a foundation for building systemic capacity in these organizational settings.

Motivating Circumstances

Autism is occurring at an alarming rate. The Centers for Disease Control and Prevention (CDC) estimate that an ASD occurs in 1 of 150 children born in the United States (CDC, 2007). For male children, the rates are even higher, with a prevalence of 1 in 94. ASD occurs across all ethnic, social, and racial strata. Data from other countries also identify similar increases in occurrence (CDC, 2007; Fombonne, 2003; Newschaffer et al., 2007).

Some would argue that these numbers are the result of overdiagnosis. Although the definition of ASDs has broadened over the past years and funding for treatment has become more available, recent research has pointed to the increasing incidence of these disorders even when these factors are taken into account (Hertz-Picciotto & Delwiche, 2009).

Extrapolation of these data suggests that ASD will be identified in 26,670 children in the United States per year: one child every 20 minutes. About 560,000 individuals between the ages of 0 and 21 in the United States are on the autism spectrum, if one assumes similar prevalence rates over the last two decades (CDC, 2009).

Costs of care can be very high, with lifetime costs estimated at $3.2 million (Ganz, 2007). Significantly increased educational costs averaging $18,000 per child with autism per year (U.S. Government Accountability Office, 2005) and medical costs between 4.1 and 6.2 times greater are seen for children on the autism spectrum as compared to their peers (Shimabukuro, Grosse, & Rice, 2008). It is likely that 90% of all costs will be experienced in the individual's adult years. Early identification and treatment of the child may decrease these lifetime costs by two thirds (Jarbrink & Knapp, 2001).

LEGISLATION AND OTHER INITIATIVES

In recent years there has been a corresponding surge in awareness of these disorders. National and international efforts have been made to mobilize resources to address the needs of individuals on the spectrum in both the governmental and private sectors. At the national level, the U.S. government has developed the Interagency Autism Coordinating Committee (IACC). This group coordinates all efforts within the Department of Health and Human Services (HHS) concerning autism spectrum disorders including policy, information dissemination, research, and education (IACC, n.d.).

Paralleling this development in the private sector, groups such as Autism Speaks and the Autism Society of America have engaged in lobbying, public education, and the development of support and funding agendas for future research. This has resulted in an unprecedented effort to develop legislative support for funding through governmental and private sources.

Indeed, model legislative packages and lobbying efforts have led, as of this writing, to the passage of laws in 15 states, which require health insurance to fund autism services (Autism Votes, 2008). An overriding tenant of these legislative efforts has been the insistence on the use evidence-based practices as the standard for treatment. In most cases, applied behavior analysis treatment has been identified as the only method named with sufficient evidence of support.

STAKEHOLDER DEMAND

The demand for treatment has created a huge number of methods being promulgated to the autism community. Many of these approaches are based on limited evidence, with appeals made to families based on testimonials and promises of benefits based on little or no research. Selection of treatments most likely to be of benefit at the earliest possible time in a child's development has been identified as critical in autism (Lovaas, 1987; Luiselli, Russo, Christian, & Wilczynski, 2008). Young children who receive ineffective treatments are less likely to see gains in critical areas such as language, social behavior, and the reduction of behavioral difficulties.

In addition to families, educators and a broad range of allied health professionals seek to understand which treatments enjoy solid research support. They are often bound by legal mandates (e.g., No Child Left Behind Act of 2001; Individuals with Disabilities Education Improvement Act of 2004) and ethical guidelines such as those promulgated by the Behavior Analysis Certification Board (BACB, 2004) and the National Association of School Psychologists (NASP, 2000). However, given how expansive the autism treatment literature has now become, it is challenging for most professionals to keep well informed about the strength of evidence supporting the many different treatment options available. Collectively, with these developments and the enormous energy and momentum driving access to appropriate care, the field stands poised to make an enormous impact on the care of children and adolescents with ASD. What has been missing is a common metric by which to evaluate the evidence for effective treatments in the field and the creation of a guide that specifies which treatments are best suited to treat the cardinal and associated symptoms of ASD.

Description of Programs

This National Standards Project centered on a systematic review of the autism treatment literature spanning a 50-year period. The National Standards Project began with the development of a model for evaluating the scientific literature on the treatment of ASD. This task was completed by working groups consisting of scientists and practitioners, and required an examination of evidence-based practice guidelines from other health and psychology fields.

From the over 7,000 abstracts that were initially reviewed for consideration, a total of 775 studies meeting the inclusionary and exclusionary requirements of the National Standards Project were reviewed. Based on a process developed by 45 autism experts from around the United States, articles were evaluated in terms of the quality of the (a) research design, (b) dependent measure, (c) treatment fidelity, (d) participant ascertainment, and (d) generalization. These indicators were combined to develop the Scientific Merit Rating Scale (SMRS) score. In addition, a process for evaluating treatment effects was developed, which allowed for a treatment effectiveness rating to be assigned to each article. The Treatment Effects Rating was determined on the basis of whether the outcomes were (a) beneficial, (b) unknown, (c) ineffective, or (d) adverse. Figure 7.1 describes the process followed for the initial development of the National Standards Project. A more detailed

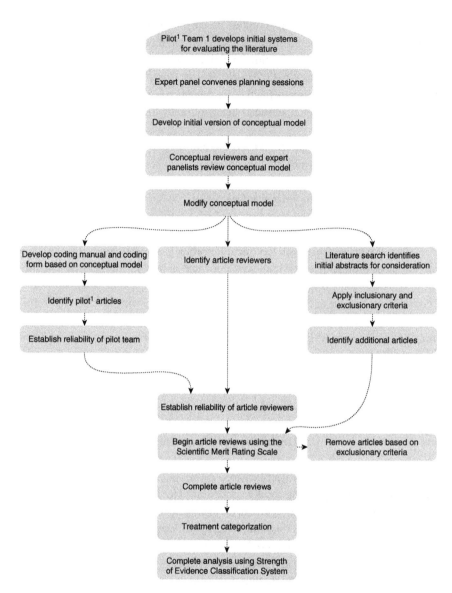

A small subset of the experts involved in the National Standards Project were involved in the initial development of the conceptual model and were known as Pilot Team 1. A second subset of experts involved in the National Standards Project helped develop the coding system and were known as Pilot Team 2. The articles for which adequate interobserver agreement was established were then sent out to reviewers. These articles were called 'pilot articles.'

FIGURE 7.1 *Process of the initial development of the National Standards Project.*

discussion of this process can be found in the *Findings and Conclusions* report (abbreviated report; NAC, 2009a) or the *National Standards Report* (full technical report) published by the National Autism Center (NAC, 2009b).

SMRS scores and Treatment Effects Ratings were aggregated across studies for each of 38 identified treatment categories. The Strength of Evidence Classification System was used to classify treatments based on the quality, quantity, and consistency of research findings. Treatments were classified as "Established Treatments," "Emerging Treatments," or "Unestablished Treatments," based on the combined outcomes of the SMRS scores and the Treatment Effect Ratings. Finally, although no treatments fell into this category, a fourth category had also been developed for Ineffective or Harmful Treatments. To fall in this category, several well-controlled studies would have to be published in peer-reviewed journals and adverse Treatment Effects Ratings would have to be rendered.

In addition to overall Strength of Evidence Classification System ratings, information about the treatment targets (e.g., communication, interpersonal, problem behaviors, etc.) and the ages and diagnostic groups for which favorable outcomes were obtained were noted in the *National Standards Report* (NAC, 2009b). In this way, parents, educators, and service providers could make more informed decisions about the level of evidence available for treatments they might consider.

Eleven different interventions were identified as Established Treatments. These intervention categories include Antecedent Package, Behavioral Package, Comprehensive Behavioral Treatment for Young Children, Joint Attention Intervention, Modeling, Naturalistic Teaching Strategies, Peer Training Package, Pivotal Response Treatment, Schedules, Self-Management, and Story-Based Intervention Package. All remaining treatments fell into the Emerging Treatments or Unestablished Treatments categories. The *National Standards Report* (NAC, 2009b) as well as the *Findings and Conclusions* report (NAC, 2009a) are available at the National Autism Center's website (http://www.nationalautismcenter.org). The interested reader is encouraged to review these sources for more detailed information about the methods employed and the findings that were obtained in this project.

Although the National Standards Project identified 11 interventions as effective, the process of treatment selection is still likely to be very complicated when applied to the individual case. Evidence-based practice requires that, in addition to research findings, treatment selection should involve input from several key stakeholders (e.g., parents, educators, service providers). Care must be taken to select the most appropriate treatment for a given child, with the child's previous response to treatments and the capacity of service providers to implement treatments with fidelity both influencing decision making.

Even if decision makers restrict their choice to the Established Treatments identified in the *National Standards Report* (NAC, 2009b), they must still select the most appropriate from an array of 11. How, then, can treatment centers or schools, those organizations most likely needing to adopt evidence-based treatments for ASD, know the best strategy for building systemic capacity for treatments with research support? Prescription of care should be made through a deliberative process including a thorough assessment of the individual case, an understanding of previous treatments, an evaluation of functional variables contributing to the problem, and the design of an adequate method to evaluate the outcomes of intervention.

FUNDING

The National Autism Center obtained support from many sources in order to complete the National Standards Project. To begin, well over a thousand hours of service were donated by volunteers to the project. These contributors include members of the expert panel, conceptual reviewers, article reviewers, computer and statistical consultants, and document commentators. In addition, financial support was provided by the May Institute, Autism Education Network, and California Department of Developmental Services.

Securing necessary resources is a challenge not only for the development of projects like the National Standards Project but also for centers that choose to adopt the treatments described in the *National Standards Report* (NAC, 2009b). Funding sources for these centers are highly variable. Schools are one of the most common service delivery agencies that are likely to provide prolonged care to children with ASD. Although a portion of funding for special education services is provided through the federal government, states and local resources also share the majority of these costs (University of Michigan, n.d.).

In addition to direct costs for special education services, many states have developed networks through their Departments of Education that are designed to support the education and training of teachers and school-based practitioners (Easter Seals Disability Services, 2009). These "collaborative" networks are often organized somewhat differently by area but often serve as a resource to school systems for children who are too difficult to manage and/or teach within specific districts.

Treatment centers or agencies also receive funding through a number of avenues. Treatment centers may receive private payment from families, may be supported through insurance reimbursement, or may be paid by schools for out-of-district placement when a more restrictive educational environment is required. In addition, treatment centers may have a development department that writes grants to secure extramural funding.

Efforts are under way in a number of states and nationally to provide treatment for ASD under health insurance. At the time of this writing, 15 states have adopted such comprehensive legislation. All have recognized the importance of empirically-supported treatments in their bills. Most have specified applied behavior analysis as the treatment of choice. The focus on applied behavior analysis is consistent with previous reviews on autism treatment. Further, the vast majority of the Established Treatments identified through the National Standards Project come directly from the behavioral literature.

Irrespective of the type of organization providing autism treatment services and the primary source of their funding, ongoing modifications to existing systems may be necessary to ensure the system engages in evidence-based practice. Staffing ratios and access to required resources and/or materials may need to be altered if all treatment targets are to be addressed and interventions are to be implemented with sufficient fidelity. For example, Comprehensive Behavioral Treatment for Young Children often requires an instructor-to-child ratio approaching 1:1, but the existing system in most schools or treatment programs is not staffed at this level.

GOALS, TARGETS, AND STANDARDS OF CARE

There were several reasons for undertaking the National Standards Project. First, the National Standards Project was intended to help parents, educators, and service providers learn more about the complicated process of evidence-based practice. Coupled with the legislative mandates, the opinions promulgated by major autism advocacy organizations, and the guidelines of major professional organizations, evidence-based practice is being increasingly recognized as the standard of care for children with ASD.

Second, the National Standards Project was completed so that the scientific community could quickly identify the areas in which further investigation is necessary. The *National Standards Report* (NAC, 2009b) identifies the extent to which favorable outcomes have been reported for treatment targets, age, and diagnosis in the literature base. The standards identify areas that have received significant research and those in which more study is needed. It is hoped that forthcoming research will address the gaps in our knowledge.

Finally, the most important purpose for the National Standards Project is to identify the level of research support for treatments that target the core and associated symptoms of ASD. The 2009 version of the National Standards Project restricted its review to individuals younger than 22 years of age; however, future reviews will cover the lifespan. Unless compelling arguments (e.g., professional judgment, data, or values and preferences of families) can be made otherwise, the Established Treatments identified through the National Standards Project should be considered the current standard of care for young individuals (younger than 22 years of age) with ASD.

The reason for completing a systematic review like the National Standards Project is ultimately to increase the likelihood individuals with ASD will gain access to interventions that will improve their skills and, as a result, their quality of life. Although knowing which treatments are associated with beneficial effects is necessary, it is insufficient for realizing this goal. It then falls to organizations serving individuals on the autism spectrum to translate research into practice. We provide recommendations on how to develop and sustain capacity to implement effective interventions to the care systems providing services to children and adolescents with ASD in the remainder of this chapter.

NEEDS ASSESSMENT/FIT TO SYSTEM NEEDS

The results of the National Standards Project speak directly to the major changes that will often need to take place in the delivery of services to individuals on the autism spectrum. The process of developing and sustaining an effective national capacity begins with self-evaluation by individual treatment centers and schools. Capacity building begins with a needs assessment paired with a set of strategies to overcome barriers to implementation. In addition, significant effort must be dedicated to identifying a training plan for all staff involved in treatment (e.g., all direct care employees).

The National Standards Project was developed with an eye to widespread implementation. Implementing treatments with a high degree of fidelity often requires significant time and energy. Long before a training plan is developed and put in place, professionals in health care, community, and educational settings must invest the time and energy required to complete a thorough needs assessment.

A needs assessment is an extensive evaluation designed to comprehensively assess needs and barriers as they are perceived by stakeholders. Needs assessments are often completed based on the use of surveys or interviews (Tobey, 2005). The goal of the needs assessment is to identify variables that will allow the system to move forward in their efforts to develop capacity to implement evidence-based treatments. It will be hard to secure adequate "buy-in" from the professionals who will be ultimately responsible for treatment implementation without investing the requisite time and energy into a needs assessment. In the absence of staff acceptance, producing meaningful long-term change is difficult (Sims & Sims, 2004).

Training of Clinicians

There is no single training requirement that is consistent across all of the Established Treatments. Some interventions (e.g., Pivotal Response Training) have a clear hierarchical training process. Others are not associated with well-known training programs but instead are described in the treatment literature (e.g., Joint Attention Interventions). For this reason, we have focused our training recommendations on the process that should be considered when developing systemic capacity to deliver Established Treatments.

For treatment centers and schools alike, there is great benefit to establishing a planning team that is responsible for systemic capacity building. This planning team should be responsible for evaluating the current capacity of the system, identifying barriers that may undermine capacity building, engaging in collaborative problem solving, clarifying the training process, developing necessary resources, and establishing a plan for sustaining capacity. In addition to the administrator, a group of professionals that represent all key organizational constituents (e.g., speech-language pathologist, therapist, teacher, support staff, etc.) should participate as members of the planning team.

The planning team should consider several training possibilities. First, what is the level of "local" expertise? For example, has the clinical training director, speech-language pathologist, or school psychologist been formally trained in an intervention? If so, have they completed a certification process, if one is available? Have they implemented the intervention with treatment fidelity? If these questions can be answered affirmatively, the local experts may be the most cost-effective trainers. Outside consultants may be a great alternative if local experts are not identified or are not in a position to dedicate the time required to develop a training program. Irrespective of whom the trainer may be, substantial groundwork must be done before training is scheduled.

The planning team must identify which staff members require training and whether or not training opportunities should be available to families of children with ASD. The planning team must also consider the format of the training. The adult learner literature suggests that simply having a didactic workshop is insufficient for developing proficiency (Fixsen, Naoom, Blase, Friedman, & Wallace, 2005). Although information is essential for developing proficiency, adults benefit greatly from experiential training as well. This experiential training should be extended into the setting(s) in which the staff member is expected to provide the intervention. Coaching, that is, on-site feedback from experts during the "real world" application of treatment strategies, should be considered not only for initial training but also for ongoing sustainability of interventions with a high degree of treatment fidelity. Without this type of multicomponent sequential planning, it is unlikely that organizations serving individuals on the autism spectrum will develop adequate capacity to implement Established Treatments.

The planning team, in collaboration with the trainer, will need to develop written documentation (e.g., guidelines, manuals) that are consistent with the methodology applied in the studies leading to the interventions classification as an Established Treatment through the National Standards Project. In addition to the procedures described in this manual, the materials required and a process for addressing accommodations (e.g., a child is diagnosed with ASD and is visually impaired) should be included (Wilczynski, 2009). According to the *National Standards Report* (NAC, 2009b), not only is it important to select appropriate treatments for children and adolescents on the autism spectrum, but also organizations and providers serving this population have a responsibility to demonstrate effectiveness on an individual case basis and they must show that they are accurately implementing the selected treatment. For this reason, the data collection procedures used to determine treatment effectiveness and treatment fidelity should be described in the procedural guideline. The responsibilities of the planning team clearly extend well beyond arranging a speaker for a one-day workshop.

In addition to the training required to teach staff how to implement treatments, training in data collection techniques may also be necessary if data are not currently used to drive intervention decisions in the service system. The planning team will need to teach staff that data collection is not restricted to measurable progress for individuals with ASD. Data will also need to be collected to establish treatment fidelity. If a treatment is not implemented with fidelity, it is not really an Established Treatment—even if the therapist, educator, or organization providing the intervention suggests this is the case.

Along with training for new treatment, it may be necessary to complete a needs assessment regarding data collection. That is, to increase the likelihood that treatment agents will collect data in order to determine if a treatment is effective and whether they are accurately implementing the treatment, it may be necessary to identify barriers to staff developing data collection capacity or using currently available data collection procedures. Strategies for overcoming these barriers can then be developed.

STRATEGIES TO TARGET BARRIERS TO ADOPTION

We would argue that organizations should focus their capacity-building training efforts on those treatments that currently enjoy the greatest research support (i.e., Established Treatments). There are many reasons treatment or advocacy organizations and/or their staff may be resistant to support an intervention, even one that enjoys strong empirical support. We describe seven of these potential barriers to the adoption of Established Treatments identified through the National Standards Project.

Barrier 1 (Awareness). In some cases, organizations or professionals are not directly resistant to change; they simply are not aware of which treatments enjoy research support. The widespread dissemination and easy accessibility of the National Standards Project should reduce this barrier to adopting empirically supported treatments. The planning team should make the *National Standards Report* (NAC, 2009b) and/or the *Findings and Conclusions* report (NAC, 2009a) readily available to staff.

Barrier 2 (Reject science). In early 21st century United States, a culture has emerged that simultaneously glorifies and violently rejects science. The ASD community is not exempt from these conflicting perspectives. Even among professionals, there are those that believe testimonials provide just as strong evidence as a well-designed study. This view sometimes stems from the perspective that a study looking at a group of individuals with ASD may not apply in a specific case. In this case, the planning team may find it helpful to show the process used to identify Established Treatments by the National Standards Project. By including single-subject research designs in the systematic review, the National Standards Project shows treatment effectiveness on a case-by-case basis. The planning team may educate staff about the importance of demonstrating a clear functional relationship between treatment and treatment outcomes. This can also serve as a foundation for applying these same methods to the individuals with ASD being served in the treatment center or school.

Barrier 3 (Do not believe the results). The results described in the *National Standards Report* (NAC, 2009b) may not be adopted by organizations if those selecting treatments do not believe the results. Previous evidence-based practice guidelines for ASD have been rejected because decisions about treatment effectiveness were perceived as being made "behind closed doors" or as being made for political reasons rather than on scientific grounds. In order to address this concern, the process used for the National Standards Project was transparent from its inception. The proposed methods were presented at dozens of national conferences and feedback was solicited from the autism community. The planning team may also point out the rigorous criteria that were met by all interventions falling into the Established Treatments category. The criteria for identifying the most effective treatments required multiple well-controlled studies demonstrating beneficial treatment effect and this should engender confidence in the findings of the National Standards Project.

Barrier 4 (Practicability). One of the most likely reasons Established Treatments may be rejected by organizations is practicality of the implementation. In some cases, the transportability of methods used in research represents the greatest challenge (Franklin & DeRubeis, 2005; Westen, 2005). However, this argument may be less tenable because of the relatively large number of Established Treatments that were identified through the National Standards Project. Certainly, not all of the 11 could be considered impractical for treatment centers or schools. In other cases, staff perceptions of effort and time represent major barriers to the adoption of effective treatments. We address these barriers below.

Effort. Irrespective of the relative complexity of an intervention, staff effort is required in order to develop expertise (Wilczynski, 2009). Instead of seamlessly delivering a familiar treatment, treatment agents must now attend to, self-evaluate, and sufficiently modify their behavior when delivering the new treatments. The added effort that is required should be acknowledged during training and ongoing coaching. In addition, resistance to change may be reduced when there are similarities between the existing treatment and new intervention (e.g., adding the strategy of self-management will require less effort when the staff are already implementing the schedule strategy because there are so many similarities between these methods).

Time. Often, organizational systems assume training time is restricted to the number of hours spent attending a formal workshop. This is not accurate, and a failure to recognize the role time may play in treatment adoption may result in systemic failure (Wilczynski, 2009). Sufficient training often requires a didactic component, an experiential component, and sustained coaching from a local expert or an outside consultant. Given the time demand, organizations may reduce staff resistance by clear expectations for staff performance and temporarily improving staffing ratios or preparing materials that are available to all staff.

Cost. Implementing treatments can be expensive. This is one reason there is such intense debate about insurance coverage in the autism community. As this issue is resolved over the next several years, organizations providing services to individuals with ASD must make difficult decisions about which treatments to provide. Certainly, some of the Established Treatments identified through the National Standards Project are more expensive than others.

There is another cost consideration that is often ignored. Treatment centers that do not demonstrate effectiveness will face increasing accountability. Schools that are able to provide improvements consistent with Individualized Education Plan goals and objectives are likely to see cost savings because they will face fewer due-process hearings. Similarly, demands for expensive consultants or out-of-district placements will be reduced. Such savings are clear incentives for embracing best practices.

Barrier 5 (Lack of understanding). Stakeholders may be resistant to the very idea of evidence-based practice because they assume that this decreases their role in the treatment selection. According to the *National Standards Report* (NAC, 2009b), evidence-based practice requires that professional judgment and data-based clinical decision making along with input from families must be considered alongside research findings when treatments are selected. The planning team may choose to educate staff about these components of evidence-based practice before adopting any treatments.

Barrier 6 (Organizational variables). Organizational variables may undermine the likelihood that empirically-supported treatments will be adopted. For example, it is easy to ignore the excitement surrounding the "new" treatment if you think it is just another fad. Treatment agents may be skeptical that a treatment is actually going to be implemented *and* sustained in the organization over a long period of time. The *National Standards Report* (NAC, 2009b) may assist organizations wishing to improve their use of evidence-based practice for individuals on the autism spectrum by improving treatment selection and enhancing compliance with legal issues and ethical guidelines that require the adoption of treatments with evidence of effectiveness.

Barrier 7 (Treatment acceptability). Treatment acceptability is another reason a treatment may not be adopted. Treatment acceptability can be determined by using any number of different treatment acceptability instruments (Carter, 2007). There are a variety of reasons treatment acceptability may not occur. If the treatment agents base their opinion on inaccurate or incomplete information, they should be educated about the exact nature of the treatment. If, on the other hand, treatment agents believe the treatment is unacceptable because it is unethical or contrary to institutional policy, efforts should be expended to determine if this could, in fact, be the case. If it is not believed to be the case, the issue must be respectfully addressed with the treatment agent.

OUTCOME EVALUATION/DATA

The *National Standards Report* (NAC, 2009b) was released in September of 2009. The extent to which large organizational systems will use this document to build sustainable capacity for the delivery of effective interventions for ASD remains to be seen. In an effort to support these organizational systems, the National Autism Center is presently developing an accreditation process for treatment centers and schools.

The accreditation process would provide voluntary review of service delivery organizations in terms of the following four factors. First, do these systems use interventions that have demonstrated evidence of effectiveness? Second, have they developed a system to incorporate professional judgment and data-based clinical decision making in the treatment selection process? Additionally, how are data used to guide decisions regarding the maintenance or modification of a treatment?

Third, to what extent do the treatment centers or schools assess and incorporate the values and preferences of families? In addition, are efforts made to consider the preferences of the individual with ASD if he or she is capable of participating in this process? Fourth, have they developed the capacity to implement the treatment with a high degree of fidelity? If so, have ongoing training and coaching needs been built into the organizational infrastructure that is required to sustain capacity?

As with any good accrediting process, participating organizational systems will receive the benefits of having well-established practices consistent with prevailing professional norms, experience success in incorporating a number of important sources of information into the treatment selection process, and enjoy better outcomes by implementing treatments with fidelity.

Future Directions and Conclusion

The number of individuals diagnosed with and requiring treatment for ASD has increased exponentially in recent decades. Legal mandates and ethical guidelines require practitioners to provide interventions that have demonstrated evidence of effectiveness. The capacity of many large organizational systems to do so has been undermined by the lack of clear, concise evidence-based practice guidelines that identify the strength of evidence available for a broad range of ASD interventions.

The National Standards Project is the most comprehensive and systematic review of the ASD treatment literature conducted to date. Treatment centers and schools should be better positioned to develop capacity to implement effective interventions armed with the information provided in the *National Standards Report* (NAC, 2009b). To that end, the National Autism Center has made their reports available as free downloadable documents from their website. They will also continue to (a) contribute information about the project through popular news outlets and professional publications and (b) deliver presentations at parent and professional conferences.

The National Autism Center seeks continued collaboration with autism experts from across the country to update their reports. The experts involved in the current version will be asked if they are interested in continuing their participation in the next version, but additional experts will be included as well. For example, professionals representing additional fields of study and/or additional populations (e.g., adults) can be expected to contribute to the next version of the National Standards Project. The report is expected to be updated once every 3 years. In this way, treatment centers and schools will be able to continue building capacity to implement treatments that enjoy research support. The National Standards Project will hopefully pave the way for a standard of care based on science and a network of practitioners capable of providing quality care consistent with these standards.

Capacity building can be a long and highly detailed process. It is cost-effective and time efficient to develop a plan for the initial adoption and sustenance of treatments over a prolonged period of time. This will most likely occur when a team of professionals, including administrators, commit to the process of building systemic capacity. By completing a thorough needs assessment, identifying strategies to overcome resistance, and carefully crafting a training plan, the planning team will more likely produce their intended goals. Although the National Standards Project is helpful in informing this process, much additional work is necessary. For example, although the National Standards Project identifies which treatments have evidence of effectiveness, the onus of responsibility continues to lie with practitioners to clearly identify and implement the intervention components that are essential for treatment fidelity.

With the completion of the National Standards Project, the National Autism Center next expects to support treatment centers and schools through the development of an accreditation process. This process will include both a self-study and outside evaluation to ensure that adequate attention is being given to each of the four components of evidence-based practice. By demonstrating their use of research findings, their incorporation of professional judgment and data-based clinical decision making, their careful consideration of the values and preferences of families, and their systemic efforts to build and sustain capacity, treatment centers and schools can clearly show they engage in evidence-based practice. It will be to the advantage of treatment centers and schools to have their services examined by an independent organization whose mission is to promote evidence-based practice for individuals with ASD. The National Autism Center will be well positioned to identify organizations providing evidence-based practice for individuals with ASD. This will further support individuals with ASD and the people who share their lives.

REFERENCES

Autism votes: An Autism Speaks initiative. (2008, August). *Autism Speaks state initiatives.* Retrieved from http://www.autismvotes.org/site/c.frKNI3PCImE/b.3909861/k.B9DF/State_Initiatives.htm

Behavior Analysis Certification Board. (2004, August). *Behavior Analyst Certification Board guidelines for responsible conduct.* Retrieved from http://www.bacb.com/maint_frame.html

Carter, S. L. (2007). Review of recent treatment acceptability research. *Educational and Training in Developmental Disabilities, 42,* 301–316.

Centers for Disease Control and Prevention. (2007). *MMWR surveillance summaries: Prevalence of autism spectrum disorders-autism and developmental disabilities monitoring network, 14 sites, United States, 2002* (56 S S01, 12–28). Retrieved from Centers for Disease Control and Prevention online via www.cdc.org

Easter Seals Disability Services. (2009). *2009 Autism state profiles.* Retrieved from www.easterseals.com/site/PageServer?pagename=ntlc8_autism_state_profiles

Fixsen, D. L., Naoom, S. F., Blase, K. A., Friedman, R. M., & Wallace, F. (2005). *Implementation research: A synthesis of the literature* (Publication No. 231). Tampa, FL: University of South Florida, Louis de la Parte Florida Mental Health Institute, The National Implementation Research Network.

Fombonne, E. (2003). Epidemiological surveys of autism and other pervasive developmental disorders: An update. *Journal of Autism and Developmental Disorders, 33,* 365–382.

Franklin, M. E., & DeRubeis, R. J. (2005). Efficacious laboratory-validated treatments are generally transportable to clinical practice. In J. C. Norcross, L. E. Beutler, & R. F. Levant (Eds.), *Evidence-based practices in mental health: Debate and dialogue on the fundamental questions* (pp. 375–383). Washington, DC: American Psychological Association.

Ganz, M. L. (2007). The lifetime distribution of the incremental societal costs of autism. *Archives of Pediatric Adolescent Medicine, 161,* 343–349.

Hertz-Picciotto, I., & Delwiche, L. (2009). The rise in autism and the role of age at diagnosis. *Epidemiology, 20,* 84–90.

Individuals with Disabilities Education Improvement Act of 2004, Pub. L. 108–466.

Interagency Autism Coordinating Committee (n.d.) Retrieved from http://iacc.hhs.gov/

Jarbrink, K., & Knapp, M. (2001). *London School of Economics study: The economic impact on autism in Britain, 5,* 7–22.

Lovass, O. I. (1987). Behavioral treatment and normal educational and intellectual functioning in young autistic children. *Journal of Consulting and Clinical Psychology, 55,* 3–9.

Luiselli, J. K., Russo, D. C., Christian, W. P., & Wilczynski, S. M. (2008). *Effective practices for children with autism: Educational and behavioral support interventions that work.* New York: Oxford University Press.

National Association of School Psychologists. (2000). *Ethical and professional practices committee procedures.* Retrieved from http://www.nasponline.org/standards/ethics/eppcommittee.aspx

National Autism Center. (2009a). *Findings and conclusions of the National Standards Project: Addressing the need for evidence-based practice guidelines for autism spectrum disorders.* Randolph, MA: National Autism Center, Inc.

National Autism Center. (2009b). *National Standards Report: National Standards Project - Addressing the need for evidence-based practice guidelines for autism spectrum disorders.* Randolph, MA: National Autism Center, Inc.

Newschaffer, C. J., Croen, L. A., Daniels, J., Giarelli, E., Grether, J. K., Levy, S. E., et al. (2007). The epidemiology of autism spectrum disorders. *Annual Review of Public Health, 28,* 235–258.

No Child Left Behind Act of 2001, 20 U.S. C. 6301 et seq. (2002).

Shimabukuro, T. T., Grosse, S. D., & Rice, C. (2008). Medical expenditures for children with an autism spectrum disorder in a privately insured population. *Journal of Autism and Developmental Disorders, 38,* 546–552.

Sims, S. J., & Sims, R. R. (2004). *Managing school system change: Charting a course for renewal.* Greenwich, CT: Information Age Publishing.

Tobey, D. (2005). *Needs assessment basics.* Alexandria, VA: ASTD press.

U.S. Government Accountability Office. (2005). *Special education: Children with autism.* Report to the Chairman and Ranking Minority Member, Subcommittee on Human Rights and Wellness, Committee on Government Reform, House of Representatives.

University of Michigan. (n.d.). *Special needs education: Funding for special needs education.* Retrieved from http://sitemaker.umich.edu/delicata.356/funding_for_special_needs_education

Westen, D. I. (2005). Transporting laboratory-validated treatments to the community will not necessarily produce better outcomes. In J. C. Norcross, L. E. Beutler, & R. F. Levant (Eds.), *Evidence-based practices in mental health: Debate and dialogue on the fundamental questions* (pp. 383–393). Washington, DC: American Psychological Association.

Wilczynski, S. M. (2009). Building and sustaining capacity to deliver treatments that work. In S. M. Wilczynski & E. G. Pollack (Eds.), *Evidence-based practice and autism in the schools* (pp. 145–181). Randolph, MA: National Autism Center, Inc.

8

The Dissemination of Evidence-Based Practices by Federal and State Mental Health Agencies

Jeanne C. Rivard, Vijay K. Ganju, Kristin A. Roberts, and G. Michael Lane, Jr.

This chapter reviews federal and state initiatives to disseminate evidence-based practices (EBPs) into public mental health systems in the United States. All states and U.S. territories have designated state mental health agencies (SMHAs) that are responsible for ensuring the provision of mental health services for adults with severe mental illnesses and children with serious emotional disturbances (Lutterman, Berhane, Phelan, Shaw, & Rana, 2009). There is much variation in how SMHAs are organized within state governments, in the specific types of services that are delivered, and in how services are delivered and funded. Some SMHAs are located within larger health and/or human service agencies; some are independent agencies within state government. SMHAs may deliver services through a network of public community mental health agencies, or they may contract with private mental health agencies for direct service provision. Funding for public mental health services comes from state general revenues and federal sources including Medicaid and the Community Mental Health Block Grant. Most SMHAs are responsible for providing an array of traditional outpatient and inpatient services. Incorporating EBPs into the service arrays of public mental health systems has become a priority of SMHAs to ensure that consumers receive services that have been proven to be effective (Lutterman et al., 2009).

The first section of this chapter describes federal funding initiatives of the Substance Abuse and Mental Health Services Administration (SAMHSA) and the National Institute of Mental Health (NIMH) to stimulate state efforts to promote the adoption and implementation of EBPs, and summarizes cumulative lessons learned after 6 years of federal funding. Turning to state-level initiatives, the second section describes public–academic partnerships that are becoming a core element of the infrastructure needed to sustain and institutionalize the use of EBPs. The third section of the chapter presents trends in the uptake of EBPs by SMHAs and concludes with a discussion of the continuing challenges faced by states in moving toward statewide dissemination and sustainability of EBPs.

The Stimulus of Federal Initiatives

SUMMARY OF FEDERAL INITIATIVES

Over the last decade, EBPs have emerged as a priority for mental health policymakers and administrators. Prompted by the Surgeon General's Report on Mental Health (U.S. Department of Health and Human Services, 1999), which alerted the public mental health system to the gap between science and mental health practice, and the report of the President's New Freedom Commission on Mental Health (2003), which designated use of EBPs as a core principle of system transformation, EBPs have been promoted by a series of activities at federal and state levels. Federal initiatives reflected the logic that interventions proven to produce certain outcomes should be incorporated into arrays of services purchased or provided by federal, state, and local agencies. The basic challenge was how to translate research into practice. Much of the initial effort focused on the development of training materials and models to facilitate the uptake of EBPs. One of the first major initiatives was the National Implementing Evidence-Based Practices Project in which implementation resource kits (or "toolkits") were developed for six EBPs for adults with severe mental illnesses and were piloted in demonstration sites across the nation. Several parallel activities included a SAMHSA Center for Mental Health Services (CMHS)-funded EBP Training and Evaluation initiative in which states were funded to implement and adapt the toolkits, a joint NIMH–CMHS initiative that provided grants to states to plan for EBP implementation, and the funding of technical assistance activities at the national level.

The National Implementing Evidence-Based
Practices Project

The purpose of the National Implementing Evidence-Based Practices Project was to develop, test, and refine the implementation of six toolkits on effective interventions for adults with schizophrenia and other severe mental illnesses, a population for whom a large gap existed between known effective treatments and routine service provision in public mental health systems (Drake, Bond, & Essock, 2009; Torrey, Lynde, & Gorman, 2005). The EBPs that would be the subject of the toolkits were selected through the work of an expert panel, composed of leading mental health services researchers and other key stakeholders, which was funded by the Robert Wood Johnson Foundation in 1998 to identify the most effective interventions for this population (Torrey et al., 2005). The EBPs selected were Assertive Community Treatment (Burns & Phillips, 2002; Phillips et al., 2001), Supported Employment (Becker & Bond, 2002; Bond et al., 2001), Integrated

Treatment for Co-Occurring Mental Health and Substance Abuse (Brunette & Drake, 2002; Drake et al., 2001), Family Psychoeducation (Dixon et al., 2001; McFarlane & Dixon, 2002), Illness Management and Recovery (Mueser & Gingerich, 2002; Mueser et al., 2002), and Medication Management (Mellman et al., 2001). Each toolkit includes extensive references that report the evidence for each intervention.

Led by the New Hampshire-Dartmouth Psychiatric Research Center, the toolkits were developed between 2000 and 2002; implementation activities were carried out from 2002 to 2005. The toolkits were constructed with components directed to state mental health authorities, provider organizations, clinicians/ service providers, consumers, and family members. The toolkits were tested in local communities of eight states (Indiana, Kansas, Maryland, New Hampshire, New York, Ohio, Oregon, and Vermont), with two EBPs being implemented by three to five agency sites in most of these states. These packages were tested and refined in the multistate initiative so that the final versions could be used to address implementation issues at each of the relevant levels. The multiuser approach was a fundamental shift from previous models of implementing innovative practices in mental health systems. It recognized that the individual clinician's or service provider's willingness, knowledge, and skills alone would not result in broad-based implementation of EBPs. It also acknowledged that for sustained uptake, structural arrangements and changes in policies, regulations, administrative procedures, and financing would be needed in combination with consumer and family member education and choice.

The training materials in each of the toolkits consisted of reviews of the research evidence for each EBP, information sheets for each user group, an introductory video, a skills demonstration video, a workbook for practitioners and clinical supervisors, a website, implementation tips, outcomes information, a fidelity scale, and a General Organizational Index, which was intended to assess the overall organizational readiness of provider organizations for implementing the EBP (Torrey et al., 2005). Training activities and consultation were also provided as a critical component of the project. Project trainers/consultants worked with site implementation leaders for a year to assist agencies in assessing and adapting policies and procedures to facilitate implementation, training staff, modeling effective clinical supervision of the EBP, evaluating fidelity and outcomes, and using results for feedback to the project as a whole and for continuous quality improvement (Torrey et al., 2005).

At a 2003 meeting of the national and state demonstration teams, site leaders, trainers/consultants, evaluation monitors, and consumers elaborated on strategies that they adopted to facilitate their implementation efforts (National Association of State Mental Health Program Directors Research Institute, Inc. [NRI], 2003). With respect to training, the most notable strategies focused on promoting an internal mentoring process within agencies, training at different levels based on varying degrees of staff knowledge and expertise, training in an interactive manner, engaging the more seasoned practitioners to share knowledge and be open to learning new skills and behaviors, constantly assessing the audience and getting feedback from each session to inform the next session, role playing and videotaping clinicians practicing skills, and using quizzes to assess levels of learning. An essential ingredient that enabled the transfer of learning into practice was for the project trainers/ consultants to rely on agency leaders to stimulate the critical integration of the EBP into the agency's array of services. The presence of a strong agency EBP steering committee, which met on a regular basis to problem solve and pay attention to incremental successes and emerging needs, lent support and reinforcement to the project staff's efforts. At the direct interface of transferring learning into practice were the key components of having structured supervision, having trainers present in supervision to increase supervisors' effectiveness, working one on one with practitioners in the field, having peer supervision in addition to regular supervision, new trainees shadowing practitioners with advanced skills in the EBP, and making booster trainings available as needed. From the consumers' point of view, listening to consumers that were receiving the practice provided a constant reality check and involving consumers in training activities added power and credibility to implementation (NRI, 2003). The original toolkits are available online at http://store.samhsa. gov/pages/searchResult/EBP and have been refined based on the multiuser assessments of the demonstration project.

State Training and Evaluation of
Evidence-Based Practice Grants

While the National Implementing Evidence-Based Practices Project was coming to a close, SAMHSA provided new funding in 2003 for eight states (California, Hawaii, Illinois, Indiana, Kentucky, New York, Ohio, and Vermont) to provide state-of-the-art training and continuing education to state mental health service providers and other stakeholders who were implementing the toolkits. The project also funded activities to evaluate the implementation of selected EBPs in two or more communities within the state. For those states that had also participated in the original demonstration project, this grant was intended to support the implementation of new EBPs.

State Evidence-Based Practice Planning Grants

Around the same time in 2003, another federal program was initiated, this time with joint funding from NIMH and SAMHSA, to assist SMHAs in planning activities that would promote the implementation of EBP in local practice settings. The grant also funded exploratory research studies focused on the implementation of EBPs in these settings (Chambers, Ringeisen, & Hickman, 2005). The nine states involved in this initiative were Arkansas, Maine, Maryland, Michigan, New York, North Carolina, Ohio, Texas, and Washington. Whereas the first two grant programs concentrated on the dissemination of EBPs for adults with schizophrenia and other severe mental illnesses, states could elect in this grant program to focus on the original six adult EBP toolkits or on EBPs for special target populations, including adults with other disorders and children. Table 8.1 shows the states that were involved in these three federal initiatives and the EBPs that were the subject of their grants.

Knowledge Transfer and Technical Assistance Activities

While a relatively small number of states participated in the federal programs described above, from 2003 to 2006 SAMHSA also funded another initiative to reach out to other states searching for approaches to integrate EBPs into their state mental health systems. A contract with the NRI was aimed at providing technical assistance and synthesizing and disseminating specific lessons being learned by the National Implementing Evidence-Based Practices Project as well as knowledge being gained from the larger field of mental health. Through NRI's Center for Mental Health Quality and Accountability, a range of strategies were utilized to transfer knowledge between science and service, and to create a nexus between policy and practice that would foster sustainability. The strategies included:

1. Forging partnerships between federal agencies, states, policymakers, foundations, universities, researchers, professional associations, advocates, consumers and families, and other technical assistance initiatives
2. Convening forums for information sharing and technical assistance in the form of special topical conferences and meetings (e.g., EBPs in adult mental health, EBPs in children's mental health, EBPs in older adults' mental health, EBPs in rural mental health, consumer and family voices and choices in EBPs, planning and financing models, policy and infrastructure needs and strategies, lessons learned in implementing specific EBP toolkits and needs for enhancement, and creating a culture of evidence-based practice)
3. Delivering direct technical assistance to states related to planning and implementation of EBPs, and developing EBP technical assistance and information resources for states and counties in the form of websites and monographs
4. Surveying states and conducting site visits to gather information about specific state-level strategies being undertaken to disseminate EBPs
5. Tracking and monitoring the uptake of EBPs by states over time

Reports and other products developed through the course of these technical assistance activities can be found at www.nri-inc.org/reports_pubs.

TABLE 8.1 States Participating in the Three Major Federal Evidence-Based
Practice Initiatives

State	SAMHSA National Implementing EBP Project	SAMHSA EBP Training/ Evaluation Grants	NIMH-SAMHSA Planning Grants
AS	—		Medication Management
CA	—	Integrated Treatment for Co-Occurring Disorders	—
HI	—	Illness Management and Recovery; Integrated Treatment for Co-Occurring Disorders	—
IL	—	Integrated Treatment for Co-Occurring Disorders	—
IN	Assertive Community Treatment; Integrated Treatment for Co-Occurring Disorders	Illness Management and Recovery	—
KS	Supported Employment; Integrated Treatment for Co-Occurring Disorders	—	—
KY	—	Medication Management	—
ME	—	—	Adults and Children
MD	Family Psychoeducation; Supported Employment	—	Children
MI	—	—	Children
NH	Illness Management and Recovery; Family Psychoeducation	—	—
NY	Assertive Community Treatment; Illness Management and Recovery	Family Psychoeducation	Children
NC	—	—	Assertive Community Treatment
OH	Integrated Treatment for Co-Occurring Disorders; Illness Management and Recovery	Supported Employment	Adults and Children
OR	Supported Employment	—	—
TX	—	—	Cognitive Behavioral Therapy
VT	Illness Management and Recovery; Family Psychoeducation	Integrated Treatment for Co-Occurring Disorders	—
WA	—	—	Adults and Children

KNOWLEDGE ON DISSEMINATION GAINED FROM THE FEDERAL EVIDENCE-BASED PRACTICE INITIATIVES

Three sources of information can be drawn upon to summarize the overall results of the federal EBP grant programs to states. The first source is composed of a series of published articles describing results of the National Implementing Evidence-Based Practices Project. The second source is a compilation of results of a study, conducted by the MacArthur Foundation Network on Mental Health Policy Research, examining the roles of state mental health agencies in facilitating the implementation of EBPs. The third is a report of the lessons learned from the experiences of states that participated in the three grant programs gathered from a conference in 2006 convened by NRI's Center for Mental Health Quality and Accountability.

Results of the National Implementing Evidence-Based Practices Demonstration Project

Results of the National Implementing Evidence-Based Practices Project have been published in numerous articles. These papers describe the process of implementing the individual EBPs within the various sites that participated in the project and present results on fidelity measurement, consumer involvement, staffing issues, and general factors that facilitated or inhibited implementation of the specific EBPs (Drake et al., 2009; Swain, Whitley, McHugo, & Drake, 2010). Looking across these studies, Drake and colleagues (2009) found that common factors that influenced the quality of EBP implementation were the leadership of state mental health agencies, funding, practice standards, skilled mentoring by trainer-consultants, administrative support, clinical supervision, systematic monitoring of fidelity and outcomes, and staff turnover. Further discussion of these factors is presented later in the chapter in a summary of lessons learned across all of the federally funded EBP projects.

Two studies have documented the results across all of the EBPs and across all of the participating sites. McHugo and colleagues (2007) examined variation in fidelity, using data on fidelity measurement that were collected as part of the demonstration project. Fidelity rating scales for each EBP had been developed and tested by researchers involved with the demonstration project and by those that developed and/or tested the interventions. The process of measuring fidelity involved two assessors conducting interviews with key personnel and clients, reviewing charts, observing program operations and critical components of each EBP, and then independently rating the various fidelity domains and reconciling differences (McHugo et al., 2007). Analyses of these data at five points in time (baseline and 6, 12, 18, and 24 months) across 49 sites in the participating states found that 55% of the sites had high fidelity implementation (i.e., score of 4.0 or greater on a 5-point scale) at the 24-month point (McHugo et al., 2007). Scores generally leveled off between 12 and 24 months. Sites implementing Supported Employment and Assertive Community

Treatment had significantly higher scores at baseline and over time than Illness Management and Recovery and Integrated Dual Disorders Treatment. Results suggested the need to incorporate booster trainings for sites not attaining high fidelity to stimulate gains and support sustainability.

Investigating the sustainability of EBPs, 49 sites that completed the first 2 years of implementation were surveyed 24 months later (Swain et al., 2010). Results showed a high sustainability rate of 80% of the sites continuing to implement the EBP for 2 years after the initial implementation period, with the other 20% discontinuing use of the EBP in their agencies. The 10 agencies that did not sustain the use of the EBPs were fairly evenly spread across all of the EBPs (one or two agencies), but the highest dropout rate involved Illness Management and Recovery, in which four agencies discontinued use. Factors that contributed to discontinuing the use of the EBPs included inadequate funding or supported training, lack of commitment from agency leadership, nonsupportive staff or agency culture, staff turnover, and competing EBPs (Swain et al., 2010). Adequately dealing with these potential barriers differentiated the agencies that sustained EBPs. A somewhat controversial factor that distinguished the sites that sustained use of EBPs was that most of the successful sites adapted the EBPs to meet state and local needs. This brings into question the actual fidelity of the EBPs that were being sustained and reinforces the need for more research on adaptation.

Roles of State Mental Health Agencies in Disseminating Evidence-Based Practices

As the National Implementing Evidence-Based Practices Demonstration Project was being carried out, researchers at the MacArthur Foundation Network on Mental Health Policy Research made site visits to the eight states participating in the project to study the roles of SMHAs in implementing the EBPs (Isett et al., 2007). Two site visits were made to each state between 2002 and 2004. Network team members used grounded case study methods to learn about the barriers and facilitators of implementation at policy and administrative levels. Results showed that specific state-level activities facilitated implementation: realigning regulations to support the new practices, identifying or establishing financing that compensated providers for start-up and ongoing implementation, having leadership that oriented the system toward effective treatment, providing training for high fidelity implementation, and linking training efforts to quality assessments and infrastructure needs (Isett et al., 2007). With respect to training, it was found that the role of the SMHA in sponsoring the 1-year training program was critical to the implementation process. The combination of skills training, feedback, and ongoing consultation was judged to be essential in supporting implementation and sustainability with a high degree of fidelity adherence (Isett et al., 2008). Further, state-level policy and administrative mechanisms that integrated fidelity measurement and standards into certification and licensure regulations provided fiscal incentives and thus greater leverage to move the system toward higher quality of care. As training needs became a priority, it became more of an imperative to partner with universities to provide the training needed or to create special training centers (Isett et al., 2008).

Lessons Learned by States, Providers, Consumers, and Evaluators across the Three Federal Grant Programs

One of the culminating technical assistance activities of NRI's Center for Mental Health Quality and Accountability was a 2006 conference titled "Lessons Learned: Embedding EBPs in Statewide Transformation." The major objective of the conference was to collect and document lessons learned from the various federally sponsored EBP initiatives. Implicit in these lessons was the recognition that interventions are needed at different levels (at the level of the program, the provider organization, and the state) and involve different sets of actors (consumers and family members, providers, local administrators, and state administrators and policymakers). Also, there was recognition that while there has been considerable effort and investment in developing first-generation knowledge and tools to support EBP implementation, models for effective implementation, especially for a sustained, statewide effort, are lacking.

The conference itself was organized around topics that had been identified as areas in which implementers had sought guidance or experienced problems. These included the development of the appropriate infrastructure components (i.e., leadership, legislation, policy, financing, fidelity and outcomes, and training/workforce development), modifying and adapting EBPs, consumer involvement in EBP implementation, statewide dissemination, sustaining EBPs over time, and lessons learned related to the implementation of specific EBPs. The major lessons learned in the key areas are summarized below (Ganju, 2007).

Lesson 1: Use a quality improvement framework with change management techniques. Framing the use of EBPs as one key strategy within a larger quality improvement framework supported the incremental nature of implementation, which requires cyclical monitoring and assessment of process and outcomes with feedback and correction loops. A point that was emphasized was that such measurement should occur as much as possible in real time. This lesson is tied implicitly to the need for change management, which recognizes that behavior, attitudes, and values are critical factors in implementation and are reflected by an organizational culture that values the use of evidence.

Lesson 2: Promote leadership commitment and alignment. Without the up-front buy-in of leadership at state and local levels, at administrative and supervisory levels, and at the level of consumers and family members, EBP implementation is unlikely to make meaningful progress. Critical aspects of leadership are aligning policy and financing for EBPs, educating and engaging stakeholders, and marketing and salesmanship.

Lesson 3: Plan for funding the evidence-based practice. Both the federal and state governments have a primary role in planning how to fund EBPs, especially after grant dollars or special funds earmarked for implementation in a demonstration effort are no longer available. The role of Medicaid is significant. At the state level, this requires exploring the potential for funding through Medicaid and then developing specific procedures and codes for reimbursement. In doing so, a close working relationship with the Medicaid authority is useful. Some states have taken advantage of the flexibility in funding they have through Medicaid waiver programs with capitated case-rate methodologies. Other funding strategies were to use multiple sources for funding the various components of an EBP.

Lesson 4: Promote consumer and family member education and leadership in EBP implementation. A recurring theme was that consumer and family member involvement and leadership was fundamental to the success of EBP implementation. In many cases, embedding EBPs in a recovery orientation within an organization facilitated EBP adoption, energizing both staff and consumers. Tying EBP implementation specifically to desired outcomes and their measurement also promoted consumer and family member commitment to, and advocacy for, EBPs. Consumers and family members are potential collaborators, supporters, and partners in the EBP implementation process. Some of the specific lessons included the importance of training and educating consumers and family members at the outset alongside staff and other stakeholders. In addition, consumers and family members should assume a variety of roles in program design, training and education, and implementation and evaluation. Roles and expectations should be explicitly defined.

Lesson 5: Recognize that some organizations are not ready for EBP implementation. While many organizations are interested in implementing EBPs, they may not have the capacity or willingness to make the needed changes in agency operations to accommodate the new practices. Increasingly, readiness assessment tools and techniques are being used to gauge organizational capacity to move forward successfully and to identify specific targets and interventions for capacity building.

Lesson 6: Ensure that ongoing consultation and technical assistance are available as part of the EBP implementation effort. A major theme that emerged was that while the toolkits provided a valuable starting point, the availability of ongoing consultation and technical assistance was pivotal in changing agency operations and equipping personnel with the necessary skills to deliver effective treatments.

Lesson 7: Support the role of the supervisor in EBP implementation. Committed, knowledgeable, clinical supervision was identified as an essential component of EBP implementation. There was recognition that in many settings, supervision structures are minimal at best. Managers and administrators in mental health settings often do not create the needed time for supervision and do not support supervisors in tangible ways. In some states, specific training has been developed for supervisors. A recommendation was that the next generation of toolkits includes an explicit component related to supervision.

Lesson 8: Monitor and provide feedback based on fidelity assessment. Fidelity assessment is an integral part of implementation, but the key component is the provision of feedback and corrective action based on such assessment. Despite the importance of fidelity, there was dissatisfaction with the state of the art related to fidelity assessment. Current methodologies require a substantial investment of resources, and EBP implementation efforts are resorting to self-assessment tools even though such an approach is recognized as problematic. Most fidelity scales focus on structural elements, which, in many cases, have not been tested or proven. Critical ingredients of EBP interventions have not been identified. Even where they have been identified, it is not clear whether variations would result in differences in outcomes. New approaches to fidelity monitoring and assessment are needed.

Lesson 9: Make adaptations to EBPs with care and caution. Adaptation of EBPs is a double-edged sword. On one side, there is the issue of how much adaptation can occur while still retaining fidelity to the model. On the other, there is the challenge that the practice, in its existing form, will not have the buy-in or work for a particular community or setting. Adaptations are being made for several reasons: limited resources, cultural factors, and service settings. There is little guidance on how such adaptations should occur. A fundamental aspect of such adaptations was monitoring outcomes, which allowed the detection of any major deviations from expected results. Identification of assumed critical components of the EBP model that needed to be retained also helped adherence to the original model. A major lesson was that a willingness to listen and accept a community's perspective with respect was a major factor in the adaptation process.

Lesson 10: Develop a training infrastructure and collaborate with universities and community colleges. In many states, a training infrastructure has been developed related to EBP implementation. The train-the-trainer model was cited as one that appeared to be working well in several settings. Collaborations with universities and community colleges have proved to be productive in various aspects of EBP implementation, including training, technical assistance and consultation, and fidelity and outcomes monitoring. The relationship with universities and community colleges also allows for preservice training related to EBP implementation. There was recognition that to have a fundamental, broad-based orientation to EBPs, curricula and professional expectations through standards and licensing are also needed. Many states have developed collaborations and partnerships with universities and community colleges toward this end.

State Initiatives in Disseminating Evidence-Based Practices through Academic–Public Partnerships

Whereas federal funding provided the impetus, initial funding, toolkits, and training models for states to introduce EBPs into their service systems, changes in infrastructure are necessary to sustain the use of EBPs beyond demonstration phases.

This section focuses on one particular type of infrastructure development that directly bridges the gaps between science and practice, and between demonstration projects and broader dissemination of EBPs. Public–academic partnerships, often in the form of centers of excellence and technical assistance centers, which are widely used in medical and substance abuse fields, have also been instrumental in exerting leverage at multiple points in the life cycle of EBP dissemination in public mental health systems (NRI, 2005). A review of the literature on dissemination theory (Stirman, Crits-Christoph, & DeRubeis, 2004) suggested that public–academic collaborations provide the infrastructure for research and information/technology transfer needed for training professionals in EBPs, for monitoring fidelity and effectiveness of the interventions as they are disseminated, and for developing adaptations that may be needed for local populations. In this section of the chapter data are presented on the nature and scope of public–academic partnerships in mental health that are centered on dissemination of EBPs. Then various examples are presented of the different types of partnerships that have formed.

To view the nature and scope of collaboration between SMHAs and universities, data from the 2009 State Mental Health Agency Profiles System were used. The Profiles System is a centrally maintained compilation of descriptive information about SMHA policies, organization, financing, operation, services, and clients that is collected at least every 2 years (NRI, 2011). A particular set of survey items inquires specifically about how SMHAs partner with universities for training, research, and evaluation of EBPs. The data collected are primarily descriptive. Out of 47 states that responded to the 2009 Profiles, Table 8.2 displays some of the questions asked and the number of states that responded in the affirmative to these items. The most frequently reported type of collaboration was ongoing provider training through contracts with universities, but not through organized research or training institutes (72%). More structurally organized arrangements to provide training through research or training institutes were established by 40% of the states. Fifty-seven percent of states reported that their collaboration with academia involved curriculum development. There was overlap in these areas where states had multiple types of collaboration with different universities.

In open-ended questions, the Profiles survey also asks SMHAs to describe the specific initiatives and activities in which they are engaged. The next section provides examples of the specific collaborations reported by some states in the 2009 data. Where additional information was available through published articles or websites, the descriptions were enhanced with this information.

Connecticut. The SMHA in Connecticut reported working with Dartmouth University on Integrated Dual Diagnosis Treatment (IDDT), the University of Connecticut School of Social Work on Family Psychoeducation, and Yale University on recovery-based mental health care. They also established a partnership with Southern Connecticut State University to start an intensive weekend cohort program with a focus on co-occurring disorders in their Master's of Social Work program. With the University of Connecticut School of Social Work and Yale

TABLE 8.2 Type and Scope of Public-Academic Relationships Related to
Evidence-Based Practices

Profiles Item	Number of Yes Responses	Percent (N = 47 States)
Collaboration with universities is used to provide ongoing training to providers related to evidence-based services.	34	72%
Establishment of research/training institute(s) is used to provide ongoing training to providers related to evidence-based services.	19	40%
Is the SMHA working with academia in curriculum development to reflect evidence-based practices, promising practices, or value-based practices?	27	57%
Does SMHA support an SMHA-operated research center/institute?	7	15%
Does SMHA support an SMHA-funded (but not SMHA-operated) research center/institute?	8	17%
Is the SMHA involved in research supported by a university research center?	17	36%

University they were developing an approach to a wider-scale dissemination of Family Psychoeducation.

Florida. The SMHA reported working on a trauma-informed care curriculum with staff at the University of South Florida's Florida Mental Health Institute.

Colorado. The SMHA was involved in ongoing consultation with the University of Colorado Health Sciences Center regarding EBP program development and monitoring.

Hawaii. The SMHA reported developing and implementing a virtual center for EBP in collaboration with the University of Hawaii, staff, consumers, and families. Faculty of the Departments of Psychiatry and Psychology have led several initiatives to assist the agency in improving service quality and outcomes through the use of research (see Chapter 9, this volume). Rather than just emphasizing the use of EBPs in children's mental health, Hawaii's Child and Adolescent Mental Health Division's strategies have focused on maximizing the use of different types of evidence stemming from services and intervention research, case-specific historical evidence, and aggregate practice-based evidence (Daleiden & Chorpita, 2005). A multidisciplinary EBP Services Committee developed, and periodically updates, a review of the research literature on EBPs and puts this into a user-friendly version that clinicians can refer to when matching child and family need to specific interventions. Using such research resources is then incorporated into interagency performance standards and practice guidelines.

Iowa. The SMHA reported having a long-standing relationship with the University of Iowa through a contract with the Iowa Consortium for Mental Health. The primary focus of the consortium was on the dissemination of EBPs in Iowa. Through the consortium, the SMHA sponsored a wide variety of training programs targeted to the workforce as well as consumers and family members. They produced a video conference series, that covered all of the SAMHSA-sponsored EBPs for adults, which was attended by an average of more than 400 providers, consumers, family members, and policymakers across 60 sites statewide. A similar series was done for child EBPs. In addition they conducted statewide trainings in co-occurring disorders, Supported Employment, Illness Management and Recovery, and numerous emerging best practices in children's mental health.

Indiana. Through a contract with the SMHA in Indiana, the implementation of Assertive Community Treatment (ACT) was facilitated by the ACT Center of Indiana that is located within the Psychology Department at the Indiana–Purdue University Indianapolis. The center was created in 2001 to provide direct training and technical assistance to the state and local providers. Over time, the center's activities have expanded to include disseminating written materials and videotapes; advising the SMHA on ACT certification standards, financing mechanisms, and policies; publishing a newsletter and facilitating a listserv providing consultation; and collecting data on fidelity and outcomes (Rapp et al., 2005; Salyers et al., 2007).

Massachusetts. The SMHA worked with the University of Massachusetts to develop curricula for the implementation of an individualized model of Supported Employment for the start-up of community-based flexible services.

Maryland. The Child and Adolescent Mental Health Institute, a partnership of the SMHA, University of Maryland, Johns Hopkins University, and the Maryland Coalition of Families for Children's Mental Health, developed a curriculum in early childhood mental health. They also worked with academia to include the concept of EBPs in their curricula and assisted a number of academic programs in adding a Vocational Aspects of Disabilities Course to their program, which contains content on supported employment.

Michigan. The SMHA worked with five different universities in the state primarily on fidelity monitoring of a range of EBPs.

Minnesota. The SMHA conducted joint training with the University of Minnesota on trauma-informed assessment and treatment, and with the Center for Excellence in Children's Mental Health. The center worked closely with experts, community providers, and policymakers to improve mental health practice for Minnesota's children through seminar series and publications showcasing current research and its practical applications. For more information see the center's website at http://www.cmh.umn.edu/index.html.

North Carolina. The SMHA worked with universities to modify curricula in relevant courses (e.g., psychology, social work) to reflect EBPs and promising practices. For example, the SMHA funded the University of North Carolina at Greensboro to modify curricula in psychology and other areas to incorporate system-of-care principles and practices.

New Hampshire. The SMHA worked closely with the Dartmouth EBP Center, which was the lead organization in providing technical assistance and evaluation for the National Implementing Evidence-Based Practices Project.

New Jersey. The SMHA reported having a contract with the University of Medicine and Dentistry of New Jersey School of Health Related Professions, Department of Psychiatric Rehabilitation to provide Illness Management and Recovery and Integrated Dual Disorder Treatment training in state psychiatric hospitals and community-based provider agencies. The SMHA also funded their Integrated Employment Institute that provides statewide training in Supported Employment.

New York. The SMHA in New York partnered with the Columbia University Department of Psychiatry in establishing the Evidence Based Treatment Dissemination Center in 2006 to facilitate social and emotional well-being and resiliency among children and youth by increasing the availability of evidence-based treatments. They provide annual training and consultation programs at several locations across the state in a statewide initiative to disseminate and research the implementation of a range of EBPs for children and adolescents. For more information see their website at http://www.omh.state.ny.us/omhweb/ebt/. Another center, the Evidence-Based Practices Technical Assistance Center at the Columbia University New York State Psychiatric Institute worked with the SMHA and the state alcohol and substance abuse services authority on a distance learning initiative. This project focused on integrated treatment for co-occurring mental health and substance use disorders and offered online training modules, webinars, and supports designed to help practitioners, clinical supervisors, and agency managers and administrators implement integrated treatment in their settings. For more information on this initiative see the website at http://www.omh.state.ny.us/omhweb/News/2009/pr_ebp_tac.html.

Ohio. The SMHA funded residency and training programs at several universities' departments of psychiatry, psychology, nursing, and social work. Ohio's SMHA has also been a leader in establishing multiple Coordinating Centers of Excellence (CCOE), focused on an array of adult and child EBPs, to promote best-practice approaches in the state and to provide training, technical assistance, consultation, and research. One example of these is the Ohio Supported Employment Coordinating Center of Excellence, which is a collaboration with Case Western Reserve University to assist in implementing and evaluating Supported Employment for adults with severe mental illnesses (Biegel, Swanson, & Kola, 2007). The center provides direct clinical training to clinicians and supervisors, administrative consultation on design and management of Supported Employment programs, and ongoing case consultation; disseminates information on research; and conducts research on fidelity measurement, model adaptations, and client outcomes. The center's administrative, clinical, and interagency educational/consulting approach has helped to overcome barriers to EBP implementation (Biegel et al., 2007).

Oregon. The SMHA partnered with the Oregon Health and Science University Department of Public Health and Preventive Medicine's North West Frontier Addiction Technology Transfer Center, which had several initiatives to infuse EBPs into the community college addiction programs. The SMHA also co-sponsored continuing education credit offerings by several Oregon universities.

Washington. In the state of Washington, new legislation in children's mental health created an Evidence-Based Practices Institute at the University of Washington to collaborate across university departments, the state, the children's hospital and regional medical center, and the Washington State Institute for Public Policy to evaluate and promote the use of evidence-based practices in children's mental health treatment.

The foregoing descriptions, as reported in the 2009 Profiles are not an exhaustive list of all of the collaborative activities between SMHAs and universities. States may have elected not to respond to these qualitative items, or they may have provided information about these arrangements in previous Profiles data submissions but not repeated them for the current fiscal year. However, as can be seen in these brief descriptions of 17 states' relationships with universities and colleges, the scope of these public-academic partnerships is broad. On one end, the activities performed by academia include contracting to perform discrete tasks such as developing curricula, training providers, and monitoring fidelity of and evaluating specific adult and child EBPs. More intense partnerships have formed that involve funding special initiatives to disseminate EBPs statewide, for example, through distance learning technologies. On the other end of the continuum, these partnerships are becoming institutionalized through integrating EBPs into existing university curricula and through the establishment of university-based institutes or centers that have multiple functions in synthesizing research to make knowledge more accessible and usable; reaching out to providers through various forums, ongoing training and consultation, conducting research and development activities; and using technology to facilitate statewide dissemination of EBPs.

State Trends in Dissemination of Evidence-Based Practices

The third section of the chapter covers trends in the uptake of EBPs by SMHAs by viewing two different indicators of dissemination—the number of programs being implemented by states and the number of persons receiving EBPs. Data on the number of discrete EBP programs operated by states were obtained from the State Mental Health Agencies Profiles System for 2003, 2005, 2007 and 2009 (NRI, 2011). Data on the number of adults and children receiving EBPs were obtained from the Uniform Reporting System (URS) of the SAMHSA-funded Mental Health Block Grant for years 2005 to 2008 (SAMHSA, 2008).

NUMBER OF EVIDENCE-BASED PRACTICE
PROGRAMS BEING IMPLEMENTED

The Profiles System contains data on the number of states/programs that reported providing a range of adult and child EBPs. Table 8.3 shows the total number of states that were implementing seven different EBPs for adults and three EBPs for children across the 4 years. Shown in each year is also the number of programs that were being implemented across all of the states that reported implementing the EBPs. The EBPs selected for presentation in Table 8.3 are those for which there is the most historical data.

Focusing mainly on the number of programs in Table 8.3, some of the greatest increases between 2003 and 2009 in the number of programs were in Assertive Community Treatment, Supported Employment, Illness Management and Recovery, and Integrated Treatment for Mental Health and Substance Abuse. The dissemination of Medication Management, Family Psychoeducation and the three children's EBPs between 2003 and 2009 appears to be more limited in scope in comparison to the four mentioned above. Some of the decreases in the number of programs between 2003 and 2005 (e.g., Supported Employment, Medication

TABLE 8.3 Total Number of States Implementing Evidence-Based Practices and the Number of Evidence-Based Practice Programs Being Implemented 2003–2009

	2003		2005		2007		2009	
	States	Programs	States	Programs	States	Programs	States	Programs
Adult EBP								
Assertive Community Treatment	37	485	39	663	46	747	41	709
Supported Employment	37	650	39	415	46	622	44	940
Medication Management for Schizophrenia	23	93	19	63	25	115	16	90
Medication Management for Bipolar Disorder	14	46	10	41	13	40	16	82
Family Psychoeducation	24	136	27	160	26	222	29	210
Illness Management and Recovery	27	274	29	163	32	255	34	446
Integrated Treatment for Mental Health/ Substance Abuse	34	341	34	287	48	417	50	568
Child/Adolescent EBPs								
Therapeutic Foster Care	25	140	31	142	34	196	31	113
Multisystemic Therapy	26	81	23	96	31	129	28	129
Functional Family Therapy[a]	--	--	18	46	24	62	24	70

[a]Functional Family Therapy was not listed on the survey as a discrete category until 2005.

Management for Schizophrenia, Illness Management and Recovery, and Integrated Treatment for Mental Health/Substance Abuse) may be explained by the fact that during this period the methods that states used to report on the number of EBP programs operated came under review, and the issue of fidelity monitoring came into the foreground. Although it is not possible for most states to measure the fidelity of their local EBP programs directly, new reporting guidelines were developed for states to use to ensure that the number of EBP programs reported were those adhering to the essential components of the fidelity measurement methods required for the individual EBPs. In response to these guidelines, states had to, in turn, establish new procedures for their regional mental health authorities and local mental health centers to follow in measuring and monitoring fidelity. It is possible that in the 2005 reporting period, states' reporting practices were impacted by the guidelines with the result of their counting EBPs more conservatively, thus reducing the total number of EBPs reported. The increases shown in the 2007 reporting period should be reflecting a rise in the dissemination of EBPs that adhere to the models that were originally found to be effective.

The types of children's EBPs that were reported have historically been limited to only the three presented in Table 8.3. At the time that EBPs were added to states' reporting requirements, prior to 2003, Multisystemic Therapy (Henggeler, Mihalic, Rone, Thomas, & Timmons-Mitchell, 1998), Functional Family Therapy (Alexander et al., 1998), and Multidimensional Treatment Foster Care (Chamberlain & Mihalic, 1998) were some of the more widely known interventions, largely due to the active dissemination efforts of the researchers of the interventions. Recent initiatives to develop toolkits for EBPs in children's mental health and to more accurately depict the scope of dissemination of EBPs in children's mental health have resulted in plans to add a much broader array of children's EBPs to federal reporting systems. For example, the 2009 Profiles survey includes these additional EBPs: Incredible Years, Parent-Child Interaction Therapy, Parent Management Training–Oregon, Brief Strategic Family Therapy, Problem Solving Skills Training, Coping Power, Cognitive Behavior Therapy for Depression, Cognitive Behavior Therapy for Anxiety, Trauma-Focused Cognitive Behavior Therapy, and Interpersonal Therapy for Depression. These EBPs were selected for inclusion based on brief surveys of states to find out what other EBPs were being provided, the input of an expert panel, and knowledge of future toolkit development that focuses on some of these EBPs for children with disruptive behavior disorders. For reviews of the evidence on these EBPs, see the special issue of the *Journal of Clinical Child & Adolescent Psychology* edited by Silverman and Hinshaw (2008).

NUMBER OF PERSONS RECEIVING EVIDENCE-BASED PRACTICES

The number of EBP programs being implemented by states is just one national indicator of dissemination. States are also required to annually report, through the Uniform Reporting System (URS) of the Mental Health Block Grant (SAMHSA,

2008), the number of individuals that receive EBPs. Table 8.4 shows the number of persons that received most of the same EBPs for adults and children as shown earlier. State totals are summed in the table to yield national totals within each cell for the state fiscal years 2005 through 2008. Across most EBPs there was an overall increase in the number of persons that received EBPs between 2005 and 2008, though the patterns show some leveling off between 2006 and 2007. Supported Housing (Rosenheck, Kasprow, Frisman, & Liu-Mares, 2003; Tsemberis & Eisenberg, 2000) is an exception where there was an increasing trend until 2007, but then a sharp decrease back to the 2005 level in 2008. The pattern for Therapeutic Foster Care was somewhat erratic, showing more than twice as many children receiving it in 2006 than in 2007, but then an upward trend in 2008. This could have been related to changes in reporting practices of some states to conform with the reporting guidelines mentioned above for Table 8.3. The greatest and most steady growth can be seen for Medication Management, where 100,000 more people were receiving it across the nation in 2008 than in 2005.

Below each set of adult and child EBPs, the table also displays the total number of adults and children served by SMHAs. This number includes persons receiving any type of services, not just the EBPs reported in the table cells. The total SMHA population served steadily increased over these time periods. Looking roughly at the proportions of the population served by SMHAs that received EBPs,

TABLE 8.4 Total Number of Persons Receiving Evidence-Based Practices through State Mental Health Agencies 2005–2008

	2005	2006	2007	2008
Adult EBPs				
Assertive Community Treatment	36,563	48,491	56,833	58,502
Supported Employment	32,421	42,440	43,090	40,387
Medication Management	153,086	170,927	195,894	253,414
Family Psychoeducation	12,541	10,724	14,875	25,127
Illness Self-Management	128,820	116,699	118,513	147,089
Dual Diagnosis Treatment	25,472	27,701	39,143	46,706
Supported Housing	65,799	79,105	81,673	65,797
Total adults with SMI served by SMHA[a]	1,640,595	1,744,630	2,061,562	2,568,326
Proportion of adults served receiving any EBPs	28%	28%	27%	25%
Child/Adolescent EBPs				
Therapeutic Foster Care	9,671	25,468	12,462	16,291
Multisystemic Therapy	5,431	3,219	4,685	8,126
Functional Family Therapy	2,036	2,950	6,204	7,027
Total children with SED served by SMHA[a]	434,707	466,485	477,156	781,981
Proportion of children served receiving any EBPs	4%	7%	5%	4%

Notes. SMI = serious mental illness; SED = serious emotional disturbance.

[a]Total number of adults and children served by SMHAs include those receiving any type of services, not just the EBPs reported in the table cells.

approximately one quarter of the adult population served received EBPs during these reporting periods, but very small proportions of the child population received EBPs. These small proportions may reflect the fewer number of child EBPs for which the states are required to report. As was noted earlier for the Profiles, efforts are also under way to allow states to report on a much broader array of child EBPs in future URS data submissions. Another caveat in viewing these data is that using the denominator of all persons served by SMHAs implies that all persons need these specific EBPs, which may not be the case. Substantial numbers of persons may be making sufficient progress with medications and other therapeutic, supportive, or case management services. However, these data from the URS system serve as approximate indicators of patterns of EBP dissemination in the United States. As refinements are made in both the Profiles and the URS systems to add relevant child EBPs and other adult EBPs as the science emerges and to enhance reporting methods, these data can be a continuing important source of information on progress being made in public mental health systems to bridge the gap between science and practice.

Conclusions

Just as in any other field of knowledge, advances in the behavioral sciences will inevitably result in changes in mental health practices and in the array of mental health services that will be made available. As the content of this chapter indicates, the challenge is how to accelerate the uptake process so that the time lag between the development of knowledge and implementation is significantly reduced. A major learning that has been reinforced substantially through the experiences reported above is that uptake and sustainability may be more likely when EBPs are embedded in organizational cultures that value and use evidence, and that have infrastructure elements that support the EBPs (i.e., training, financing, fidelity monitoring, etc.).

Ultimately, the dissemination of EBPs depends on the availability of funding and the incentives provided. Medicaid, a major source of public mental health funding, has made clarifications to the field related to how Medicaid can be used to finance EBPs. For example, in 2005 the Centers for Medicare and Medicaid developed a report describing how Medicaid has been used to fund a range of EBPs, including Medication Management, Assertive Community Treatment, Supported Employment, Family Psychoeducation, Illness Management and Recovery, and Integrated Dual Disorders Treatment (Centers for Medicare and Medicaid Services, 2005). However, implementation of policies guiding Medicaid reimbursement for various EBPs has had variations and inconsistencies across Medicaid regions.

Clearly, federal initiatives have provided both leadership and impetus to the national prioritization of EBP implementation. After the initial thrust of developing the first set of toolkits, the focus of federal EBP implementation initiatives shifted to two areas: (a) the development of new EBP toolkits, and (b) EBP implementation being subsumed under the rubric of mental health transformation. The second generation of SAMHSA-funded toolkit development has focused on adding two more toolkits for adults with schizophrenia: Supported Housing and Consumer Operated Services (Resnick & Rosenheck, 2008; Rogers et al., 2007), which had acquired more evidence of their effectiveness since the development of the original toolkits. This second generation of toolkit development has also focused on developing two additional toolkits for distinct target populations: children and adolescents with disruptive behavior disorders and older adults with depression. These latter toolkits contain information on a range of EBPs, which were reviewed and selected through two expert panels, composed of leading researchers, experts in each content area, consumers, advocates, providers, and other stakeholders. In selecting which interventions to include in the toolkit for children with disruptive behavior disorders, the panel used Hawaii's system of rating EBPs (Hawaii Department of Health, Child and Adolescent Mental Health Division, 2004), which is based on the criteria used by the American Psychological Association (for a review of the evidence of the types of EBPs covered, see Eyberg, Nelson, & Boggs, 2008). The child toolkit is available at: http://store.samhsa.gov/product/Interventions-for-Disruptive-Behavior-Disorders-Evidence-Based-Practices-EBP-KIT/SMA11-4634CD-DVD. The interventions used in the toolkit for older adults with depression were chosen because they met the American Psychological Association's criteria for evidence-based psychotherapy for older adults (Yon & Scogin, 2007) (for a review of the evidence of the types of EBPs covered, see Mackin & Arean, 2005). The older adult toolkit is available at: http://store.samhsa.gov/product/The-Treatment-of-Depression-in-Older-Adults-Evidence-Based-Practices-EBP-KIT/SMA11-4631CD-DVD.

The shift to subsuming EBP implementation as a national priority under mental health transformation recognizes the need for changes in organizational culture and infrastructure supports as an essential, critical aspect of broad EBP dissemination initiatives. A side effect, however, is that the specific national priority focus on EBP promulgation was diluted. Only a few states received federal grants for mental health transformation, and even among these, EBP implementation was emphasized more in some of these "transformation" states than others. Instead of further development of national-level EBP training and technical assistance support systems, resources were devoted to the development of the new toolkits. The implicit expectation is that each state will develop its own training and technical assistance capacity. This has been easier for some of the larger, better funded states than for the smaller or poorer ones.

Research and higher education have pivotal roles in this emerging trend. For example, a neglected area related to EBP dissemination is the one that covers the characteristics of the practice itself. Many EBPs for adults with serious mental illnesses are complex and very expensive services. Little has been done over time to refine and simplify practices (in some cases, the practice being promoted is essentially in the same form as it was originally developed decades ago). Along the same lines, technologies to monitor fidelity remain resource intensive, curtailing widespread efforts. The field also needs models of what to do when EBPs do not produce expected outcomes for specific individuals. These are areas in which knowledge development is clearly needed. At the same time, the role of higher education in producing professionals who are well versed in EBPs is emergent rather than well established. EBP training is gradually making inroads into medical, psychology, nursing, and social work graduate programs, but these are spotty and sporadic efforts rather than being broadly available. Certification of university curricula and licensing of professionals has, for the most part, not been tied to EBP training. Such initiatives could clearly have a widespread impact.

The experiences and lessons described in this chapter represent the inchoate, initial phase of a new era in mental health care resulting from giant strides in science. Public mental health systems across the country are clearly moving along the arc of increased and substantive EBP implementation. Even with resource limitations and the downturn in the economy, more states are implementing more EBPs, and that is likely to remain the ongoing trend, especially in view of health care reform proposals and their emphasis on effectiveness of interventions. The dissemination of EBPs goes hand-in-glove with the management of change at all levels—clinical, administrative, and financial. Without addressing infrastructure needs, the implementation of EBPs will remain an embattled, uphill climb. The luxury of time, however, has a cost, both in terms of dollars and in terms of human lives.

REFERENCES

Alexander, J., Barton, C., Gordon, D., Grotpeter, J., Hansson, K., Harrison, R., et al. (1998). Functional family therapy: Blueprints for violence prevention, book three. In D. S. Elliott (Series Ed.), *Blueprints for Violence Prevention Series*. Boulder, CO: Center for the Study and Prevention of Violence, Institute of Behavioral Science, University of Colorado.

Becker, D. R., & Bond, G. R. (Eds.). (2002). *Supported Employment implementation resource kit*. Rockville, MD: Center for Mental Health Services, Substance Abuse and Mental Health Services Administration. Retrieved September 30, 2011, from http://store. samhsa.gov/product/Supported-Employment-Evidence-Based-Practices-EBP-KIT/ SMA08-4365

Biegel, D. E., Swanson, S., & Kola, L. A. (2007). The Ohio Supported Employment Coordinating Center of Excellence. *Research on Social Work Practice, 17*(4), 504–512.

Bond, G. R., Becker, D. R., Drake, R. E., Rapp, C. A., Meisler, N., Lehman, A. F., et al. (2001). Implementing supported employment as an evidence-based practice. *Psychiatric Services, 52*, 313–322.

Brunette, M., & Drake, R. (Eds.). (2002). *Integrated Dual Disorders Treatment implementation resource kit*. Rockville, MD: Center for Mental Health Services, Substance Abuse and Mental Health Services Administration. Retrieved September 30, 2011, from http://store.samhsa.gov/product/Integrated-Treatment-for-Co-Occurring-Disorders- Evidence-Based-Practices-EBP-KIT/SMA08-4367

Burns, B., & Phillips, S. (Eds.). (2002). *Assertive Community Treatment implementation resource kit*. Rockville, MD: Center for Mental Health Services, Substance Abuse and Mental Health Services Administration. Retrieved September 30, 2011, from http://

store.samhsa.gov/product/Assertive-Community-Treatment-ACT-Evidence-Based-Practices-EBP-KIT/SMA08-4345

Centers for Medicare and Medicaid Services. (2005). *Medicaid support of evidence-based practices in mental health programs.* Retrieved September 30, 2011 from http://www.cms.hhs.gov/PromisingPractices/Downloads/EBP_Basics.pdf

Chamberlain, P., & Mihalic, S. F. (1998). Multidimensional Treatment Foster Care: Blueprints for violence prevention, book eight. In D. S. Elliott (Series Ed.), *Blueprints for Violence Prevention Series.* Boulder, CO: Center for the Study and Prevention of Violence, Institute of Behavioral Science, University of Colorado.

Chambers, D. A., Ringeisen, H., & Hickman, E. E. (2005). Federal, state, and foundation initiatives around evidence-based practices for child and adolescent mental health. *Child and Adolescent Psychiatric Clinics of North America, 14*, 307–327.

Daleiden, E. L., & Chorpita, B. F. (2005). From data to wisdom: Quality improvement strategies supporting large-scale implementation of evidence-based services. *Child and Adolescent Psychiatric Clinics of North America, 14*, 329–349.

Dixon, L., McFarlane, W. R., Lefley, H., Lucksted, A., Cohen, M., Falloon, I., et al. (2001). Evidence-based practices for services to families of people with psychiatric disabilities. *Psychiatric Services, 52*, 903–910.

Drake, R. E., Bond, G. R., & Essock, S. M. (2009). Implementing evidence-based practices for people with schizophrenia. *Schizophrenia Bulletin, 35*, 704–713.

Drake, R. E., Essock, S. M., Shaner, A., Carey, K. B., Minkoff, K., Kola, L., et al. (2001). Implementing dual diagnosis services for clients with severe mental illness. *Psychiatric Services, 52*, 469–476.

Eyberg, S. M., Nelson, M. M., & Boggs, S. R. (2008). Evidence-based psychosocial treatments for children and adolescents with disruptive behavior. *Journal of Clinical Child & Adolescent Psychology, 37*, 215–237.

Ganju, V. (2007, May). *Report of the conference: Lessons learned on embedding EBPs in statewide transformation.* Alexandria, VA: National Association of State Mental Health Program Directors Research Institute, Inc.

Hawaii Department of Health, Child and Adolescent Mental Health Division. (2004). *Evidence-Based Services Committee 2004 biennial report: Summary of effective interventions for youth with behavioral and emotional needs* (EBS 011). Retrieved September 30, 2011, from http://hawaii.gov/health/mental-health/camhd/library/pdf/ebs/ebs011.pdf

Henggeler, S. W., Mihalic, S. F., Rone, L., Thomas, C., & Timmons-Mitchell, J. (1998). Multisystemic Therapy: Blueprints for violence prevention, book six. In D. S. Elliott (Series Ed.), *Blueprints for Violence Prevention Series.* Boulder, CO: Center for the Study and Prevention of Violence, Institute of Behavioral Science, University of Colorado.

Isett, K. R., Burnman, M. A., Coleman-Beattie, B., Hyde, P. A., Morrissey, J. P., Magnabosco, J., et al. (2007). Implementation issues for evidence-based practices: The state policy context. *Psychiatric Services, 58*, 914–921.

Isett, K. R., Burnman, M. A., Coleman-Beattie, B., Hyde, P. S., Morrissey, J. P., & Magnabosco, J. L. (2008). The role of state mental health authorities in managing change for the implementation of evidence-based practices. *Community Mental Health Journal, 44*, 195–211.

Lutterman, T., Berhane, A., Phelan, B., Shaw, R., & Rana, V. (2009). *Funding and characteristics of state mental health agencies, 2007* (DHHS Publication No. SMA 09–4424). Rockville,

MD: Center for Mental Health Services, Substance Abuse and Mental Health Services Administration. Retrieved September 30, 2011, from http://store.samhsa.gov/product/ Funding-and-Characteristics-of-State-Mental-Health-Agencies-2007/SMA09-4424

Mackin R. S., & Arean P. A. (2005). Evidence-based psychosocial interventions for geriatric depression. *Psychiatric Clinics of North America, 28,* 805–820.

McFarlane, W., & Dixon, L. (Eds.). (2002). *Family Psychoeducation implementation resource kit.* Rockville, MD: Center for Mental Health Services, Substance Abuse and Mental Health Services Administration. Retrieved September 30, 2011, from http://store. samhsa.gov/product/Family-Psychoeducation-Evidence-Based-Practices-EBP-KIT/ SMA09-4423

McHugo, G. M., Drake, R. E., Whitley, R., Bond, G. R., Campbell, K., Rapp, C. A., et al. (2007). Fidelity outcomes in the National Implementing Evidence-Based Practices Project. *Psychiatric Services, 58,* 1279–1284.

Mellman, T. A., Miller, A. L., Weissman, E. M., Crismon, M. L., Essock, S. M., & Marder, S. R. (2001). Evidence-based pharmacologic treatment for people with severe mental illness: A focus on guidelines and algorithms. *Psychiatric Services, 52,* 619–625.

Mueser, K. T., Corrigan, P. W., Hilton, D. W., Tanzman, B., Schaub, A., Gingerich, S., et al. (2002). Illness management and recovery: A review of the research. *Psychiatric Services, 53,* 1272–1284.

Mueser, K., & Gingerich, S. (Eds.). (2002). *Illness Management and Recovery implementation resource kit.* Rockville, MD: Center for Mental Health Services, Substance Abuse and Mental Health Services Administration. Retrieved September 30, 2011, from http:// store.samhsa.gov/product/Illness-Management-and-Recovery-Evidence-Based-Practices-EBP-KIT/SMA09-4463

National Association of State Mental Health Program Directors Research Institute, Inc. (2003, April). *Notes of Meeting on Implementing Evidence-Based Practices Project: National review of effective implementation strategies and challenges.* Alexandria, VA: Author.

National Association of State Mental Health Program Directors Research Institute, Inc. (2005, August). *Results of a survey of state directors of adult and child mental health services on implementation of evidence-based practices.* Alexandria, VA: Author.

National Association of State Mental Health Program Directors Research Institute, Inc. (2011). *State Mental Health Agency Profiles System 2003 to 2009* [Data file]. Retrieved September 30, 2011 from NRI website, http://www.nri-inc.org/projects/Profiles/data_ search.cfm

Phillips, S. D., Burns, B. J., Edgar, E. R., Mueser, K. T., Linkins, K. W., Rosenheck, R. A., et al. (2001). Moving assertive community treatment into standard practice. *Psychiatric Services, 52,* 771–779.

President's New Freedom Commission on Mental Health. (2003). *Achieving the promise: Transforming mental health care in America. Final Report* (DHHS Publication No. SMA-03–3832). Rockville, MD. Retrieved September 30, 2011, from http://store. samhsa.gov/shin/content/SMA03-3831/SMA03-3831.pdf

Rapp, C. A., Bond, G. R., Becker, D. R., Carpinello, S. E., Nikkel, R. E., & Gintoli, G. (2005). The role of state mental health authorities in promoting improved client outcomes through evidence-based practice. *Community Mental Health Journal, 41,* 347–363.

Resnick, S. G., & Rosenheck, R. A. (2008). Integrating peer-provided services: A quasi-experimental study of recovery orientation, confidence, and empowerment. *Psychiatric Services, 59,* 1307–1314.

Rogers, E. S., Teague, G. B., Lichenstein, C., Campbell, J., Lyass, A., Chen, R., et al. (2007). Effects of participation in consumer-operated service programs on both personal and organizationally mediated empowerment: Results of a multi-site study. *Journal of Rehabilitation Research and Development, 44*, 785–800.

Rosenheck, R., Kasprow, W., Frisman, L., & Liu-Mares, W. (2003). Cost effectiveness of supported housing for homeless persons with mental illness. *Archives of General Psychiatry, 60*, 941–951.

Salyers, M. P., McKasson, M., Bond, G. R., McGrew, J. H., Rollins, A. L., & Boyle, C. (2007). The role of technical assistance centers in implementing evidence-based practices: Lessons learned. *American Journal of Psychiatric Rehabilitation, 10*, 85–101.

Silverman, W. K., & Hinshaw, S. P. (Eds.). (2008). The second special issue on evidence-based psychosocial treatments for children and adolescents: A 10-year update [Special issue]. *Journal of Clinical Child & Adolescent Psychology, 37*, 62–104, 105–130, 156–183, 215–237.

Stirman, S. W., Crits-Christoph P., & DeRubeis, R. J. (2004). Achieving successful dissemination of empirically supported psychotherapies: A synthesis of dissemination theory. *Clinical Psychology: Science and Practice, 11*, 343–359.

Substance Abuse and Mental Health Service Administration, Center for Mental Health Services (SAMHSA). (2008). *Uniform Reporting System output tables 2005 to 2008* [Data file]. Retrieved from SAMHSA website, http://mentalhealth.samhsa.gov/cmhs/MentalHealthStatistics/

Swain, K., Whitley, R., McHugo, G. J., & Drake, R. E. (2010). The sustainability of evidence-based practices in routine mental health agencies. *Community Mental Health Journal, 46*, 119–129.

Tsemberis, S., & Eisenberg, R. F. (2000). Pathways to housing: Supported housing for street-dwelling homeless individuals with psychiatric disabilities. *Psychiatric Services, 51*, 487–493.

Torrey, W. C., Lynde, D. W., & Gorman, P. (2005). Promoting the implementation of practices that are supported by research: The National Implementing Evidence-Based Practice Project. *Child and Adolescent Psychiatric Clinics of North America, 14*, 297–306.

U.S. Department of Health and Human Services. (1999). *Mental health: A report of the Surgeon General.* Rockville, MD: U.S. Department of Health and Human Services, Substance Abuse and Mental Health Services Administration, Center for Mental Health Services, National Institutes of Health, National Institute of Mental Health.

Yon, A., & Scogin, F. (2007). Procedures for identifying evidence-based psychological treatments for older adults. *Psychology and Aging, 22*, 4–7.

9

Sustaining Hawaii's Evidence-Based Service System in Children's Mental Health

Brad J. Nakamura, Charmaine K. Higa-McMillan, and Bruce F. Chorpita

Introduction and Motivating Circumstances

Hawaii is a place unlike many others, characterized by an extraordinary level of diversity and geographic isolation. Its capitol city, Honolulu, is one of the largest cities in the United States, with more than 1 million people in its greater metropolitan area. Outside the city, Hawaii is composed primarily of isolated towns in rural areas spread across eight islands. Beginning with its history in colonialism and commercial development, a theme of diversity has permeated many aspects of the state's ethos, including ethnicity, culture, and lifestyle, to create a unique community that is geographically isolated and ethnically different from the rest of the nation. Not surprisingly, Hawaii's local culture strongly prioritizes interpersonal relationships and local trust when doing business, and there is healthy skepticism regarding external impositions and innovations. It is within this sociopolitical environment that significant changes to its direct service system were introduced in the mid-1990s (Chorpita & Donkervoet, 2005).

In 1994, the state of Hawaii settled a class action lawsuit concerning education and mental health system inadequacies for youth with special needs. In short, this settlement, known as the Felix Consent Decree (named for the index plaintiff), mandated the state to build a statewide system of care in accordance with Child and Adolescent Service System Program (CASSP) principles (Stroul & Friedman, 1986). In short, these child-centered and family-focused principles are a well-defined set of axioms for providing mental health services to children and adolescents with emotional disturbances in the least restrictive or intrusive service settings. Charged with federal oversight for implementing externally imposed changes, local leadership carefully executed numerous strategic plans for balancing this change stimulus with a vision for sustaining progress after oversight withdrawal. In other words, acknowledging that federal funding and oversight would eventually end, leadership leveraged temporary federal support to apply principles of dissemination and implementation science (Rogers, 2003) toward the ultimate goal of sustaining an evidence-based service delivery system in children's mental health (Daleiden & Chorpita, 2005). As an example of just one start-up strategy, Stroul and Friedman's (1986) original CASSP principles were "reinvented" in collaboration with local "opinion leaders" to fit Hawaii's needs and values while remaining true to the original principles (Chorpita & Donkervoet, 2005; Rogers, 2003). This process of reinvention through collaboration ensured respect for local knowledge and compatibility with local values and language preferences.

The example above is but one of many strategies employed between 1994 and the mid-2000s, during which time temporary federal support and oversight helped to build Hawaii's CASSP-consistent system of care. Much has been written about these start-up strategies, building Hawaii's evidence-based service delivery system in children's mental health, and associated positive outcomes (Chorpita, 2003; Chorpita & Donkervoet, 2005; Chorpita et al., 2002; Daleiden, Chorpita, Donkervoet, Arensdorf, & Brogan, 2006; Schiffman & Donkervoet, 2008). Hawaii's system of care now finds itself in the "post-Felix" era, with mandated federal oversight now gone and state legislative appropriations decreasing. Moreover, like the rest of the nation, the state faces unprecedented financial hardships. In addition, there have been changes in key leadership positions in the state mental health system, as well as significant staff turnover between 1994 and today. Given these conditions, this chapter will focus on how Hawaii is maintaining successful initiatives in children's mental health within this rather challenging context.

HAWAII'S CHILDREN'S PUBLIC MENTAL HEALTH SERVICE SYSTEM

Within Hawaii, two branches of state government coordinate together to provide most of its public sector youth mental health services. These include the Hawaii State Department of Health, Child and Adolescent Mental Health Division (CAMHD) and the Hawaii State Department of Education (DOE). Generally speaking, DOE-registered youth are thought to require less intensive services and frequently are treated in school-based settings, whereas CAMHD-registered youth tend to exhibit more impairment and are served across an array of settings ranging from intensive in-home to hospital-based residential care. Fully acknowledging the synergistic nature of this interdepartmental collaboration for creating a continuum of care, for the purposes of this chapter, since most of the work described below focuses on CAMHD initiatives, the term "system" or "evidence-based service system" used hereafter refers to CAMHD. In order to provide a relevant background for discussing targeted adoption and sustainment strategies, three core aspects of Hawaii's evidence-based service system will first be described, namely, funding support for initial start-up, quality improvement initiatives for services and standards of care, and therapist training.

Funding Support for Initial Start-Up

Initially, funding for system change came from increases in state appropriations mandated by federal court. The federal court requirements included that CAMHD develop a practice improvement office, which was initially called the Felix Staff and Services Development Institute and later became the Practice Development Office of the CAMHD. This office had three primary foci: (a) standard setting for the state, (b) procuring and overseeing the implementation of evidence-based "package programs" (e.g., Multisystemic Therapy [MST]; Henggeler & Borduin, 1990), and (c) providing training to front-line clinicians in evidence-based approaches. At the time, it was not clear whether all of these evidence-based approaches could or would be drawn from existing programs, or whether some approaches would be adapted and developed locally. Over time, the system focused on a blended approach of implementing formal evidence-based programs along with training in a broader model of applying evidence from the children's mental health literature (Chorpita et al., 2002), regularly reviewing child outcomes using a data-driven information system (Daleiden & Chorpita, 2005), and building partnerships with university experts in evidence-based treatments (e.g., Chorpita & Mueller, 2008).

The increase in government oversight helped set high standards for public mental health services, including such practices as formalizing care coordination through regional family guidance centers, formalizing family partnerships and consumer involvement, and establishing a wide service array ranging from school-based mental health services to hospital-based residential services. Collectively, these efforts helped create Hawaii's system of care and increased youth and family access to treatment services. For example, between 1996 and 1998, the number of system-registered youth went from 1,938 to 8,343, representing an increase of 330% (Chorpita & Donkervoet, 2005).

Quality Improvement Initiatives for Services and Standards of Care

It became clear around 1999 that despite increased service delivery and associated expenditures, services being provided were not fully meeting the needs of Hawaii's children and families. Efforts then began focusing more intensively on the quality and effectiveness of youth services, not just their coordination, accessibility, and availability. At that time, CAMHD and the DOE partnered to develop the *Interagency Performance Standards and Practice Guidelines* (IPSPG; http://hawaii. gov/health/mental-health/camhd/library/webs/ipspg/ipspg.html, State of Hawaii, 2006). The IPSPG is designed to define service content standards and to improve the efficiency and effectiveness of the school-based behavioral health services and the array of intensive mental health services provided by CAMHD. The IPSPG has gone through multiple revisions since 1999, and plans for a fourth edition are currently under way.

In addition, in 1999 the system formed the Empirical Basis to Services (EBS) Task Force, an interdisciplinary task force that brought administrators, researchers, therapists, educators, and families together to identify the most promising treatments for Hawaii's youth (Chorpita et al., 2002). Building from the latest research at that time (e.g., Lonigan, Elbert, & Bennett Johnson, 1998; Task Force on Promotion and Dissemination of Psychological Procedures, 1995), the EBS Task Force adapted and expanded practice definitions along a number of parameters such as (a) units of analyses when comparing treatments (e.g., moving away from an emphasis on specific brand named therapy manuals to methodologies that emphasized commonalities across those manuals), (b) level of treatment support (e.g., shifting from a two-level to a five-level efficacy system), and (c) effectiveness parameters (e.g., coding and aggregating generalizability, feasibility, and cost-effectiveness findings) to best fit Hawaii's youth. In 2002 the task force became a standing quality committee of the CAMHD. Findings have been regularly disseminated in the form of two major technological innovations, the "Blue Menu" (a one-page efficacy level x problem area matrix, named for the blue paper on which it was printed and distributed) and the Biennial Report (a more detailed report on best practice outlining additional information such as practice element profiles and effectiveness information, which is published approximately every other year) (Child and Adolescent Mental Health Division, 2002, 2004; Chorpita & Daleiden, 2007).

By the year 2000, using its newly created Blue Menu and its first Biennial Report, state leadership conceptualized quality and effectiveness efforts as falling largely into one of two categories: (a) importing or implementing an empirically demonstrated approach to a specific mental health challenge and (b) improving the technology for both decision-support tools and the feedback loop about performance and outcomes for therapists and supervisors. Regarding the first category, leadership recognized that sometimes evidence-based package programs, such as MST, provided a good fit with important youth characteristics within Hawaii's system of care. Indeed, data on system-registered youth characteristics indicate that a typical youth in CAMHD is approximately 14 years old, male, and exhibiting disruptive behavior concerns (Higa-McMillan, Daleiden, & Kimhan, 2009). During these instances, programs as a whole were imported into the system. Since 2000, in addition to MST, Hawaii has implemented Functional Family Therapy (FFT; Alexander & Parsons, 1973) and Multidimensional Treatment Foster Care (MTFC; Chamberlain & Reid, 1998).

Many times, however, youth characteristics did not provide a good fit with existing evidence-based package programs, youth did not achieve as much progress as desired in the program, and/or the system did not have fiscal and training resources proportional to the intended impact of a specific program to justify its adoption. For these and other reasons, leadership increased the system's focus on improving decision-support tools and the feedback mechanisms about performance and outcomes. Toward this goal, local leadership made significant efforts toward fostering and developing a culture of data-driven decision making. At the forefront of this effort was CAMHD's "Supervision Decision Making Framework" (see Figure 9.1). This model has been fully elaborated elsewhere (Daleiden & Chorpita, 2005), but

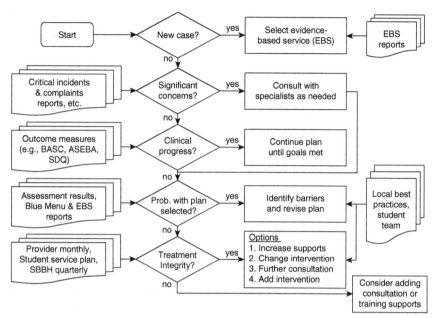

FIGURE 9.1 *The "Supervision Decision Making Framework" flowchart.*

Note. ASEBA = Achenbach System of Empirically Based Assessment; BASC = Behavior Assessment System for Children, 2nd edition; EBS = Evidence-Based Services; SBBH quarterly = School-Based Behavioral Health quarterly progress reports (documentation of Individualized Education Plan progress); SDQ = Strengths and Difficulties Questionnaire. Adapted from Daleiden, E. L., & Chorpita, B. F. (2005). From Data to Wisdom: Quality Improvement Strategies Supporting Large-scale Implementation of Evidence-Based Services. *Child and Adolescent Psychiatric Clinics of North America, 14,* 329–349.

generally involves prioritizing recent case-specific evidence (i.e., up-to-date patient-specific treatment outcome data) as being the highest priority for decision making. In other words, if clinical progress could be demonstrated through objective measurement, the model dictated no need for further review (regardless of whether or not the intervention implemented was an evidence-based treatment, however defined). It was only in the absence of documented progress that one needed to ask whether the intervention was appropriate, for which the Blue Menu and Biennial Reports were potential tools, and if so, whether that intervention was delivered with integrity.

Given the importance of case-specific and local data for steering decisions in the Supervision Decision Making Framework, the state initiated and established infra-structure for administering several objective measures on a regular basis. First, administration of objective measures of symptoms and functioning (Achenbach System of Empirically Based Assessment, Achenbach & Rescorla, 2001; Child and Adolescent Functional Assessment Scale [CAFAS], Hodges & Wong, 1996) for all system-registered youth (including those receiving the package program interventions indicated above) began occurring on a quarterly basis. Additionally, a standardized measure for determining level-of-care judgments (Child and Adolescent Level of Care Utilization System, American Academy of Child, Adolescent Psychiatry & American Association of Community Psychiatrists, 1999) was also put into place for administration every quarter. Finally, an idiographic measure for youth treatment targets, clinical progress, and intervention practices (Monthly Treatment and Progress Summary [MTPS]; http://hawaii.gov/health/mental-health/camhd/library/pdf/paf/paf-002.pdf; Child and Adolescent Mental Health Division, 2003; Daleiden, Lee, & Tolman, 2004; Nakamura, Daleiden, & Mueller, 2007; Orimoto, Higa-McMillan, Mueller, & Daleiden, 2009) was initiated in June 2003 for monthly administration. More specifically, concerning treatment targets, clinicians are asked to specify up to 10 target concerns, which were the focus of treatment during the reporting month. The targets are selected from a list of 53 predefined targets (e.g., hyperactivity, depressed mood, anxiety, etc.) and two additional open-response fields. For each target selected, clinicians provide a progress rating relative to the child's baseline level of functioning and the goal specified for the target. Progress ratings are provided on a 7-point (0 to 6) scale, with higher numbers indicating greater improvement. Finally, with regard to intervention practices, clinicians are asked to indicate all treatment techniques used during the reporting period. Discrete practices are selected from a list of 63 predefined elements (e.g., cognitive, modeling, exposure, etc.) and three additional open-response fields. Since replacing unstructured provider narrative reports (i.e., traditional progress report notes) in June 2003, the MTPS has been built into CAMHD's core business structure, such that providers must fill out this brief form on a monthly basis for all individual clients for billing reimbursement. This system allows for transparent and repeated surveillance of not only idiographic treatment progress but also, and just as important, the extent to which self-reported practices align with problems or concerns as prescribed by the literature. For example, if a therapist reports treating the target concern of anxiety, does he or she also report using exposure and cognitive techniques (rather than techniques like catharsis or hypnosis)?

With tools for choosing interventions, a clinical decision-making model, and standardized and idiographic measurement models in place, the system focused its energies toward strengthening the feedback loop between interventions and outcomes (and other performance indicators) to assist therapists, supervisors, and administrators in making data-driven clinical decisions. A primary strategy to increase evidence-based decision making was the development of on-demand, user-friendly, graphics-based reports in the Child and Adolescent Mental Health Management Information System. Through an analogy with the instrument panel for driving a car, these reports became known as the "dashboards" for driving decision making (Daleiden & Chorpita, 2005). Numerous dashboards were put into place across a wide range of ongoing clinical and operational procedures, all toward the unified goal of increasing the availability of up-to-date data for informing and supporting decision making. For example, at the direct service delivery level for an individual patient, a one-page clinical dashboard (i.e., termed the "Clinical Reporting Module" or "CRM") was established to graphically display any desired combination of patient-specific data (e.g., outcome data, therapeutic practices, level of care, etc.) in a standardized format. It should be noted that although the CRM has historically been used to implement this feedback concept, it has had varying degrees of implementation success within CAMHD. Under recent new leadership, CAMHD is currently moving toward replacing its Child and Adolescent Mental Health Management Information System (mentioned above) with an electronic health record, which will have the potential to integrate feedback tools such as the CRM in a more effective manner than in the past. As examples at the systems operational level, ongoing user-friendly reporting schemes were put into place for summarizing patterns of service utilization, fiscal spending, and consumer satisfaction. Others have written about Hawaii's innovative reporting schemes (e.g., Chorpita & Daleiden, in press; Chorpita & Donkervoet, 2005; Daleiden & Chorpita, 2005), so the main point here is that significant changes were put into place at the day-to-day infrastructure level for organizing and reporting data in live and user-friendly ways for supporting evidence-based decision making.

Therapist Training

The third core aspect noteworthy of discussion surrounds therapist training initiatives. Therapist training goes hand in hand with service selection and standards of care. In other words, the next logical step after selecting an evidence-based intervention involves training providers to deliver those interventions. These training efforts took one of two major forms, falling along the lines of the two practice development strategies mentioned above. When a package program such as MST, FFT, or MTFC was implemented, the state purchased trainings directly from treatment developers. For the majority of the time, however, training capacity was developed internally through its Practice Development Office, structuring training efforts around CAMHD's Supervision Decision Making Framework and its innovative ways of pulling practice information from the general children's mental health literature (e.g., Chorpita & Daleiden, 2010). For example, therapist training efforts have focused, and continue to focus, on prioritizing recent case-specific treatment outcome data for clinical decision making. More specifically, Practice Development Office staff explicitly train on the Supervision Decision Making Framework (see Figure 9.1), stressing the importance of ongoing data collection with, and interpretation of, the standardized and idiographic instruments mentioned above for steering treatment decisions. As mentioned above, case-specific data are of highest priority, and if clinical progress is demonstrated through repeated assessment, the model indicates no need for further case review. With regard to the delivery of these training services, Hawaii's state mental health practice guidelines dictate ongoing education and trainings for all credentialed clinicians, and Practice Development Office staff facilitate this process by routinely providing free in-service training workshops for clinicians throughout the state.

The content of these therapist trainings hosted by the Practice Development Office are continuously maturing over time, trying best to capitalize on advances in and summaries of the treatment outcome literature (e.g., the Biennial Report mentioned above). For example, therapist training has focused on the "practice element" or "common elements" approach to treatment. A practice element can be defined as a discrete clinical technique or strategy (e.g., time-out, relaxation, etc.) used as part of a larger intervention plan such as a manualized treatment program (Chorpita, Becker, & Daleiden, 2007; Chorpita & Daleiden, 2009; Chorpita, Daleiden, & Weisz, 2005). Through coding and identifying discrete techniques and procedures that make up evidence-based protocols within specific problem areas (e.g., anxiety, depression, disruptive behavior, etc.), Chorpita and colleagues (2005) demonstrated high commonalities with regard to treatment techniques among evidence-based treatments. For example, the vast majority of evidence-based protocols for anxiety problems use the techniques or practice elements of exposure, cognitive restructuring, and psychoeducation. In other words, this model conceptualizes evidence-based treatments at a lower level of analysis than simply their treatment manuals, and training efforts focus on common elements across protocols, without prescription of any one brand name. For instance, expanding upon the example above on the commonalities between evidence-based protocols for anxiety problems, the Practice Development Office would focus on teaching and demonstrating the general techniques of exposure, cognitive restructuring, and psychoeducation, rather than training therapists on a specific treatment manual.

More recently, looking to advancements in the dissemination and implementation literature bases (e.g., Fixsen, Naoom, Blase, Friedman, & Wallace, 2005), training efforts are gradually moving toward a growing focus on teaching methods that utilize behavioral rehearsal strategies (e.g., role play and trainer feedback) for skill acquisition, in addition to traditional lecture-based methods. For instance, the most recent series of trainings offered by the Practice Development Office involve both traditional lecture-style instruction and information handouts as well as time for therapist role play and trainer feedback. In these trainings, the overall number of therapists allowed per training is limited to a maximum of approximately 30, so that the two to three trainers per training have time to sufficiently circulate and provide feedback on therapist role plays. In its latest training project, the Practice Development Office has offered a core series of four types of trainings over the last 18 months, each devoted to a different focus area, that include (a) an introduction to Hawaii's evidence-based service system in children's mental health (14 trainings completed); (b) common practice elements for delinquency behaviors (5 trainings completed); (c) common practice elements for internalizing behaviors (6 trainings completed); and (d) motivational interviewing techniques (6 trainings completed). In all, approximately 450 participants from 21 differing child-serving agencies across the state have attended one or more of these trainings, and evidence-based practice attitudes (i.e., Evidence-Based Practice Attitude Scale: Aarons, 2004; Attitudes Towards Evidence-Based Practice Scale: Borntrager, Chorpita, Higa-McMillan,

Weisz, & the Research Network on Youth Mental Health, 2009) and knowledge (i.e., Knowledge of Evidence-Based Services Questionnaire: Stumpf, Higa-McMillan, & Chorpita, 2008) are surveyed prior to and after each training. This training project and its associated data collection are currently coming to a close, and data are currently being analyzed.

TARGETED STRATEGIES FOR BARRIERS TO ADOPTION AND SUSTAINMENT

Like other mental health service delivery systems, CAMHD has faced, and continues to face, difficulties all too common in the public sector. These threats to sustainability include, but are not limited to, frequent and significant staff turnover, financial constraint, and evolving program requirements. In Hawaii's experience, efforts for sustaining and maintaining an evidence-based service system in such a climate has centered around five major themes: (a) empirical epistemology and performance evaluation, (b) infrastructure development and standardization, (c) building and maintaining partnerships, (d) financial planning and creativity, and (e) increased coordination for dissemination and implementation strategies.

Empirical Epistemology and Performance Evaluation

Inherent within its name, an evidence-based service system relies on various forms of observable evidence for steering a wide range of decisions. Such a system acknowledges the relationship between interventions and associated outcomes as reciprocally dynamic and ongoing. Within this repeated assessment paradigm, local and immediate evidence tends to be prioritized over more distal forms of information when evaluating the effectiveness of an intervention, with the weight and role of expert judgment increasing inversely as a function of the availability of relevant and valid evidence (Chorpita & Daleiden, 2010; Daleiden & Chorpita, 2005). Leadership within CAMHD view this philosophy as a central decision-making tenant, cutting across all internal operations.

All quality improvement committees within CAMHD are accountable to performance indicators unique to their specific tasks and functions. Currently there are six such committees that report to an overarching Quality Steering Committee, which oversees all improvement initiatives. Toward the goal of providing high-quality evidence-based services in fiscally responsible ways, these committees address the core areas of (a) provider credentialing services, (b) youth safety and risk management, (c) service utilization management, (d) consumer grievance and appeals, (e) agency compliance with protocols and procedures, and (f) evidence-based services within the system of care.

As an example of one such committee, the Evidence-Based Services (EBS) Committee strives to provide relevant, easily understood, and up-to-date knowledge to key stakeholders in order to support evidence-based decision making and the system's mission of providing timely and effective services. In working toward this mission, the committee has traditionally had five goals with associated observable performance indicators and benchmarks for success, repeatedly assessed over time. Toward its first goal of identifying interventions for a broad range of problems, the committee reviewed at least three different target problem areas (e.g., depression, delinquency, anxiety, etc.) per quarter. Second, in efforts toward exposing committee members to the latest scientific findings and providing feedback to the CAMHD community, the committee sought to review at least 12 new research papers or treatment protocols per quarter. Third, in order to ensure that the Blue Menu and Biennial Report were disseminated (i.e., twice per year and every other year, respectively), the committee reviewed and distributed these decision-support tools. Toward its fourth goal of facilitating discussions on how to develop training and dissemination materials regarding best practices, committee members took turns presenting the procedural details of specific clinical practices consistent with the practice element model or approach (e.g., demonstrating "relaxation" or "cognitive restructuring" to the committee). At least three specific clinical practices were demonstrated per quarter. Finally, when requested by CAMHD leadership, the committee provided brief reports based on the literature for special topics related to evidence-based services within 90 days of the initial request. This example is just one illustration of the six quality improvement committees mentioned above, but it demonstrates the main ideas of transparency and accountability and determining courses of action in ways consistent with an empirical epistemology (e.g., repeated and ongoing data collection, benchmarking, data-driven recommendations, etc.).

As Daleiden and Chorpita (2005) suggest, the risk of such guided decision making is the potential for becoming overburdened with data collection and feeling hindered rather than supported by the evidence. The cost of data gathering, analysis, and delivery must be weighed against the benefits of improved decision making. This is a never-ending issue for CAMHD leadership, who, in defining policy, must regularly balance this cost–benefit ratio. Of significant note, however, is that in balancing this cost–benefit ratio, leadership do not rely solely on human judgment; they look to measurable outcomes associated with use of various data-support strategies. In other words, the core ideas of empirical epistemology and performance evaluation are meta-level overarching philosophies that steer even decisions for whether or not collecting, analyzing, and delivering certain data are worth their costs for the potential added benefit of providing timely and effective services to children.

This idea can be demonstrated by the following example. Looking to data on the costs and associated benefits for maintaining the number and structure of CAMHD's quality improvement committees, CAMHD leadership recently reduced the number of overall committees from nine to six, and decreased the frequency with which all committees convene together for one overarching meeting. Moving forward, the system will keep track of standardized key performance indicators (e.g., fiscal outcomes, rate of youth improvement, number of out-of-home placements, etc.) to evaluate the effects of this decision in a reciprocally ongoing fashion.

Infrastructure Development and Standardization

It is important to recognize that many behavioral health organizations operate on what has been called a "credentialed practitioner model" (Fixsen et al., 2005). In this model, individual therapists with the appropriate academic and licensing credentials are hired, and clinical practice stems from their unique education and training experiences. This staffing model results in an eclectic treatment approach in which an organization's programs and practices are amorphous and diffuse. Compounding this problem is the fact that behavioral health organization staff frequently turn over, resulting in inconsistencies even within the smallest units of analyses. In other words, in this model, important practice decisions hinge on the unique personal experiences of whoever is employed at any given time.

Given these concerns, CAMHD leadership has made concerted and ongoing efforts to invest in a system that articulates explicit models for implicit processes. Explicit specification and mapping of important and complex decisions such as clinical supervision often take the form of diagrams and flowcharts (Chorpita & Daleiden, 2010). One such example, the Supervision Decision Making Framework flowchart, appears in Figure 9.1 and explicitly outlines the implicit process of clinical supervision. This model is articulated within the IPSPG and has been discussed in depth elsewhere (e.g., Chorpita & Daleiden, 2010; Daleiden & Chorpita, 2005), but broadly speaking, this flowchart heavily prioritizes immediate case-specific evidence over more distal forms of data for steering clinical decisions within the supervision context. Its mention here is mainly to serve as one example for demonstrating the point that it is our view that giving explicit visibility to implicit processes reduces the likelihood of problems (e.g., procedural unreliability and nonstandardization compounded by training drift or staff turnover) classically associated with the credentialed practitioner model.

Behavioral health care seems to be moving slowly away from the model in which a clinician's unique experiences determine the treatment approach (Dulcan, 2005). Slowly emerging in its place is an industrialized model calling for greater standardization of training and treatment procedures, as well as more attention to treatment fidelity and quality assurance (Becker, Nakamura, Young, & Chorpita, 2009; Hayes, Barlow, & Nelson-Gray, 1999). Examples of successful treatment approaches that have stepped away from the credentialed practitioner model toward a business model with high standardization within behavioral health care contexts include MST (Henggeler & Borduin, 1990) and Parent-Child Interaction Therapy (McNeil, Eyberg, Einstadt, Newcomb, & Funderburk, 1991).

Toward the goal of sustaining and maintaining its evidence-based system, CAMHD has invested significant resources for specifying and mapping complex decisions to contexts other than clinical decision making including, but not limited to, service utilization management, consumer grievance and appeals, youth safety and risk management, and even the change processes for creating or modifying these explicitly visible protocols.

Building and Maintaining Partnerships

Building and maintaining partnerships between administrative leadership, service agency staff, researchers, consumers, and other system stakeholders are viewed as very important initiatives for sustaining Hawaii's evidence-based system. Of its many differing initiatives within this domain, the two specific examples below seem to be particularly successful and are discussed to highlight some characteristics thought important for maintaining and furthering an evidence-based system.

First, at the broad community level, significant efforts continue for socially engaging various community stakeholders in meaningful and ongoing dialogues about defining evidence (Daleiden & Chorpita, 2005), evidence-based decision making in general, and disseminating information on evidence-based practices. Research suggests that innovation diffusion is largely a social process, with community buy-in and support necessary for changes to occur (Rogers, 2003). Sitting at the forefront of this social initiative is CAMHD's interdisciplinary EBS Committee composed of administrators, direct service providers, educators, family members, social workers, and nurses from varying settings. Working together for over 10 years now, the committee has reviewed research literature findings together in order to discuss collaboratively theoretical and practical issues relevant to evidence-based services in Hawaii. One example of how this committee has fostered social engagement is through a monthly presentation called "EBS in my life," during which at least one committee member shares how evidence-based services play a role in his or her professional or personal life. EBS in my life has encouraged discussions on topics such as system selection of EBS programs, training on EBS in the community, implementation challenges, and the impact of EBS on family and parenting.

Outside the context of monthly meetings, EBS members serve as "purveyors" (Fixsen et al., 2005) in their respectively differing settings of not only their decision-support tools (e.g., Blue Menu) but also the broader message that data are needed when making decisions for serving Hawaii's youth. Members are transparent in their message that empiricism and other core scientific values are paramount in decision making and take precedence over allegiance to any specific type of treatment (e.g., cognitive behavioral therapy). This sophisticated view on evidence-based practices is conveyed through an open-door policy to anyone in the system to share concerns about decision-support tools, attend a committee meeting as a guest, join the committee as a member, or ask the committee to investigate the research literature for any certain type of treatment that may not be indicated as evidence-based by the committee's standards.

Second, an example of a partnership between CAMHD and the University of Hawaii is the Research and Evaluation Training Program, a health science and service learning collaboration that aims to provide leadership on systems-of-care research and evaluation, create service learning opportunities in research and evaluation, and provide leadership and support for scientific literacy and data-driven decision making within CAMHD and across its child-serving agencies.

The program represents over 10 years of formal partnership, which is mutually beneficial to both parties involved. For example, researchers learn about real-world concerns regarding the implementation of evidence-based practices in direct service settings, inspiring new research questions. And at the same time, researchers help to develop scientific literacy in CAMHD service staff while completing specialized evaluation projects for local and immediate-result application in service delivery settings (Chorpita & Mueller, 2008).

Across both examples shared above, several points are noteworthy toward the goal of maintaining an evidence-based system amidst a number of sustainability threats. First, consistent with the theme of "Infrastructure Development and Standardization" mentioned above, both EBS and Research and Evaluation Training Program units have been formalized or institutionalized, such that collaborations are not built around specific individuals or political alliances that can be transitory in nature. Second, both collaborations are transparent in the sense that there are no hidden agendas, and involved parties openly know what the other stands to gain. Finally, and perhaps most important, both emphasize the importance of input and approval from personnel and the role of social connections and mutually beneficial relationships.

Financial Planning and Creativity

As mentioned above, initial funding for many of the previously described programs and activities came as a result of mandated federal oversight with state funding for implementing the Felix Consent Decree. State legislative appropriations increased 350% from the late 1990s at $23.6 million to $106.5 million in 2003 (Higa-McMillan et al., 2009). However, since 2005, when federal oversight officially ended, inflation-adjusted legislative appropriations have decreased at an average rate of 13%. This section focuses on financial planning and creative strategies employed by system leadership for moderating the effects of financial constraint and cutbacks.

One core theme underlying several financial planning efforts is the notion of balancing temporary change stimuli with a vision for long-term effects and maintaining and sustaining an evidence-based system. As an example, when Felix Consent Decree implementation efforts first began in 1994, Hawaii leadership acknowledged that mandated federal oversight would eventually end, and that use of temporary federal support should be used to not only build an evidence-based system but also create internal supports within the system for long-term sustainment. Internal support efforts occurred not only through investing in the infrastructure development and partnership initiatives mentioned above but also through actively seeking other funding streams long before federal oversight for state funding ended. In other words, as the system matured between 1994 and 2005, federal funding was pursued as a way to supplement and slowly replace receding state funding. Funding from federal grants through the Substance Abuse and Mental Health Services Administration such as the Community Mental Health Services Block Grant, the State Mental Health Data Infrastructure Grant, the Systems of Care

Grant, and the Alternatives to Restraint and Seclusion State Incentive Grant were used not only to support their primary aims but also to boost the overall system commitment to evidence-based services for children and adolescents. Emphasis was less on bringing up specific evidence-based programs and was more on developing an evidence-based system of care that routinely used national and local evidence to inform practice. Additionally, federal funding through Medicaid was pursued for the service provision of specific evidence-based programs (e.g., Multisystemic Therapy).

The theme of balancing temporary change stimuli with a vision for long-term effects is especially important during this current time of acute financial constraint. Faced with the reality of financial cutbacks, leadership is forced to make very difficult decisions about reducing and/or terminating certain initiatives, committees, and programs. In doing so, keeping an eye to the future as well as relying on data to inform financial decisions may serve as a wise investment, as cutting certain types of initiatives too deeply may save money in the short term at the expense of significant cost escalation in the long term. One example of how the system has relied on data to inform financial decisions is through a cost-effectiveness analysis conducted by the Research and Evaluation Office at CAMHD. As service costs can be viewed as an investment in outcomes, Higa-McMillan, Daleiden, and Kimhan (2009) examined youth outcomes on the CAFAS and the MTPS per dollar spent within each of CAMHD's most commonly used intensive mental health service programs (i.e., Hospital Residential, Community Residential, Therapeutic Group Home, Multidimensional Treatment Foster Care, Therapeutic Foster Care, Multisystemic Therapy, Intensive In-Home Therapy, and Functional Family Therapy). They found that of the services with adequate sample sizes, all services demonstrated statistically significant improvements per dollar on at least one outcome measure, except for Therapeutic Group Homes. Thus, one potential area for cost savings may be either through improving the quality of services provided by group homes or by removing these programs altogether. One lesson regarding sustainability, then, is that all services and approaches may need continual scrutiny to identify and address areas of inefficiency in the system. Otherwise, in times of hardship, systems may simply employ a "recency bias"—cutting their latest innovations and most recently implemented flagship programs, simply because they were the last to come on board and because their costs are well known. Such a heuristic could quickly lead to the dissolution of evidence-based practice within many systems.

Another concept noteworthy of brief mention is the idea of cost sharing, where Hawaii demonstrates financial creativity during fiscally lean times. Over the past several years, the major analytic and writing responsibilities for two of Hawaii's major evidence-based decision-support tools (i.e., the Blue Menu and the Biennial Report) slowly shifted from a model using CAMHD staff, its EBS Committee, and work-for-hire through private consultants to a model that outsourced much of the analytic and reporting work to a private corporation specializing in these analytics (PracticeWise, LLC). Along with this change came both short- and long-term costs and benefits. First, having an outsourced team of professional coders and researchers complete the analytic and writing responsibilities for these decision-support tools allowed knowledge accumulation to occur at a much faster pace than when previously performed by of a team of committee volunteers and staff with other clinical responsibilities. Second, delegating these professional services freed up committee time to address both theoretical (e.g., partnering to provide conceptual input for refining decision-support tools) and practical (e.g., how study findings should affect best practices in Hawaii) issues relevant to evidence-based services (see EBS Committee performance indicators mentioned above). Third, given that other states, agencies, and individuals have sought similar analyses and reporting regarding the children's mental health evidence base, the costs of intensive coding and reporting are now distributed across a variety of organizations and individuals, creating economies of scale. These savings have allowed for an extraordinary level of innovation and development that would not have been sustainable at the individual state level; for example, PracticeWise recently created an extremely detailed interactive online reporting application, with metrics similar to those of the Blue Menu and the Biennial Report.

Increased Coordination for Dissemination and Implementation Strategies

As discussed up until now, with the help of federal oversight and coordinated strategic planning, CAMHD has put forth significant efforts to create an evidence-based system. Along the way, multiple partnerships have spawned numerous innovative ideas and practices in the areas of evidence-based practices and systems of care, many of which have been recognized at the national level. These innovations include, but are not limited to, CAMHD's clinical decision-support tools (e.g., the Biennial Report), Supervision Decision Making Framework, clinical reporting modules, and the innovative MTPS reporting scheme. Traditionally speaking, efforts for disseminating and implementing these innovations in direct service settings across all of CAMHD's service-providing agencies have been small and informal. Recently, however, with the vision of new leadership, and with the help of the Practice Development Office and EBS Committee, CAMHD has formally increased its focus on coordination, dissemination, and implementation efforts.

Over the years, the quality improvement committees discussed above as well as other child-serving agencies in Hawaii sometimes found themselves performing in "silos." Indeed, at times agencies outside Hawaii knew more about Hawaii's evidence-based practice initiatives than local agencies. Fixsen and colleagues (2005) suggested that this problem can be a common pattern found in peak-performing manufacturing teams, with a potential solution being cross-fertilization between teams for keeping staff aware of innovations and exposed to a diversity of ideas. Along these lines, efforts are now being made toward more strategically coordinating information within *and* between committees and agencies within the system.

Coordination efforts for disseminating and implementing evidence-based practices have taken several forms. First, the EBS Committee has recently decided to begin shifting its focus from that of knowledge accumulation for evidence-based practices (see its five performance indicators above under "Empirical Epistemology and Performance Evaluation") to disseminating and implementing various EBS products and the Supervision Decision Making Framework *within* Hawaii's system of care. Focusing primarily on reviewing over 350 articles over the past 10 years, it seemed that the committee did in fact become a "silo." Its small core membership of approximately 30 people learned more and more nuanced details about the randomized controlled trial literature, while many stakeholders in Hawaii's system continued their unawareness about even the existence of some of the most basic EBS products mentioned above. The committee has therefore formulated several new goals, many of which focus on increasing knowledge of and positive attitudes toward EBS products (cf. Fixsen et al.'s [2005] "exploration and adoption phase") for those stakeholders unfamiliar with them. These new goals and their associated performance indicators were still in development at the time this chapter was written. However, consistent with its past history of accumulating knowledge for data-driven decision making, the committee has begun reviewing dissemination and implementation articles from the scientific literature for informing its forthcoming strategies.

Several other coordination, dissemination, and implementation efforts are well under way. Unlike EBS Committee efforts that focus on early stages of implementation, these other efforts are focused on later stages such as "initial implementation" and "full operation" (Fixsen et al., 2005) at the level of the direct service provider. First, CAMHD's specialized Practice Development Office has increased its efforts in training direct service providers. As mentioned above, innovative trainings focused on practice elements common across many evidence-based treatments (rather than specific manual brand names) with increased role-playing activities for behavioral rehearsal opportunities (rather than pure didactic lecturing) are sponsored by the state on a frequent and ongoing basis. Second, the Research and Evaluation Training Program hosts regular "data parties" for direct service providers and supervisors, during which feedback is provided on how their self-reported intervention practices (as reported by their MTPS forms described above) align with practices from the evidence-based services literature as well as with what other providers in the state are using for similar youth (Higa-McMillan, Powell, Daleiden, & Mueller, 2011). For example, data on the frequency with which an agency reports using practices drawn from evidence-based versus non–evidence-based approaches (e.g., exposure vs. catharsis in the context of youth with anxiety disorders) is graphically displayed and is compared to the state average use of these practice elements (e.g., how often do all state agencies use exposure for anxiety?). The feedback environment is collaborative in nature, with feedback going two ways between researchers and service providers.

Like other public behavioral health service systems, Hawaii has and continues to face significant threats to sustaining gains for delivering evidence-based services within its system of care. With Hawaii's period of mandated federal oversight officially ending in 2005, factors such as financial constraint and frequent and significant staff turnover are examples of such threats that have become especially salient within the last several years. Hawaii's efforts to sustain and maintain its evidence-based system has thus far focused on the five major themes of (a) empirical epistemology and performance evaluation; (b) infrastructure development and standardization; (c) building and maintaining partnerships; (d) financial planning and creativity; and (e) increased focus on coordination, dissemination, and implementation strategies.

RESULTS AND CONCLUSIONS SO FAR

CAMHD measures outcomes of evidence-based services in multiple ways. Given the hybrid system of evidence-based package programs (e.g., Functional Family Therapy) and the practice elements approach to treatment (mentioned above) as well as the desire to provide both continuous outcome evaluation and comprehensive program evaluation, the system of care has implemented several ways of evaluating outcomes. Package programs are continuously monitored through a combination of treatment developer standardized measures (e.g., the Therapist Adherence Measures for MST) as well as youth, parent, clinician, and case manager reports of clinical improvement. On the developer side, individual cases are managed through highly structured supervision and national consultation with direct care providers where both clinical progress and treatment model adherence are monitored. On the system side, case managers and program monitors routinely evaluate clinical progress and practice through multiple measurement tools (e.g., see measurement systems mentioned above in the section on quality improvement initiatives for services and standards of care).

Package programs are also evaluated at the aggregated group level in more traditional program evaluation fashion. The CAMHD produces an annual evaluation report that includes an evaluation of outcomes by service program. In fiscal year 2008, youth in the three evidence-based programs implemented in CAMHD (MST, FFT, and MTFC) demonstrated significantly improved treatment progress ratings by therapist report, and youth in MST demonstrated significantly reduced functional impairment by case manager report (Higa-McMillan et al., 2009). Although FFT and MTFC did not demonstrate statistically significant change in functional impairment, this was likely due to the fact that there was a small sample size because the services are relatively new to the system. Further support for MST in Hawaii was evidenced by Tolman, Mueller, Daleiden, Stumpf, and Pestle (2008). Tolman and colleagues found that although effect sizes were smaller than those reported by developers of the program in randomized controlled trials, effects were similar and within the 95% confidence interval.

The implementation of elements commonly used in evidence-based treatments is evaluated on a continuous individual case-by-case basis as well as at the aggregated group level. Direct service providers in the state submit monthly treatment summaries, which include a list of the individual practice elements they used in their treatment. This information is tracked at the individual level and is displayed on a dashboard (e.g., CRM mentioned above), where case managers and clinical supervisors monitor practices. Treatment team members are thus encouraged to monitor treatment practices and to suggest alternative practice elements when treatment is not progressing as indicated by outcome measures. At the group level, routine monitoring of youth outcomes and use of evidence-based treatment practice elements are aggregated by program within provider agencies and are compared to statewide benchmarks as well as the evidence-based literature as described above (Higa-McMillan et al., 2011).

Additionally, longitudinal outcomes of practice elements employed by direct care providers in the state are currently being evaluated. Studies under way are exploring whether the use of specific practice elements predict faster rates of improvement over the course of treatment. Initial findings suggest that greater use of elements commonly used in evidence-based treatments is associated with increased rates of youth functional improvement for attention-deficit/hyperactivity disorder (Mueller, Daleiden, Chorpita, Tolman, & Higa-McMillan, 2009).

Under mandated federal oversight, many innovative strategies were employed in Hawaii to create a system of care. Over time, through leadership and collaboration, Hawaii's system evolved into a highly functioning evidence-based service system. Five core strategies were utilized by CAMHD to sustain and maintain its evidence-based service system. Across all five, two concepts seem apparent and noteworthy of mention. First, when faced with major difficulties such as rapidly receding funding, an emphasis should be placed on sustainment and maintenance of existing initiatives rather than creating new ones. However, because a system's needs and goals are never static and change over time, it is noteworthy that the term "sustainment" here does not necessarily refer to continuation of the same policies and procedures. Utilized here, sustainment refers to an ongoing commitment to a set of principles for helping children and families. In other words, although CAMHD's day-to-day operations continue to evolve, its dedication to evidence-based principles has not. Second, the synergistic marriage of practice and science in the public health sector setting is not easy, and is a humbling experience for all involved. The journey on the path of providing evidence-based treatments to youth and their families began many years ago, and the path is proving longer and more challenging than originally anticipated. Sustaining this commitment to progress and to science-driven practice should thus be viewed as a fluid and ongoing process, rather than a single task or initiative. Given the expectation of continuing innovation in the treatment outcome literature and the constant evolution and uncertainty of public mental health, this is the only view that makes sense.

REFERENCES

Aarons, G. A. (2004). Mental health provider attitudes toward adoption of evidence-based practice: The evidence-based practice attitude scale (EBPAS). *Mental Health Services Research, 6*, 61–74.

Achenbach, T. M., & Rescorla, L. A. (2001). *Manual for ASEBA school-age forms & profiles.* Burlington, VT: University of Vermont, Research Center for Children, Youth, & Families.

Alexander, J. F., & Parsons, B. V. (1973). Short-term behavioral intervention with delinquent families: Impact on family process and recidivism. *Journal of Abnormal Psychology, 81*, 219–225.

American Academy of Child, Adolescent Psychiatry & American Association of Community Psychiatrists. (1999). *Child and adolescent level of care utilization system: User's manual.* Pittsburgh: American Association of Community Psychiatrists.

Becker, K. D., Nakamura, B. J., Young, J., & Chorpita, B. F. (2009). What better place than here, what better time than now? ABCT's burgeoning role in the dissemination and implementation of evidence-based practices. *The Behavior Therapist, 32*, 89–96.

Borntrager, C. F., Chorpita, B. F., Higa-McMillan, C., Weisz, J. R., & the Research Network on Youth Mental Health. (2009). Provider attitudes toward evidence-based practices: Are the concerns with the evidence or with the manuals? *Psychiatric Services, 60*, 1–5.

Chamberlain, P., & Reid, J. B. (1998). Comparison of two community alternatives to incarceration for chronic juvenile offenders. *Journal of Consulting and Clinical Psychology, 66*, 624–633.

Child and Adolescent Mental Health Division. (2002). *Evidence-based services committee - Biennial report - Summary of effective interventions for youth with behavioral and emotional needs.* Honolulu, HI: Hawaii Department of Health, Child and Adolescent Mental Health Division.

Child and Adolescent Mental Health Division. (2003). *Instructions and codebook for provider monthly summaries.* Honolulu, HI: Hawaii Department of Health, Child and Adolescent Mental Health Division.

Child and Adolescent Mental Health Division. (2004). *Evidence-based services committee - Biennial report - Summary of effective interventions for youth with behavioral and emotional needs.* Honolulu, HI: Hawaii Department of Health, Child and Adolescent Mental Health Division.

Chorpita, B. F. (2003). The frontier of evidence-based practice. In A. E. Kazdin & J. R. Weisz (Eds.), *Evidence-based psychotherapies for children and adolescents* (pp. 42–59). New York: Guilford Press.

Chorpita, B. F., Becker, K. D., & Daleiden, E. L. (2007). Understanding the common elements of evidence-based practice: Misconceptions and clinical examples. *Journal of the American Academy of Child and Adolescent Psychiatry, 46*, 647–652.

Chorpita, B. F., & Daleiden, E. (2007). *Evidence-based services committee - Biennial report - Effective psychological interventions for youth with behavioral and emotional needs.* Honolulu, HI: Hawaii Department of Health, Child and Adolescent Mental Health Division.

Chorpita, B. F., & Daleiden, E. L. (2009). Mapping evidence-based treatments for children and adolescents: Application of the distillation and matching model to 615 treatments from 322 randomized trials. *Journal of Consulting and Clinical Psychology, 77,* 566–579.

Chorpita, B. F., & Daleiden, E. L. (2010). Building evidence-based systems in children's mental health. In J. R. Weisz and A. E. Kazdin (Eds.) *Evidence-based psychotherapies for children and adolescents* (2nd ed.) (pp. 482–499). New York: Guilford Press.

Chorpita, B. F., Daleiden, E., & Weisz, J. R. (2005). Identifying and selecting the common elements of evidence based interventions: A distillation and matching model. *Mental Health Services Research, 7,* 5–20.

Chorpita, B. F., & Donkervoet, C. (2005). Implementation of the Felix Consent Decree in Hawaii: The impact of policy and practice development efforts on service delivery. In R. G. Steele & M. C. Roberts (Eds.), *Handbook of mental health services for children, adolescents, and families* (pp. 317–332). New York: Kluwer Academic/Plenum Publishers.

Chorpita, B. F., & Mueller, C. W. (2008). Toward new models for research, community, and consumer partnerships: Some guiding principles and an illustration. *Clinical Psychology: Science and Practice, 15,* 144–148.

Chorpita, B. F., Yim, L. M., Donkervoet, J. C., Arensdorf, A., Amundsen, M. J., McGee, C., et al. (2002). Toward large-scale implementation of empirically supported treatments for children: A review and observations by the Hawaii empirical basis to services task force. *Clinical Psychology: Science and Practice, 9,* 165–165.

Daleiden, E., & Chorpita, B. F. (2005). From data to wisdom: Quality improvement strategies supporting large-scale implementation of evidence based services. *Child and Adolescent Psychiatric Clinics of North America, 14,* 329–349.

Daleiden, E. L., Chorpita, B. F., Donkervoet, C., Arensdorf, A. M., & Brogan, M. (2006). Getting better at getting them better: Health outcomes and evidence-based practice within a system of care. *Journal of the American Academy of Child & Adolescent Psychiatry, 45,* 749–756.

Daleiden, E., Lee, J., & Tolman, R. (2004). *Child and Adolescent Mental Health Division: 2004 annual report.* Honolulu, HI: Child and Adolescent Mental Health Division.

Dulcan, M. K. (2005). Practitioner perspectives on evidence-based practice. *Child and Adolescent Psychiatric Clinics of North America, 14,* 225–240.

Fixsen, D. L., Naoom, S. F., Blase, K. A., Friedman, R. M. & Wallace, F. (2005). *Implementation research: A synthesis of the literature* (FMHI Publication #231). Tampa, FL: University of South Florida, Louis de la Parte Florida Mental Health Institute, The National Implementation Research Network.

Hayes, S. C., Barlow, D. H., & Nelson-Gray, R. O. (1999). *The scientist practitioner: Research and accountability in the age of managed care.* Needham Heights, MA: Allyn & Bacon.

Henggeler, S. W, & Borduin, C. M. (1990). *Family therapy and beyond: A multisystemic approach to treating the behavior problems of children and adolescents.* Pacific Grove, CA: Brooks/Cole.

Higa-McMillan, C., Daleiden, E., & Kimhan, C. K. (2009). *Child and Adolescent Mental Health Division: 2008 annual report.* Honolulu, HI: Child and Adolescent Mental Health Division.

Higa-McMillan, C. K., Powell, C. K. K., Daleiden, E. L., & Mueller, C. W. (2011). Pursuing an evidence-based culture through contextualized feedback: Aligning youth outcomes and practices. *Professional Psychology: Research and Practice, 42,* 137–144.

Hodges, K., & Wong, M. M. (1996). Psychometric characteristics of a multidimensional measure to assess impairment: The Child and Adolescent Functional Assessment Scale. *Journal of Child and Family Studies, 5*, 445–467.

Lonigan, C. J., Elbert, J. C., & Bennett Johnson, S. (1998). Empirically supported psychosocial interventions for children: An overview. *Journal of Clinical Child Psychology, 27*, 138–145.

McNeil, C. B., Eyberg, S., Einstadt, T. H., Newcomb, K., & Funderburk, B. (1991). Parent-Child Interaction Therapy with behavior problem children: Generalization of treatment effects to the school setting. *Journal of Clinical Child Psychology, 20*, 140–151.

Mueller, C. W., Daleiden, E. L., Chorpita, B. F., Tolman, R. T., & Higa-McMillan, C. (2009, August). EBS practice elements and youth outcomes in a statewide system. In A. Marder (Chair), *A demonstration of mapping and traversing the science-practice gap*. Symposium conducted at the annual convention of the American Psychological Association, Toronto, Canada.

Nakamura, B. J., Daleiden, E. L., & Mueller, C. W. (2007). Validity of treatment target progress ratings as indicators of youth improvement. *Journal of Child and Family Studies, 16*, 729–741.

Orimoto, T. E., Higa-McMillan, C. K., Mueller, C. W., & Daleiden, E. L. (2011). Measurement and organization of therapeutic practice elements in a youth community mental health setting. Manuscript in preparation.

Rogers, E. M. (2003). *Diffusion of innovations* (4th ed.). New York: Free Press.

Schiffman, J., & Donkervoet, T. (2008). Improving services through evidence-based practice elements. In E. Stroul & G. Blau (Ed.), *The system of care handbook: Transforming mental health services for children, youth and families* (pp. 437–468). Baltimore, MD: Paul H Brookes Publishing Company.

State of Hawaii. (2006). *Interagency performance standards and guidelines*. Honolulu, HI: Hawaii Departments of Child and Adolescent Mental Health Division and Education.

Stroul, B. A., & Friedman, R. (1986). *A system of care for children and youth with severe emotional disturbances* (Revised edition.). Washington, DC: Georgetown University Child Development Center, CASSP Technical Assistance Center.

Stumpf, R. E., Higa-McMillan, C. K., & Chorpita, B. F. (2008). Implementation of evidence-based services for youth: Assessing provider knowledge. *Behavior Modification, 33*, 48–65.

Task Force on Promotion and Dissemination of Psychological Procedures, Division of Clinical Psychology, American Psychological Association. (1995). Training in and dissemination of empirically-validated psychological treatments: Report and recommendations. *The Clinical Psychologist, 48*, 3–23.

Tolman, R. T., Mueller, C. W., Daleiden, E. L., Stumpf, R. E., & Pestle, S. L. (2008). Outcomes from Multisystemic Therapy in a statewide system of care. *Journal of Child and Family Studies, 17*, 894–908.

{10}

Dissemination and Implementation of Dialectical Behavior Therapy
AN INTENSIVE TRAINING MODEL
Sara J. Landes and Marsha M. Linehan

Dialectical Behavior Therapy (DBT) is a comprehensive cognitive behavioral treatment originally developed to treat suicidal patients that evolved into a treatment for suicidal patients with borderline personality disorder (BPD). It has since been adapted for the treatment of patients with BPD and presenting problems other than suicidal behaviors. To date, there have been 11 published randomized controlled trials (RCTs) on DBT (Koons et al., 2001; Linehan, Armstrong, Suarez, Allmon, & Heard, 1991; Linehan et al., 1999, 2002, 2006; Lynch, Morse, Mendelson, & Robins, 2003; McMain et al., 2009; Safer, Telch, & Agras, 2001; Telch, Agras, & Linehan, 2001; van den Bosch, Verheul, Schippers, & van den Brink, 2002; Verheul et al., 2003) and five controlled trials (Barley et al., 1993; Bohus et al., 2000; Koerner & Dimeff, 2000; Stanley, Ivanoff, Brodsky, & Oppenheim, 1998; Trupin, Stewart, Beach, & Boesky, 2002). At present, DBT is considered the front-line treatment for BPD, suicidal behavior, and severe behavioral dyscontrol. The Substance Abuse and Mental Health Services Administration's (SAMHSA) National Registry of Evidence-based Programs and Practices independently rated DBT as a well-researched treatment effective at reducing suicide attempts, non-suicidal self-injury, drug use, and symptoms of eating disorders and improving psychosocial adjustment and treatment retention (SAMHSA, 2006).

Given the effectiveness of DBT in a difficult-to-treat population with high utilization of services and therefore high expense, as well as high societal cost (Geller, 1986; Surber et al., 1987; Swigar, Astrachan, Levine, Mayfield, & Radovich, 1991; van Asselt, Dirksen, Arntz, & Severens, 2007; Widiger & Weissman, 1991; Woogh, 1986), DBT dissemination and training has been in high demand. In response to the initial demand, DBT treatment developer Marsha Linehan first provided lectures and workshops on the new treatment and disseminated the treatment manual to interested providers. Before long, however, the demand for DBT training outstripped her group's available time. Through a succession of training organizations (the University of Washington Linehan Training Group; the Behavioral Technology Transfer Group; Behavioral Tech, LLC; the nonprofit Marie Institute for Behavioral Technology; the

University of Washington Behavioral Research and Therapy Clinics), she sought to increase opportunities for training by bringing together graduate students, former students, and colleagues trained in DBT as additional trainers and DBT consultants. Over time, training by these individuals has been aimed at graduate students and psychology and psychiatry residents in training, individual providers, clinical treatment teams, private and public mental health outpatient clinics, psychiatric inpatient units, residential treatment centers, county and state mental health care systems, adult forensic and juvenile justice systems, and various other systems looking for effective interventions for high-risk, high-danger, and out-of-control clients. Historically, DBT training has been based on an "early adopter model" in which interested groups who demonstrate high levels of interest seek training. The focus of this chapter is to describe the DBT Intensive Training Model developed by Linehan and first implemented in 1993. This model was developed once it became clear that training with 1- or 2-day workshops would not be sufficient for teaching both basic concepts of cognitive behavioral therapy and specific concepts unique to DBT. The chapter will also describe how this model fits with other implementation models, data about its effectiveness, and future directions.

EFFECTIVENESS OF STANDARD WORKSHOP TRAINING

The standard method of transferring evidence-based treatments (EBTs) for mental disorders to the clinical community has been and still is brief clinical workshops, ordinarily lasting 1 or 2 days. All professional organizations offer these workshops at annual meetings, and licensing boards do not require more in-depth training to satisfy required continuing education credits. Although this method has been in use for years, there is little evidence that it is effective in advancing evidence-based treatment implementation. Davis and colleagues (1999) reviewed a number of RCTs of formal didactic and/or interactive continuing medical education (CME) interventions and reported that although there is some evidence that interactive CME sessions can effect change in professional practice and, on occasion, health care outcomes, didactic sessions do not appear to be effective in changing physician performance. Sohn, Ismail, and Tellez (2004) examined 11 systematic reviews and concluded that the evidence showed that formal CME and distributing educational materials do not effectively change primary care providers' behaviors. While changes in mental health provider knowledge are consistently demonstrated after training in EBTs as well as other continuing education topics (Bootzin & Ruggill, 1988; Freiheit & Overholser, 1997; Miller & Rollnick, 1991; Sholomskas et al., 2005), only six studies have demonstrated that practitioners (outside of research therapists trained for efficacy trials) can conduct a psychotherapy EBT after training based on observed therapist behavior (Crits-Christoph et al., 1998; Henry, Strupp, Butler, Schacht, & Binder, 1993; Sholomskas et al., 2005), and only three studies found that psychotherapy EBT training resulted in improved client outcomes (Milne, Baker, Blackburn, James, & Reichelt, 1999; Russell, Silver, Rogers, & Darnell, 2007; Strosahl, Hayes,

Bergan, & Romano, 1998). Many larger studies that have investigated therapist training have not reported therapist participant dropout rate (Crits-Christoph et al., 1998; Henry et al., 1993; Milne et al., 1999; Sholomskas et al., 2005). However, studies investigating training in Motivational Interviewing have reported attrition rates, functionally defined as rates of completion of research measures after training. These studies reported 91% to 100% completion of study measures at posttraining, 76% to 100% completion at 4-month follow-up, 54% completion at 8-month follow-up, and 45% completion at 12-month follow-up (Miller & Mount, 2001; Miller, Yahne, Moyers, Martinez, & Pirritano, 2004).

HISTORY AND DEVELOPMENT OF THE DIALECTICAL BEHAVIOR THERAPY INTENSIVE TRAINING MODEL

The first steps in DBT dissemination were incorporated into the original treatment manual (Linehan, 1993a). In particular, Linehan was interested in why treatments that work in efficacy trials often do not work in community settings. While some work has been done on just this topic, what has largely been ignored is an examination of whether the treatment manuals used to disseminate treatments include all of the relevant treatment characteristics applied in clinical trials. Two characteristics of clinical efficacy trials are almost never included in descriptions of the treatments themselves—the use of regular therapist meetings to support and maintain adherence to the manual and the evaluation of clinical outcomes at regular intervals in the treatment. In writing the DBT treatment manual, these two characteristics were included as essential characteristics of the treatment rather than characteristics of the research enterprise. Therapist treatment teams that meet regularly as well as regular and systematic evaluation of treatment outcome are considered essential elements of DBT.

The DBT Intensive Training Model (ITM) was developed by Linehan in response to the demand for DBT training following the publication of the first RCT in 1991 demonstrating the efficacy of DBT (Linehan et al., 1991) and the DBT treatment manuals (Linehan, 1993a, 1993b) in 1993. The DBT ITM is an outcome of an evolution of efforts by Linehan to develop a method for transporting DBT from university to community clinical settings. Like DBT itself, the ITM was developed through iterative attempts to respond to the needs of community providers to learn the treatment and implement and adapt it to their own mental health settings.

Initial limitations of standard continuing education formats led to a number of modifications that are now important features of the ITM: (a) the training schedule was expanded to include two 5-day training segments separated by a 6-month self-study and trial implementation, (b) the structure of the ITM and practice and homework exercises were reorganized to target team building and mutual responsibility for learning and implementing DBT, (c) a substantial set of contingency management procedures were instituted, and (d) content and coaching on how to use DBT strategies to target barriers to full implementation and maintenance of DBT programs within providers' organizations was added. The first DBT Intensive Training Course (ITC) was held in 1993 with six teams attending.

DIALECTICAL BEHAVIOR THERAPY INTENSIVE TRAINING COURSE

Intensive Training Course Structure

The ITC is provided in two 5-day trainings (Parts I and II) separated by 6 months of self-study. In accordance with Michaelsen's (1983) recommendations, training is based on team learning. Team members are seated together at a round table to facilitate discussion, and physical placement of teams within the overall training group is changed daily.

Part I

The first 5-day training (Part I) covers the main content areas of DBT, with structure and elements of DBT taught, modeled with video and/or role play, and practiced within teams. Each day includes mindfulness practice, chain analyses of participants who were late that session or engaged in any other training-interfering behavior, review of feedback from the previous day, and teaching on new topics with team-based exercises and viewing of recorded therapy sessions. Trainers have the flexibility in the training schedule to tailor the experiences to specific needs of the group and ensure they target both practicing new concepts and building team behavior. Therefore, while the content covered in each intensive training remains the same, one intensive training course may have topics fall on different days than others (e.g., spending more time to clarify contingency management leads to finishing the topic on the following day). On most days, team homework assignments are given and then presented the next morning.

Day 1 orients teams to training and concentrates on the foundation (e.g., the biosocial theory, research on DBT) and structure of DBT. As each part of the structure is taught, teams begin to plan the organization of their DBT team, receive consultation from trainers, and conceptualize implementation problems that could arise. During each teaching section, there is at least one experiential exercise, as well as team-based exercises and team homework assignments over lunch periods and evenings. These exercises are designed to challenge the team to problem solve possible issues. For example, during the first teaching section on day 1, the DBT consultation team agreements are taught. Teams are given time to go through these in depth and determine if any of the agreements are going to prove difficult for any of the team members. Active debate is encouraged during such exercises with a focus on finding the synthesis and troubleshooting difficulties before they occur. Day 2 continues with the structure of DBT and, after discussing targeting in treatment, addresses the assessment and treatment of suicidal behavior in DBT. Teams learn how to build these suicidal behavior protocols and practices into their programs. Day 3 focuses on dialectics and validation. As dialectics is a key to management of a DBT team and program, teams complete several practice exercises on what to do when team members are polarized, when therapists are polarized with clients, and when the team is polarized with administration. Day 4 concentrates on behavior therapy, which includes behavioral analysis, skills training, problem solving, contingency management, orienting to treatment, and obtaining commitment to treatment. Team members watch video samples and practice with role-play exercises. Day 5 addresses stylistic strategies, case management, and the consultation team. Finally, ITC self-study (i.e., homework) for Part II is distributed as a packet. Trainers orient teams to the self-study and answer questions. Teams are given time to review the self-study and create a plan for completing the assignments. Trainers ask teams to commit to a plan and either set a date for their first study group or assign a member of their team as the responsible person for setting up the study group. Problem-solving strategies are used to aid teams in creating a plan for successful completion of the self-study.

Two hours of training are devoted specifically to walking trainees through steps for implementing their DBT clinical program in their home setting. Topics covered include the following implementation issues: (a) who to treat, and how to target who to treat; (b) how to navigate/restructure the system as it currently exists if necessary; (c) how to overcome challenges to setting up all modes of DBT; (d) how to hold onto a DBT frame in the midst of a system with a different orientation and approach to treatment; (e) how to explain DBT's approach to case management that can often conflict with treatment as usual (TAU); (f) how to contend with union, salary, legal, billing, and staffing issues surrounding phone availability; (g) how to integrate DBT suicide crisis protocols when they run counter to standard legal/medical protocols; and (h) how to resist pressures to combine staff/administrative time with the "consult meeting" time. Several training modes are used, such as didactic presentation including examples from trainers' experience implementing DBT, team-based exercises (e.g., matching their current DBT program and future DBT plans with the modes and functions of DBT), small group discussions among the teams with consultation from the trainers, homework assignments that explicitly address these issues (e.g., program presentation at Part II, explicit documentation of inclusion and exclusion criteria), and contingency management including positive reinforcement of all adaptive behaviors by trainees (e.g., demonstration of problem solving, troubleshooting, etc.) and potential aversive contingency of presentation of the homework at Part II (which can be embarrassing if not complete).

Intensive Training Course Self-Study

Michaelsen (1983) suggests that new learning occurs when teams work together inside and outside of class. Between Parts I and II, a self-study is completed by the team and individual members practicing DBT principles and strategies. Individuals must complete the DBT take-home exam (first as a closed book exam, second as open book, and third by review in team). The team is instructed to review the exam and ensure everyone understands the correct answers given in a sealed envelope to the team leaders. Following completion of the 22 individual self-study assignments (e.g., explaining biosocial theory, completing a diary card, doing chain analyses), each participant completes a DBT Individual Homework Score Sheet. The team self-study is composed of 15 assignments, including agreeing on any program adaptations for their own setting, writing a program description, developing program inclusion and exclusion criteria, determining program outcome measures, writing a detailed case formulation, practicing strategies, and putting together a poster describing their program and program adaptations.

To create skills and a contingency for learning suicide risk assessment and DBT crisis call protocols, one member of each team receives a "suicide call" from a trainer before Part II. The trainer poses as a suicidal client and allows the participant to respond freely. Afterward, the trainer calls the participant again and reviews the call, highlighting positive aspects and giving feedback on what was missing and aspects to be strengthened. The participant discusses the call with the team at their next meeting.

Part II

During Part II all teams present their self-study. The morning of day 1 is dedicated to reviewing assignments and the DBT exam and answering questions. Teams present case formulations, complete with role plays, and their programs. Trainers structure consultation on cases and program descriptions to ensure teams receive valid positive reinforcement and constructive feedback from other teams and the trainers. Additional training on areas teams appear weak on is provided didactically or through exercises or role plays. At the beginning of day 1, each team leader completes a score sheet with input from the team members. This team score sheet summarizes the individual self-study and the completion of the team self-study. At the end of day 4, the team with the highest score is given a prize, usually a mindfulness bell or DBT videos or CDs.

A major focus of Part II is to consult with each team about barriers to implementation in their clinical settings. During these individualized consultations, all teams are invited to provide input and coaching such that a shared set of implementation strategies are developed. A course e-mail list is set up so teams can consult with each other about solving implementation problems. After Part II, teams can join the international listserv of teams who have completed the ITC. The listserv is quite active; posts include practical questions about how others implement different aspects of DBT (e.g., what do teams do with diary cards?), theoretical questions (e.g., how can a given problem be viewed dialectically?), inquiries about adaptations or uses with different populations or in different settings (e.g., are different skills used for adolescents?), and queries for referrals in different locations (e.g., a client is moving to another state and would like to continue with DBT). Members of the listserv are responsive to posts and interesting discussions often occur. I (SJL) recently posted a request for a referral in another state and received six detailed and helpful replies within 3 days, including offers of additional assistance if needed. Others have expressed thanks in listserv posts for plentiful, helpful, and supportive responses.

Consultation to Teams

Between Parts I and II, trainers act as consultants to teams. Each team is given a letter at the end of Part I telling them how to get in touch with trainers. In addition, trainers check in with team leaders during the homework period to ensure all consultation issues are addressed. In general, teams are not expected to average more than two calls per team between Parts I and II.

Contingency Management of Teams

Trainers play close attention to contingencies in the ITC. Teams are reinforced with praise or validation for completing tasks and changing attitudes/behaviors. All assignments are publicly reviewed and all teams are expected to complete assignments. Noncompletion of assignments and other training-interfering behaviors (e.g., lack of attention) are targeted with behavioral chain analyses, problem solving, and contingency management strategies. A prize is given to the team with the highest cumulative score for completion of assignments. If teams do not complete the exam, case presentation, or program descriptions and presentations, they do not receive the team certificate attesting to attendance and completion of assignments. Under some circumstances, teams are given additional time to complete assignments. Although names of team members attending the ITC are listed on certificates, the actual certificates attest to a team completing the training, not to individuals.

Funding of Training Efforts

Funding for teams to attend the ITC occurs in a variety of ways. Teams working within an agency or institution may have training funds available to use to attend trainings. Sometimes the agencies apply for small grants from state or foundation funders to pay for training. Other participants, such as teams working in private practice, may pay for their attendance to the ITC with personal contributions.

Individual states may contract and pay for the training of several teams at once. In this case, the state will request applications from the relevant agencies that have potential DBT teams and want to attend the training. Requesting applications for the training enhances the likelihood of having motivated individuals (opinion leaders and early adopters) who are interested in learning the treatment attend the training.

If no opinion leaders are apparent, the system often arranges for a more extensive DBT "implementation training" that includes additional training and support prior to and after the ITC. At the start of the implementation, there is a 2-day kickoff event with the goal of communicating what DBT is to as many people as possible in the system before training. Following this kickoff, a third day is devoted to interaction with agency administrators and their direct staff supervisors to discuss the intensive training model and how to identify early adopters on their staff who are most enthused about DBT and most likely to make it stick, and to answer questions about the resources needed to implement DBT and its likely impact on the agency. Orienting and commitment strategies are used with potential teams and management, parallel to how they are used in the beginning of treatment with a client, to ensure that only voluntarily motivated teams come to the training. Orienting the system at this level is designed to bring teams closer to being early adopters, like those who seek out standard ITCs. Note that in system implementations extra training is also provided after the ITC is completed to help ensure DBT continues and expands given that the teams selected by this method—even with the ITC's focus on how to be an opinion leader—are less likely to succeed since they did not come to the training at a time that was ideal for their agency and with experience in DBT but instead grabbed a training opportunity offered by their system at an essentially arbitrary time.

CONCEPTUAL MODELS OF IMPLEMENTATION
OF EVIDENCE-BASED PRACTICE

While the intensive training model (ITM) was developed before conceptual models for successful implementation such as those by Simpson (Simpson, 2002, 2004; Simpson & Flynn, 2007), Fixsen (Fixsen, Naoom, Blase, Friedman, & Wallace, 2005), and Glisson (Glisson, Dukes, & Green, 2006; Glisson & Schoenwald, 2005) were developed, the ITM substantially reflects the principles in these models. The Program Change Model developed by Simpson (2002) and expanded by Simpson and Flynn (2007) emphasizes the implementation process and divides it into four crucial features that are characteristic of the ITM. (See Table 10.1 for a comparison of ITM and the Program Change Model.)

First, *exposure to a new treatment* via *training* includes didactic information but also hands-on practice with feedback and rewards for progress, realistic views of skill requirements and limitations, team building, peer support, and empirical evaluation of results. The ITM includes not only didactic presentations but also hands-on practice with feedback and reinforcement during the training sessions and via practice exercises given to the teams as homework between the initial and follow-up trainings. The key aspect of training according to Simpson is that it is relevant, accessible, and accredited, all of which are true of the ITM as it has developed over the past 17 years. (See also "Conceptual Models of Training" below for further discussion of training research and the ITM.)

The second stage is *adoption,* which is used by Simpson and Flynn (2007) to indicate a trial process of implementation involving decision making and action taking. Decision making is based on leadership support, the perceived quality and utility of the intervention in the real-world setting, and its perceived adaptability for the specific nuances of the treatment setting. The Part I 5-day training course of the ITM closely matches this process as specific didactic presentations, exercises,

TABLE 10.1 Relationship of Dialectical Behavior Therapy Intensive Training to Simpson Model of Stages of Change and Organizational Readiness and Context

Stages of Change	DBT Intensive Training Component
Stage 1: Exposure	
a. Lecture	75% of individuals likely will have attended previous DBT lectures or 2-day workshops
b. Self-study	Self-study assigned at screening until Part I and at the end of Part I for 6 months until Part II
c. Workshop	Two 5-day training workshops (Part I, Part II)
d. Consultation	Consultation occurs during Part I and Part II and is available during the Self-Study
Stage 2: Adoption	
a. Individual decisions	Individual application questions trigger such decisions. Day 1 of Part I: Teams coached in DBT commitment strategies to elicit and strengthen commitments from each team member to learn DBT and contribute to its implementation
b. Group decisions	Team leader application and interview questions trigger decisions to implement as a team. Day 2 of Part I: Team exercises to develop DBT implementation plan
c. Exploratory use	Initial program development and homework assignments between Part I and Part II
Stage 3: Implementation	
Stage 4: Practice improvement	
Characteristics of Organizational Readiness (Simpson)	DBT Training Component Targeting Organizational Characteristics
1. Motivation to Learn and Use New Treatment	
a. Motivated treatment providers	Contingencies for practicing, learning, and implementing DBT
b. Motivated program managers	Training in using DBT strategies with program managers to increase their motivation
c. Sufficient institutional resources	Training in using DBT strategies to find and obtain institutional resources
2. Reception and (Perceived) Utility of New Treatment	
a. Adequate training	The DBT exam and implementation assess this outcome
b. Easy to use and fits in context	Training in how to adapt DBT for specific settings
c. Fit with abilities of providers	Part I: Team exercises to organize provider roles in accord with provider abilities

(Continued)

TABLE 10.1 Relationship of Dialectical Behavior Therapy Intensive Training to Simpson Model of Stages of Change and Organizational Readiness and Context (*Continued*)

Stages of Change	DBT Intensive Training Component
3. Organizational Climate for Change	
a. Clarity of mission and goals	Parts I and II: Team exercises to clarify team mission and goals
b. Staff cohesion/teamwork	Parts I, II, and consultation: Team-building exercises and consultation
c. Clinical autonomy	Training in using DBT skills with program managers to increase autonomy
d. Communication	Training in using DBT interpersonal skills to improve communication within team and with colleagues and program managers
e. Openness to change	Training in DBT skills for openness to change and in "marketing" DBT within organization
4. Institutional Supports	
a. Monitoring	Training in outcomes assessment as essential part of DBT
b. Feedback and reinforcement	Formal and informal reinforcement during training; training in provision of feedback and reinforcement to team members as part of DBT teams and to agency administration
5. Staff Attributes	
a. Efficacy, adaptability	
b. Influence	Training in "marketing" DBT; provision of teaching materials and information designed to demonstrate value of DBT to organization

(Lehman, Greener, & Simpson, 2002; Simpson, 2002, 2004; Simpson & Flynn, 2007)

and team discussions are focused on ensuring the team can see the quality, utility, and adaptability of DBT to their setting. In addition, DBT strategies are taught not only by lecture but also by team-specific consultation to directly address barriers to full leadership support at home. Action taking involves a trial implementation of the innovation that allows adopters to form opinions about applications. The key issues in this trial period are the capacity and proficiency of the innovation to meet expectations, produce satisfactory preliminary results, and manage resistance. In the ITM, this trial period is engineered into the homework required by the teams in the 6 months between the Part I and II trainings. Specifically, the homework requires trainees to implement a DBT program, collect outcome data, and present the program at the Part II training along with specific difficulties they have encountered. Anecdotal experience and data presented by trainees indicate that this 6-month trial period, combined with consultation provided to each program during the Part II training, can satisfactorily address trainees' concerns.

The third major stage in the Simpson and Flynn Program of Change model is called *implementation* and "reflects an attitude shift from one of 'let's see how this might work' to a longer view of putting it to work" (Simpson & Flynn, 2007, p. 114). Success in this phase is based on perceived effectiveness, feasibility, and sustainability of the innovation. In the ITM, full implementation is expected to follow the Part II training. However, many teams actually come to the ITC having been through the adoption stage (i.e., decided to try DBT and had a trial period of using DBT based on the manuals alone). In this case, the trial period engineered between the Part I and II trainings serves the purpose of full implementation and they return to the Part II focused on the effectiveness, feasibility, and sustainability of DBT. Either way, to maximize the chance of full implementation by each team, the Part II training involves the presentation of each team's program as well as case presentations of DBT. This allows for focused consultation for each team as well as a chance to learn from the difficulties of other teams. This vicarious learning is consistently reported to be very helpful in troubleshooting issues teams have not yet had to address themselves.

The fourth and final stage is *practice improvement,* which presumes full implementation and focuses on outcomes, services, and budget and is an outcome of the ITM rather than a part of it. Simpson and Flynn (2007) also note that prior to implementation there is a Strategic Planning and Preparation process in which it is decided to pursue the implementation process. In the ITM, this generally starts prior to the ITC application, is facilitated by the trainers' review of the applications, and is strengthened during Parts I and II of the training.

Other models of implementation are similar to Simpson and Flynn. Fixsen and colleagues (2005) share the general approach of awareness through exploration, decision making, implementation, and sustainability, but does not imply a trial period, instead focusing on two stages of program installation and then initial implementation and distinguishing this from full operation when the program has been successfully implemented. They also highlight that following full operation is a stage of innovation in which adaptations specific to the site are achieved prior to sustainability. By contrast, the Availability, Responsiveness, and Continuity (ARC) organizational intervention strategy developed by Glisson and colleagues (2005) focuses much less attention on the actual training and implementation stages and much more on the development of the setting to be ready for an innovation and support from the trainers throughout the process. This differs substantially from the ITM in that it does not presume that those participating in the implementation will be able to facilitate the implementation themselves. By contrast, the ITM presumes that teams can be taught to take the lead on these steps themselves and thus the ITM is not intended for population-based interventions across a system but instead for "innovators" and "early adopters" who are trained in the ITC to be "opinion leaders."

INNOVATORS, EARLY ADOPTERS, AND OPINION LEADERS

When an innovation is disseminated, there are a range of individuals to whom it will be disseminated. These individuals are often divided into categories, with the first to adopt a new innovation being categorized as innovators (2.5%), who are distinguished by their interest in new ideas and willingness to connect with others outside of the community in order to learn. Because they are not focused on their community, they may be seen as mavericks or heavily invested in a particular special topic. Next are the early adopters (13.5%), who are also willing to take risks but are more connected within their home community rather than outside of it and are often opinion leaders who are watched by others (Berwick, 2003; Rogers, 1995). The DBT ITM is based on training this group of innovators and early adopters rather than the population as a whole. ITC teams are generally a combination of innovators and early adopters. Often the innovators have discovered or learned something about DBT in their larger professional community and have sold it to the early adopters at their site.

The goal of the ITM is to invest in these innovators and early adopters to mobilize implementation (Berwick, 2003; Rogers, 1995) by being opinion leaders (Kelly, 2004; Valente & Davis, 1999). Opinion leaders are influential individuals in their social context who can improve the uptake of an intervention (Kelly, 2004) or the implementation of a health care innovation (Berwick, 2003). Kelly (2004) used opinion leaders as the basis for his safer sex interventions and identified key elements that are needed to train opinion leaders to have a positive impact on the larger community including training in groups, role-play practice, homework that is reviewed by the trainers, and personal endorsement of the intervention by the opinion leaders. These strategies, which are supported by other training models, are all part of the ITM. A review of methods for selecting opinion leaders categorized methods into 10 categories: celebrities, self-selection, self-identification, staff selection, positional approach (i.e., history of leadership positions), judge's ratings, expert identification, snowball, sample sociometric, and sociometric (Valente & Pumpuang, 2007). They do not find one method more effective than others, but recommend the use of multiple methods to maximize identification. Generally in the DBT ITCs, opinion leaders consist primarily of individuals selected by self-selection, self-identification, staff selection, and positional selection.

Thus, the goal with the DBT ITM is to provide training to innovators and early adopters who have become interested in DBT from the manuals, other trainings, or word of mouth and who have begun using DBT in their setting. The training ensures they understand DBT thoroughly and have practiced all the important strategies (hopefully with clients in their program but, if not, as role plays during the training and as part of their homework). It is also designed to increase their interest in and motivation to practice DBT. These well-trained opinion leaders then expand their own DBT programs as well as model the benefits of DBT and advocate for adherent DBT in their communities, which will likely encourage others to learn and implement DBT.

CONCEPTUAL MODELS OF TRAINING AND
THEIR EMPIRICAL SUPPORT

Like opinion leader training, the DBT ITM is highly experiential, is team-focused, and incorporates systematic feedback and contingencies to motivate new behaviors. Because many of the teams are working within much larger institutions, the training also provides specific training and consultation on institutional implementation strategies. Each of these training components has a strong theoretical and empirical base.

Focus on Teams

The ITM utilizes a team-based learning focus. There is a large body of research indicating that team learning formats, in contrast to individual-focused learning formats, lead to greater learner engagement as well as greater content and procedural mastery (Guzzo & Dickson, 1996; Haidet, Morgan, O'Malley, Moran, & Richards, 2004; Haidet, O'Malley, & Richards, 2002; Johnson, Johnson, Stanne, & Garibaldi, 2001; Kelly et al., 2005; Levine et al., 2004; Michaelsen, 1983; Moreland & Myaskovsky, 2000; Wegner, 1987). Michaelsen (1983) examined team learning courses where students were on a stable team of three to eight members throughout the course. When engaged in solving contextually relevant and consequential problems, teams outperformed their most proficient team member 97% of the time; 40% of the process gains could not be explained by either the average or the most knowledgeable group member scores. Team-based learning is particularly prevalent in business school settings but in recent years has been increasingly incorporated into medical education (Haidet & Fecile, 2006), including psychotherapy training programs (Touchet & Coon, 2005). Team learning can also enhance commitment to the group, provide an opportunity to organize team activities and work plans, and allow team members to resolve problems that can limit performance such as anxiety about acceptance, interpersonal conflicts, and uncertainty about group norms (Tuckman, 1965; Wittenbaum, Vaughan, & Strasser, 1998). Learning is enhanced when team-building exercises are added to either individual training or team training (Moreland, 1999; Moreland, Argote, & Krishnan, 1996, 1998). This latter finding is particularly important because it suggests that for teams who plan to continue working together, it is important to be trained together as a team. This point is strengthened by findings indicating that the benefits of team-based learning may be lost if training groups are disrupted (Prichard, Bizo, & Stratford, 2006). This latter finding appears to highlight the importance of training teams in the skills of working as a team, a finding also reported by Gillies (2004).

Contingency Management

There is ample evidence that contingencies per se have powerful effects on behavior in general and in education. When teams are structured such that the entire team's performance is rewarded, performance improves (Fandt, 1991; Johnson & Johnson, 1989; Johnson et al., 2001). In classroom studies, for example, it has been shown repeatedly that group contingencies result in better performance than individual contingencies (Cohen, 1994; Fraser, Beaman, Diener, & Kelem, 1997; Gillies, 2004; Johnson & Johnson, 1999). Similar outcomes have also been found in nonclassroom settings. For example, De Dreu (2006) conducted a cross-sectional field study involving 46 management teams and found that the more team members perceived outcome interdependence, the better they shared information, the more they learned, and the more effective they were.

DATA ON THE INTENSIVE TRAINING MODEL

Data are limited but promising on ITM effectiveness. Little research has been conducted on DBT training methods. Only one study has directly addressed client outcomes of DBT training (Trupin et al., 2002). Providers in two juvenile justice residential units attended either a DBT 2-day workshop or an ITC. Clients treated by those attending the ITC training showed significant reductions in intentional self-injury, aggression, and class disruptions and staff showed reduced use of punitive actions. In contrast, following the 2-day workshop, clients showed no reduction in behavior problems and staff showed increased use of punitive procedures, perhaps suggesting that they misunderstood key components of the treatment. However, conclusions from this study are limited because there was not random assignment to training. To date, no carefully controlled studies of the effectiveness of the ITM have been published.

Hawkins and Sinha (1998) evaluated the effectiveness of the ITM by evaluating participants' scores on a DBT knowledge exam and found community mental health providers from a wide variety of disciplines learned the material as reflected in exam performance. In two of the DBT RCTs published to date, all DBT treatment was provided by therapists who attended a DBT Intensive Training Course but did not otherwise receive DBT training (Verheul et al., 2003) or more than very minimal supervision (Koons et al., 2001). The findings of significantly more improvement in clients treated by therapists trained in DBT ITCs versus those not trained in DBT ITCs suggests that training is likely effective in teaching the essential characteristics of DBT. The alternative hypothesis, that early adopters of DBT are more effective therapists than non–early adopters, is also a possibility. Without further testing, we cannot be sure of our interpretations of these outcomes.

In evaluations of training across several Intensive Training Courses, nearly three quarters of teams offered three of the four standard DBT treatment modes (individual psychotherapy, group skills training, and therapist consultation team) within 1 year after receiving intensive training, and nearly half of the teams were offering the fourth mode, after-hours telephone consultation. Pre/post data indicate that the training increases knowledge of DBT principles (Linehan, Manning, & Ward-Ciesielski, 2008).

INTENSIVE TRAINING MODEL FEASIBILITY

Adoption of DBT has been widespread and the demand from providers and mental health systems remains high. Since 1993, over 600 teams in 19 countries have been trained using the DBT ITM format. Currently, 5 to 8 intensive training courses are offered annually in the United States and 9 to 10 are conducted internationally (United Kingdom, Netherlands, Switzerland, Germany, Norway, Sweden, Australia, New Zealand). There are active DBT teams in most U.S. states, almost all of whom have attended a DBT Intensive Training Course. Sixteen U.S. state implementation Intensive Training Courses have been conducted or contracted to date (S. Y. Manning, personal communication, January 20, 2010). Variations on the ITM format are beginning to be offered by other training groups as indicated by online advertisements.

In the implementation of a DBT program, there is a strong emphasis on monitoring outcomes for sustained fidelity and quality improvement (Comtois, Elwood, Holdcraft, Simpson, & Smith, 2007). This process is critical to the long-term success of training efforts to maximize effectiveness and to prevent drift. The team-based approach may provide both support and a means to facilitate continued fidelity to the treatment model and evaluation procedures.

The results of the training requirement to monitor clinical and provider outcomes have suggested that the implementation model is feasible, as is success of adoption into clinical settings. These results, along with feedback from clinical teams regarding barriers to implementation, have been used to continually improve upon the training model. Barriers to implementation can include a variety of difficulties. Linehan and colleagues (2008) found that more than 30% of team leaders reported the following as barriers to implementation: team problems (team members left, 59%; difficulty meeting regularly, 41%), administrative problems (productivity needs, 68%; no release time provided for learning and implementing a new program, 46%), theoretical/philosophical problems (nonbehavioral theoretical orientation, 36%; not willing to take phone calls or extend limits, 32%), and structural problems (lack of individual therapists, 41%).

Training in DBT is now gradually spreading into residency and graduate training programs of mental health providers. The University of Washington School of Medicine offers a DBT training program created by Kate Comtois to approximate what occurs in the ITC for psychiatry residents, psychology interns, postdoctoral fellows, and faculty (https://catalyst.uw.edu/workspace/comtois/13581/73860). The program begins with a 2-day introductory workshop. Individuals can continue training with a weekly seminar that meets for 6 months. This seminar includes a self-study of assigned readings (including the DBT text and skills manual), homework assignments, and a written DBT exam. The seminar is taught by a variety of DBT experts and practitioners. In addition to the workshop and seminar, individuals can opt to participate in clinical training as well. The clinical training includes seeing an individual client for a year, weekly one-on-one supervision from a DBT expert for an hour, and participation in weekly consultation team meetings. A skills group is also run by participants in the clinical training for the clients in the program. Separate additional supervision is provided for the leaders of the skills group.

Training in DBT in graduate programs currently takes a variety of forms, including brief seminars, courses on effective treatments including DBT, and external practica in DBT programs. Linehan has developed a 2-year clinical-scientist training program at the University of Washington that is provided in her clinical research and training center, the Behavioral Research and Training Clinics (BRTC). The training includes research and clinical skills to aid individuals in preparing for careers where they will both develop their own DBT training programs and conduct clinical research with difficult-to-treat populations.

FUTURE DIRECTIONS: CERTIFICATION
AND ACCREDITATION

Certification of individuals and accreditation of programs is currently not available, but is in development. In 2005, a workgroup for certification and accreditation was formed to "develop a comprehensive way to certify individuals in their *competency* to deliver DBT effectively and to accredit programs in their ability to deliver DBT *programmatically with fidelity to the model as it has been researched* [italics added]" (DBT Certification & Accreditation Website, 2008).

The workgroup has established a website to communicate with the public about the certification and accreditation process, as well as progress updates in the development of both. The website currently contains background regarding certification and accreditation, descriptions, workgroup membership list, a study guide and "toolkit" of exam preparation materials, updates on progress, and target dates for the next steps in the process. The workgroup intends to create registries for both certified individuals and accredited programs.

Certification

Individual certification "conveys to the public that such an individual has been examined and designated as having a special proficiency in the delivery of DBT" (DBT Certification & Accreditation Website, 2008). Certification will be available for three areas of practice: individual therapists, skills trainers, and team leads.

To be eligible for certification, an individual must have at least a master's degree or the equivalent in a behavioral health field and have a professional license. To be certified as a team lead, individuals must also be certified as either an individual therapist or a skills trainer. Other requirements will include an application, documentation of having performance-based supervision, letters of recommendation, professional references, and a practice sample in the form of three consecutive sessions recorded on DVD. One session will be chosen randomly and coded for adherence. If not at adherence, three additional sessions will be required (Korslund, 2009).

The certification process will include written and oral exams. The written exam includes DBT practices and principles, as well as general CBT practices. The oral exam will constitute a performance exam that confirms an individual is able to perform DBT practices effectively.

Accreditation

As DBT is a team-based treatment and is often delivered as a program, accreditation of DBT programs will also occur. "Accrediting an overall program's capacity to deliver the treatment in a manner most similar to the way DBT was studied in randomized controlled trials becomes an important means by which stakeholders can discern effective programs from ones in which efficacy is unknown. Accreditation, therefore, seeks to establish an objective means to insure a program's fidelity to the DBT model" (DBT Certification & Accreditation Website, 2008).

For a program to be accredited, it must provide all four primary modes of DBT (individual therapy, skills training, method for skills generalization such as phone coaching, and a consultation team). A program must have at least one team member who is certified or eligible for certification. Programs must also be currently providing clinical services.

The workgroup intends to begin accreditation with standard DBT programs only and expects to accredit other versions in the future (e.g., adapted versions). The accreditation process will include use of a Program Fidelity Scale and some form of a site visit.

Conclusion

The DBT Intensive Training Model is an excellent example of a training model that has a strong theoretical base and has evolved over time in response to perceived effectiveness of training and data on briefer trainings in general. In these ways, the training model development has mirrored the development of the treatment itself. As described previously, the ITM substantially reflects the principles of current conceptual models for successful implementation. The ITM is feasible, with trainings occurring in 19 countries, and initial data suggest that training is effective. Currently, processes for certification of individual DBT providers and accreditation of DBT programs are in development. Additional research is needed to support the model and will likely facilitate further development as needed.

REFERENCES

Barley, W. D., Buie, D. H., Peterson, E. W., Hollingsworth, A. S., Griva, M., Hickerson, S. C., et al. (1993). The development of an inpatient cognitive-behavioral treatment program for borderline personality disorder. *Journal of Personality Disorders, 7*, 232–240.

Berwick, D. (2003). Disseminating innovations in health care. *Journal of the American Medical Association, 289*, 1969–1975.

Bohus, M., Haaf, B., Stiglmayr, C., Pohl, U., Bohme, R., & Linehan, M. M. (2000). Evaluation of inpatient dialectical-behavioral therapy for borderline personality disorder: A prospective study. *Behaviour Research and Therapy, 38*, 875–887.

Bootzin, R. R., & Ruggill, J. S. (1988). Training issues in behavior therapy. *Journal of Consulting and Clinical Psychology, 56*, 703–709.

Cohen, E. G. (1994). Restructuring the classroom: Conditions for productive small groups. *Review of Educational Research, 64*, 1–35.

Comtois, K. A., Elwood, L., Holdcraft, L. C., Simpson, T. L., & Smith, W. R. (2007). Effectiveness of dialectical behavioral therapy in a community mental health center. *Cognitive and Behavioral Practice, 14*, 406–414.

Crits-Christoph, P., Siqueland, L., Chittams, J., Barber, J. P., Beck, A. T., Frank, A., et al. (1998). Training in cognitive, supportive-expressive, and drug counseling therapies for cocaine dependence. *Journal of Consulting and Clinical Psychology, 66*, 484–492.

Davis, D., O'Brien, M. A. T., Freemantle, N., Wolf, F. M., Mazmanian, P., & Taylor-Vaisey, A. (1999). Impact of formal continuing medical education: Do conferences, workshops, rounds, and other traditional continuing education activities change physician behavior or health care outcomes? *Journal of the American Medical Association, 282*, 867–874.

DBT Certification & Accreditation Website. (2008). Retrieved December 29, 2009, from http://depts.washington.edu/brtc/dbtca/

De Dreu, C. K. W. (2006). When too little or too much hurts: Evidence for a curvilinear relationship between task conflict and innovation in teams. *Journal of Management, 32*, 83–107.

Fandt, P. M. (1991). The relationship of accountability and interdependent behavior to enhancing team consequences. *Group & Organization Studies, 16*, 300–312.

Fixsen, D. L., Naoom, S. F., Blase, K. A., Friedman, R. M., & Wallace, F. (2005). *Implementation research: A synthesis of the literature.* Tampa, FL: University of South Florida, Louis de la Parte Florida Mental Health Institute, The National Implementation Research Network.

Fraser, S. C., Beaman, A. L., Diener, E., & Kelem, R. T. (1997). Two, three, or four heads are better than one: Modification of college performance by peer monitoring. *Journal of Educational Psychology, 69*, 101–108.

Freiheit, S. R., & Overholser, J. C. (1997). Training issues in cognitive-behavioral psychotherapy. *Journal of Behavior Therapy and Experimental Psychiatry, 28*, 79–86.

Geller, J. L. (1986). In again, out again: Preliminary evaluation of a state hospital's worst recidivists. *Hospital and Community Psychiatry, 4*, 386–390.

Gillies, R. M. (2004). The effects of cooperative learning on junior high school students during small group learning. *Learning and Instruction, 14*, 197–213.

Glisson, C., Dukes, D., & Green, P. (2006). The effects of the ARC organizational intervention on caseworker turnover, climate, and culture in children's service systems. *Child Abuse and Neglect, 30*, 855–880.

Glisson, C., & Schoenwald, S. K. (2005). The ARC organizational and community intervention strategy for implementing evidence-based children's mental health treatments. *Mental Health Services Research, 7*, 243–259.

Guzzo, R. A., & Dickson, M. W. (1996). Teams in organizations: Recent research on performance and effectiveness. *Annual Review of Psychology, 47*, 307–338.

Haidet, P., & Fecile, M. L. (2006). Team-based learning: A promising strategy to foster active learning in cancer education. *Journal of Cancer Education, 21*, 125–128.

Haidet, P., Morgan, R. O., O'Malley, K. J., Moran, B. J., & Richards, B. F. (2004). A controlled trial of active versus passive learning strategies in a large group setting. *Advances in Health Sciences Education, 9*, 15–27.

Haidet, P., O'Malley, K. J., & Richards, B. (2002). An initial experience with "team learning" in medical education. *Academic Medicine, 77*, 40–44.

Hawkins, K. A., & Sinha, R. (1998). Can line clinicians master the conceptual complexities of dialectical behavior therapy? An evaluation of a state department of mental health training program. *Journal of Psychiatric Research, 32*, 379–384.

Henry, W. P., Strupp, H. H., Butler, S. F., Schacht, T. E., & Binder, J. L. (1993). Effects of training in time-limited dynamic psychotherapy: Changes in therapist behavior. *Journal of Consulting and Clinical Psychology, 61*, 434–440.

Johnson, D. W., & Johnson, R. T. (1989). *Cooperation and competition: A meta-analysis of the research.* Hillsdale, NJ: Lawrence Erlbaum.

Johnson, D. W., & Johnson, R. T. (1999). Making cooperative learning work. *Theory into Practice, 38*, 67–73.

Johnson, D. W., Johnson, R. T., Stanne, M. B., & Garibaldi, A. (2001). Impact of group processing on achievement in cooperative groups. *Journal of Social Psychology, 130*, 507–516.

Kelly, J. A. (2004). Popular opinion leaders and HIV prevention peer education: Resolving discrepant findings, and implications for the development of effective community programmes. *AIDS Care: Psychological and Socio-medical Aspects of AIDS/HIV, 16*, 139–150.

Kelly, P. A., Haidet, P., Schneider, V., Searle, N., Seidel, C. L., & Richards, B. F. (2005). A comparison of in-class learner engagement across lecture, problem-based learning, and team learning using the STROBE classroom observation tool. *Teaching and Learning in Medicine, 17*, 112–118.

Koerner, K., & Dimeff, L. A. (2000). Further data on dialectical behavioral therapy. *Clinical Psychology: Science and Practice, 7*, 104–112.

Koons, C. R., Robins, C. J., Tweed, J. L., Lynch, T. R., Gonzalez, A. M., Morse, J. Q., et al. (2001). Efficacy of dialectical behavior therapy in women veterans with borderline personality disorder. *Behavior Therapy, 32*, 371–390.

Korslund, K. E. (2009, October). *Update on certification and accreditation.* Presentation at the Dialectical Behavior Therapy Strategic Planning Meeting, Seattle, WA.

Lehman, W. E. K., Greener, J. M., & Simpson, D. D. (2002). Assessing organizational readiness for change. *Journal of Substance Abuse Treatment, 22*, 197–209.

Levine, R. E., O'Boyle, M., Haidet, P., Lynn, D. J., Stone, M. M., Wolf, D. V., et al. (2004). Transforming a clinical clerkship with team learning. *Teaching and Learning in Medicine, 16*, 270–275.

Linehan, M. M. (1993a). *Cognitive-behavioral treatment of borderline personality disorder.* New York: Guilford Press.

Linehan, M. M. (1993b). *Skills training manual for treating borderline personality disorder.* New York: Guilford Press.

Linehan, M. M., Armstrong, H. E., Suarez, A., Allmon, D., & Heard, H. L. (1991). Cognitive-behavioral treatment of chronically parasuicidal borderline patients. *Archives of General Psychiatry, 48*, 1060–1064.

Linehan, M. M., Comtois, K. A., Murray, A. M., Brown, M. Z., Gallop, R. J., Heard, H. L., et al. (2006). Two-year randomial trial + follow-up of dialectical behavior therapy vs. therapy by experts for suicidal behaviors and borderline personality disorder. *Archives of General Psychiatry, 63,* 757–766.

Linehan, M. M., Dimeff, L. A., Reynolds, S. K., Comtois, K. A., Welch, S. S., & Kivlahan, D. R. (2002). Dialectical behavior therapy versus comprehensive validation plus 12-step for the treatment of opioid dependent women meeting criteria for borderline personality disorder. *Drug and Alcohol Dependence, 67,* 13–26.

Linehan, M. M., Manning, S., & Ward-Ciesielski, E. F. (2008, November). *The dialectical behavior therapy intensive training model.* Paper presented at the Association for Cognitive and Behavioral Therapies, Orlando, FL.

Linehan, M. M., Schmidt III, H., Dimeff, L. A., Craft, J. C., Kanter, J., & Comtois, K. A. (1999). Dialectical behavior therapy for patients with borderline personality disorder and drug-dependence. *American Journal of Addictions, 8,* 279–292.

Lynch, T. R., Morse, J. Q., Mendelson, T., & Robins, C. J. (2003). Dialectical behavioral therapy for depressed older adults. A randomized pilot study. *American Journal of Geriatric Psychiatry, 11,* 33–45.

McMain, S. F., Links, P. S., Gnam, W. H., Guimond, T., Cardish, R. J., Korman, L., et al. (2009). A randomized trial of dialectical behavior therapy versus general psychiatric management for borderline personality disorder. *American Journal of Psychiatry, 166,* 1365–1374.

Michaelsen, L. K. (1983). Team learning in large classes. In C. Bouton & R. Y. Garth (Eds.), *Learning in groups* (pp. 13–22). San Francisco: Jossey-Bass.

Miller, W. R., & Mount, K. A. (2001). A small study of training in motivational interviewing: Does one workshop change clinician and client behavior? *Behavioural and Cognitive Psychotherapy, 29,* 457–471.

Miller, W. R., & Rollnick, S. (1991). *Motivational interviewing: Preparing people to change addictive behavior.* New York: Guilford Press.

Miller, W. R., Yahne, C. E., Moyers, T. B., Martinez, J., & Pirritano, M. (2004). A randomized trial of methods to help clinicians learn motivational interviewing. *Journal of Consulting and Clinical Psychology, 72,* 1050–1062.

Milne, D. L., Baker, C., Blackburn, I., James, I., & Reichelt, K. (1999). Effectiveness of cognitive therapy training. *Journal of Behavior Therapy and Experimental Psychiatry, 30,* 81–92.

Moreland, R. L. (1999). Transactive memory: Learning who knows what in work groups and organizations. In L. Thompson, D. Messick, & J. Levine (Eds.), *Shared cognition in organizations: The management of knowledge* (pp. 3–31). Mahwah, NJ: Erlbaum.

Moreland, R. L., Argote, L., & Krishnan, R. (1996). Socially shared cognition at work: Transactive memory and group performance. In J. L. Nye & A. M. Brower (Eds.), *Research on socially shared cognition in small groups* (pp. 57–84). Thousand Oaks, CA: Sage.

Moreland, R. L., Argote, L., & Krishnan, R. (1998). Training people to work in groups. In R. S. Tindale, L. Heath, J. Edwards, E. J. Posavac, F. B. Bryant, Y. Suarez-Balcazar, et al. (Eds.), *Theory and research on small groups* (pp. 37–60). New York: Plenum.

Moreland, R. L., & Myaskovsky, L. (2000). Exploring the performance benefits of group training: Transactive memory or improved communication? *Organizational Behavior and Human Decision Processes, 82,* 117–133.

Prichard, J. S., Bizo, L. A., & Stratford, R. J. (2006). The educational impact of team-skills training: Preparing students to work in groups. *British Journal of Educational Psychology, 76*, 119–140.

Rogers, E. M. (1995). *Diffusion of innovations* (4th ed.). New York: Free Press.

Russell, M. C., Silver, S. M., Rogers, S., & Darnell, J. N. (2007). Responding to an identified need: A joint Department of Defense/Department of Veteran Affairs training program in eye movement desensitization and reprocessing (EMDR) for clinicians providing trauma services. *International Journal of Stress Management, 14*, 61–71.

Safer, D. L., Telch, C. F., & Agras, W. S. (2001). Dialectical behavioral therapy for bulimia nervosa. *American Journal of Psychiatry, 158*, 632–634.

Sholomskas, D. E., Syracuse-Siewert, G., Rounsaville, B. J., Ball, S. A., Nuro, K. F., & Carroll, K. M. (2005). We don't train in vain: A dissemination trial of three strategies of training clinicians in cognitive-behavioral therapy. *Journal of Consulting and Clinical Psychology, 73*, 106–115.

Simpson, D. D. (2002). A conceptual framework for transferring research to practice. *Journal of Substance Abuse Treatment, 22*, 171–182.

Simpson, D. D. (2004). A conceptual framework for drug treatment process and outcomes. *Journal of Substance Abuse Treatment, 27*, 99–121.

Simpson, D. D., & Flynn, P. M. (2007). Moving innovations into treatment: A stage-based approach to program change. *Journal of Substance Abuse Treatment, 33*, 111–120.

Sohn, W., Ismail, A. I., & Tellez, M. (2004). Efficacy of educational interventions targeting primary care providers' practice behaviors: An overview of published systematic reviews. *Journal of Public Health Dentistry, 64*, 164–172.

Stanley, B., Ivanoff, A., Brodsky, B., & Oppenheim, S. (1998, November). *Comparison of DBT and "treatment as usual" in suicidal and self-mutilating behavior.* Paper presented at the Association for the Advancement of Behavior Therapy, Washington, DC.

Strosahl, K. D., Hayes, S. C., Bergan, J., & Romano, P. (1998). Assessing the field effectiveness of acceptance and commitment therapy: An example of the manipulated training research method. *Behavior Therapy, 29*, 35–64.

Substance Abuse and Mental Health Services Administration. (2006, 2009). *National Registry of Evidence-Based Programs and Practices.* Retrieved September 21, 2009, from http://www.nrepp.samhsa.gov/

Surber, R. W., Winkler, E. L., Monteleone, M., Havassy, B. E., Goldfinger, S. M., & Hopkin, J. T. (1987). Characteristics of high users of acute psychiatric inpatient services. *Hospital and Community Psychiatry, 38*, 1112–1114.

Swigar, M. E., Astrachan, B., Levine, M. A., Mayfield, V., & Radovich, C. (1991). Single and repeated admissions to a mental health center: Demographic, clinical and use of service characteristics. *The International Journal of Social Psychiatry, 37*, 259–266.

Telch, C. F., Agras, W. S., & Linehan, M. M. (2001). Dialectical behavioral therapy for binge eating disorder. *Journal of Consulting and Clinical Psychology, 69*, 1061–1065.

Touchet, B. K., & Coon, K. A. (2005). A pilot use of team-based learning in psychiatry resident psychodynamic psychotherapy education. *Academic Psychiatry, 29*, 293–296.

Trupin, E. W., Stewart, D. G., Beach, B., & Boesky, L. (2002). Effectiveness of a dialectical behaviour therapy program for incarcerated female juvenile offenders. *Child and Adolescent Mental Health, 7*, 121–127.

Tuckman, B. W. (1965). Developmental sequence in small groups. *Psychological Bulletin, 63*, 384–399.

Valente, T. W., & Davis, R. L. (1999). Accelerating the diffusion of innovations using opinion leaders. *Annals of the American Academy of Political and Social Science, 566*, 55–67.

Valente, T. W., & Pumpuang, P. (2007). Identifying opinion leaders to promote behavior change. *Health Education & Behavior, 34*, 881–896.

van Asselt, A. D. I., Dirksen, C. D., Arntz, A., & Severens, J. L. (2007). The cost of borderline personality disorder: Societal cost of illness in BPD-patients. *European Psychiatry, 22*, 354–361.

van den Bosch, L. M., Verheul, R., Schippers, G. M., & van den Brink, W. (2002). Dialectical behavior therapy of borderline patients with and without substance use problems. Implementation and long-term effects. *Addictive Behaviors, 27*, 911–923.

Verheul, R., van den Bosch, L., Louise, M. C., Koeter, M. W., de Ridder, M. A. J., Stijnen, T., et al. (2003). Dialectical behaviour therapy for women with borderline personality disorder: 12-month, randomised clinical trial in The Netherlands. *British Journal of Psychiatry, 182*, 135–140.

Wegner, D. M. (1987). Transactive memory: A contemporary analysis of the group mind. In B. Bullen & G. R. Goethals (Eds.), *Theories of group behavior* (pp. 185–205). New York: Springer-Verlag.

Widiger, T. A., & Weissman, M. M. (1991). Epidemiology of borderline personality disorder. *Hospital and Community Psychiatry, 42*, 1015–1021.

Wittenbaum, G. M., Vaughan, S. I., & Strasser, G. (1998). Coordination in task-performing groups In R. S. Tindale, L. Heath, J. Edwards, E. J. Posavac, F. B. Bryant, Y. Suarez-Balcazar, et al. (Eds.), *Theory and research on small groups* (pp. 177–204). New York: Plenum.

Woogh, C. M. (1986). A cohort through the revolving door. *Canadian Journal of Psychiatry, 31*, 214–221.

Enhancing Dissemination Outcomes through a Population-Based Approach to Parenting Intervention

Matthew R. Sanders and Rachel Calam

As the evidence linking parenting practices to important developmental and health outcomes in children and adolescents strengthens, so has the demand for effective, readily accessible, culturally appropriate parenting programs (World Health Organization [WHO], 2009). Parenting interventions based on behavioral and social learning principles have been repeatedly demonstrated to be effective in reducing a variety of social, emotional, behavioral and health problems in young children, and to a lesser extent, in youth. Several systematic reviews (e.g., Kazdin, 2005; Eyberg, Nelson, & Boggs, 2008) and meta-analyses (e.g., Nowak & Heinrichs, 2008) have documented the efficacy of parent training, particularly with children with conduct problems.

Although parenting programs have been around for several decades (Patterson, Reid, Jones, & Conger, 1975), they are not readily available or as widely used by service providers working with families as they could be (Sanders & Prinz, 2008). Program developers and clinical researchers have historically not paid a lot of attention to whether service providers adopt evidence-based approaches. Consequently, there are relatively few examples of evidence-based child and family interventions being successfully translated into regular services in a sustainable manner. This lack of sustained application of existing knowledge about parent training is a major obstacle to the prevention and effective management of many social, behavioral, and emotional problems in children.

Although a great deal of attention has been given to the development of procedures to promote behavioral and cognitive change in parents and children, much less attention has been given to developing and testing procedures that enable programs to be successfully disseminated to professionals serving families. The effective dissemination of programs is critical for intervention research to have any significant community impact. Most of the parent training programs that have been disseminated have targeted children with diagnosed conduct problems, who are identified as high risk for such disorders, or who are identified as being abusive or neglectful—rather than being disseminated as prevention programs.

To reduce prevalence rates of family dysfunction, child maltreatment, and emotional and conduct problems in children and adolescents, a population-level approach is needed that seeks to strengthen the knowledge, skills, and confidence of parents as well as the broader ecological context of parenting (e.g., Biglan, 1995). The Triple P - Positive Parenting Program developed by Sanders and colleagues at the University of Queensland (see Sanders, 2008) is an example of a comprehensive, integrated, multilevel system of parenting and family support. Interventions within the Triple P system range from universal media strategies targeting all parents to primary care consultations specifically targeting mild to moderate behavioral and emotional problems in children. Triple P interventions also extend to intensive parent training and family intervention programs for families with multiple risk factors (e.g., relationship problems, family violence, parental adjustment problems) or children with more severe emotional and behavioral problems. The system seeks to provide the "minimally sufficient" intervention for the parent in order to promote healthy positive development and to deflect a child away from a trajectory leading toward more serious problems. This chapter explores some of the key tasks and challenges in disseminating a public health approach to parenting programs through the lens of the Triple P system.

The Triple P - Positive Parenting
Program: An Overview

Triple P began on a small scale as a home-based individually administered training program for parents of disruptive preschool children (Sanders & Glynn, 1981). It has evolved over the past 30 years into a comprehensive public health model of intervention that has been disseminated to 24 countries and to 62,000 practitioners. Inspired by examples of large-scale health promotion studies including studies conducted by the Center for Disease Prevention at Stanford University targeting behaviors such as smoking, sedentary lifestyle, and unhealthy diet (Farquhar et al., 1985) and concepts such as the need to design "living environments" for children (Risley, Clark, & Cataldo, 1976), Sanders and colleagues, primarily from the University of Queensland, set out to design a comprehensive evidence-based system that could be successfully disseminated to parents and professionals (Sanders, Cann, & Markie-Dadds, 2003). This involved designing a range of brief, cost-effective interventions (e.g., Turner & Sanders, 2006), more economical ways of delivering programs through groups (Zubrick et al., 2005), more flexible delivery formats such as telephone consultation (Connell, Sanders, & Markie-Dadds, 1997) and the media (Sanders & Prinz, 2008), and the use of epidemiological data to inform public policy decisions about how to target parenting services (e.g., Sanders, Markie-Dadds, Rinaldis, Firman, & Baig, 2007).

MOTIVATING CIRCUMSTANCES

The immediate context for the development of the different levels of the Triple P system was the recognition that existing intensive behavioral parent training programs were having little impact at a population-level on children's behavioral and emotional problems. Although impressive evidence showed group and individually administered programs could be effective in teaching positive parenting and contingency management skills to parents and thereby reducing child conduct problems, these programs were not widely used by professionals working with parents and therefore only a small number of parents benefited (Sanders et al., 2007). This lack of impact is partly explained by lack of effective mechanisms to disseminate programs to the professional workforce and partly by the fact that existing modes of delivery were not appropriate or seen as acceptable to some families. Heavy reliance on intensive group and individual programs and lack of interdisciplinary-based training ensured that evidence-based parenting interventions remained a highly specialized and, in many countries, a relatively inaccessible service.

Another limitation of parenting programs at the time was the relatively narrow age range targeted by the interventions (mainly toddlers and preschoolers). The prevailing assumption was that early intervention was important and hence the focus on the early years. However, there was a lack of acknowledgment that the parenting experience from infancy through adolescence has both continuities and discontinuities. Successful early parenting is no guarantee that parenting problems in the adolescent years can be completely avoided. Hence, there was a need to develop and test parenting programs across a wider age spectrum from infancy through adolescence. In an effort to increase the reach and impact of parenting interventions, a different emphasis was required. The adoption of a whole-population perspective offered opportunities and demanded that new programs be developed (Sanders, Cann, & Markie-Dadds, 2003).

Stakeholder Demand

There are many different stakeholders who have an interest in how children are raised including governments, psychologists, psychiatrists, social workers, teachers, child care staff, general practitioners (GPs), pediatricians, primary care providers, drug and alcohol case workers, and police and crime prevention agencies. However, the ultimate beneficiaries of high-quality parenting services are the parents and children themselves. Over the past 20 years there has been a noticeable increase in demand for parenting programs in many countries, particularly for the treatment of conduct problems. There is also evidence that parents value programs that are evidence-based and are shown to be effective (Sanders, Haslam, Calam, Southwell, & Stallman, 2011).

Policy Developments

In parallel with this recognition, national and local governments have started to commission parenting interventions not just as treatments, but as preventative early intervention strategies often targeting low-income, high-need parents (e.g. Sure Start, Family Intervention Projects). More recently there has been wider international recognition of the value of adopting a population-based approach to the delivery of parenting interventions (American Psychological Association, 2009; National Research Council and Institute of Medicine [IOM], 2009; United Nations Office on Drugs and Crime, 2009; WHO, 2009). For example, the WHO (2009) recently released a report documenting evidence-based approaches to violence prevention and clearly identified that parenting programs are needed to promote safe, stable, and nurturing relationships between children and their parents and caregivers. The U.S. IOM (2009) report on the prevention of mental, emotional, and behavioral disorders in children and youth also called on government to invest in parenting programs as part of a comprehensive prevention agenda.

Legislation or Other Incentives

In some countries a legislative response has provided an impetus to the wider dissemination of parenting programs. For example, in the United Kingdom the Respect Agenda introduced by the Blair administration included the establishment of parenting orders that required parents of children showing significant antisocial behavior to undertake parenting courses. In 2005, the New Zealand government introduced a law banning the use of corporal punishment by parents, providing an impetus to improve the provision of parenting services and the commissioning of reviews of evidence-based programs. However, in many countries calls for better access to parenting programs have not been preceded by legislative change.

Context

The sociopolitical context for the emergence of Triple P has been the existence of ongoing major concerns about the well-being and poor mental health of children and adolescents as reflected by high rates of conduct problems, antisocial behavior, juvenile delinquency, and drug and alcohol problems; high adolescent suicide rates; and high rates of child maltreatment. Most of these problems seem unlikely to be resolved without a significant parenting or family intervention-based response as part of a comprehensive prevention agenda. Fortunately, increasing evidence has shown that effective interventions are available for many of these problems, but there is a significant gap relating to how best to disseminate these programs into the community.

Description of Triple P

The overall aim of the Triple P system of intervention is to prevent the onset of severe behavioral, emotional, and developmental problems in children and adolescents by enhancing the knowledge, skills, and confidence of parents. Triple P incorporates five levels of intervention on a tiered continuum of increasing strength for parents of children from birth to age 16 (see Sanders, 2008, for an overview of

Triple P). The suite of multilevel programs in Triple P is designed to create a family-friendly environment that supports parents in the task of raising their children. It specifically targets the social contexts that influence parents on a day-to-day basis. These contexts include the mass media, primary health care services, childcare and school systems, worksites, religious organizations, and the broader political system. The multilevel strategy is designed to maximize efficiency, contain costs, avoid waste and overservicing, and ensure the program has wide reach in the community. Also, the multidisciplinary nature of the program involves upskilling a broad existing workforce in the task of promoting competent parenting.

The system targets five different developmental periods from infancy to adolescence. Within each developmental period, the reach of the intervention varies from very broad (targeting an entire population) to quite narrow (targeting only high-risk children). This flexibility enables services and practitioners to determine the scope of the intervention given their own service priorities, expertise, and funding.

Triple P teaches parents strategies to encourage their child's social and language skills, emotional self-regulation, independence, and problem-solving ability. It is hypothesized that attainment of these skills promotes family harmony, reduces parent–child conflict, fosters successful peer relationships, and prepares children for academic and occupational challenges. To achieve these child outcomes, parents are taught a variety of child management skills including monitoring problem behavior; providing brief contingent attention for appropriate behavior; arranging engaging activities in high-risk parenting situations; using directed discussion and planned ignoring for minor problem behavior; giving clear, calm instructions; and backing up instructions with logical consequences, quiet time (nonexclusionary time-out), and time-out. Parents learn to apply these skills both at home and in the community. Specific strategies such as planned activities training are used to promote the generalization and maintenance of parenting skills across settings and over time.

Triple P interventions combine the provision of information with active skills training and support. Active skills training methods include modeling, rehearsal, feedback, and homework tasks. Segments from videotapes (e.g., Sanders, Markie-Dadds, & Turner, 1996) can also be used to demonstrate positive parenting skills. Several generalization enhancement strategies are incorporated into the system of intervention (e.g., training with sufficient exemplars until parents can generalize skills to an untrained situation, and training loosely with varied target behaviors and children) to promote the transfer of parenting skills across settings, siblings, and time. Practice sessions can be conducted at home or in the clinic during which parents select their own practice goals, are observed interacting with their child and implementing parenting skills, and subsequently review their performance and receive feedback from the practitioner. For families with additional modifiable risk factors, such as parental distress or relationship conflict, or problems with anger management and violence, intervention can be expanded to include a focus on mood management, stress coping, communication or partner support skills, or cognitive therapy relating to attributional bias.

FUNDING

Triple P can be delivered by different service providers and service delivery systems (health, welfare, education, mental health). The funding model for Triple P depends on whether it is being implemented as a whole population approach or as a more targeted intervention for high-need groups. To illustrate, a state government may fund through a policy initiative the training of service providers and the materials used to implement the program. The funding for various aspects of the program varies from one jurisdiction to another depending on local funding arrangements. For example, in a population-level roll-out of Triple P the funding arrangements could consist of a state government paying for all training and implementation costs or a co-pay arrangement where training costs are paid by government but implementation resources are paid for by the agencies delivering Triple P.

The research and development model that has guided the dissemination of Triple P is outlined in Figure 11.1. The research documenting the efficacy of Triple P has been funded by nationally competitive grant schemes in Australia through the National Health and Medical Research Council and the Australian Research Council and supplemented by funding from philanthropic organizations (e.g., Telstra Foundation, Rotary Health Research Council). In other countries, Triple P research has primarily been funded by competitive grant schemes. However, the sustainability of Triple P as a population-level intervention, like all preventive

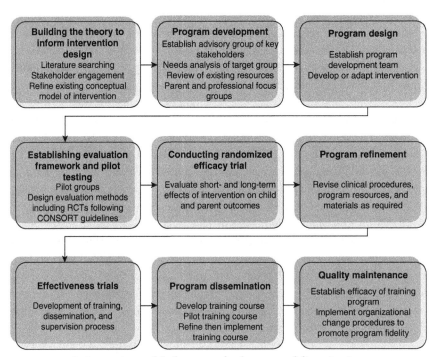

FIGURE 11.1 *An integrative model of program development and dissemination.*

interventions, depends on government priorities and having a policy framework that mainstreams services such as the delivery of parenting programs.

GOALS, TARGETS, AND STANDARDS OF CARE

What should guide governments and agencies as they make costly decisions on which parenting intervention to implement? Determining the overall aims and intended goals of the intervention is an essential first step. The National Research Council and Institute of Medicine (2009) recently published a review of interventions and summarized the family, school, and community interventions for which there is the strongest evidence. In their review, Triple P emerges as the only multilevel intervention designed as a universal, population-level strategy to improve parenting and increase positive emotional and behavioral outcomes for children and families. It is this multilevel approach that makes implementation as a public health–level strategy possible. The decision, then, for agencies and governments is whether they are aiming to address targeted disorder-specific populations or achieve public health-level benefits, or a blending of the two.

Triple P shares a number of features with other public health interventions. There is evidence, for example, that it leads to improvements in parenting when used in different formats, including self-directed variants (Sanders, Markie-Dadds, Tully, & Bor, 2000). It also works when seen in the format of a reality TV series (Sanders, Calam, Durand, Liversidge, & Carmont, 2008). Given sufficient exposure to good programming, simply viewing a well-constructed television series demonstrating families participating in a Triple P intervention has been shown to promote significant change in families, especially those with high levels of problem child behavior (Calam, Sanders, Miller, Sadhnani, & Carmont, 2008). This is analogous to the work of Sabido and colleagues (Singhal, Cody, Rogers, & Sabido, 2003), who demonstrated a public health benefit in the increase in the use of contraceptives using an engaging television-based series format. Interventions such as these, which step outside the consulting room or community center and engage the wider population, demonstrate the potential of creative alternatives to the traditional approaches to parenting intervention to bring about major public health benefits. The successful implementation of alternative modes of delivery depends on the fit with the needs, priorities, and goals of the adopting agencies and whether their funding model allows for flexible delivery of programs.

A number of reviews have compared different parenting programs (e.g., National Institute of Clinical Excellence and Social Care, 2006; O'Connell et al., 2009) and the active components within them. A recent meta-analysis (Kaminski, Valle, Filene, & Boyle, 2008) identified the active components that increase the effect sizes obtained by interventions to reduce problem behavior in children. Components of programs associated with larger effects include increasing positive interactions between parent and child, emotional communication skills, effective use of time-out, and consistency in parenting. Practicing new skills with the child during parent training sessions was also associated with larger effect sizes. It is noteworthy that some additional elements, for example, teaching parents to promote their child's cognitive or social skills, were associated with lower effect sizes. This finding suggests that the assumption that the more risk factors targeted the better may not be accurate in the context of parenting programs for child externalizing behavior.

When change at the population-or public health-level is the goal, the RE-AIM model (Glasgow, Klesges, Dzewaltowski, Estabrooks, & Vogt, 2006; Glasgow, Lichtenstein, & Marcus, 2003) provides some useful concepts to consider in maximizing the impact of an intervention. The acronym stands for *Reach*—the percentage of people accessing the intervention; *Efficacy*—the positive and negative outcomes associated with the intervention, and the measurement of these; *Adoption*—the proportion and representativeness of settings taking up the program; *Implementation*—the extent to which the program is delivered as intended by trained providers; and *Maintenance*—the degree to which trained providers continue to use the program over time. These elements all imply specific levels of measurement that can be assessed when a public health approach to parenting is employed in a particular setting.

NEEDS ASSESSMENT AND FIT TO SYSTEM NEEDS

The processes involved in establishing an evidence-based parenting program have been documented (Murphy-Brennan, 2007; Sanders & Murphy-Brennan, 2010). Understanding the organizational change aspects of the implementation of a newly introduced system of intervention and the use of effective dissemination practices increases the chances that a parenting intervention will be adopted successfully. Successful dissemination is associated with five key factors: (a) Support at the policy and funding level is essential. Secure, long-term funding has been identified by the World Health Organization as a key element in establishing new initiatives (Mittlemark, Puska, O'Byrne, & Tang, 2005). Establishing the cost-benefit of programs is a key component of this. Making links between priority concerns and the proposed intervention, based on needs assessment, should facilitate uptake and dissemination. (b) Advocacy at a high level by key stakeholders. Engaging stakeholders in consultation prior to implementation should increase their engagement and enthusiasm for the process and maximize the fit to the needs of the local system. (c) Evaluation is central to the process of monitoring the effect of a new intervention for policy implications and outcomes (Flay et al., 2005). The results of this can help to ensure that relevant needs are being met. (d) Professional training and workplace support is also essential for successful dissemination, as is the provision of ready access to all the materials required to carry out the implementation (Flay et al., 2005). This specific aspect is considered in more detail in the next section. (e) Quality assurance. It is important to consider both the fidelity of application, so that the integrity of the program is maintained, and the outcomes achieved. Concise, easily administered forms of evaluation are essential, to ensure that these are used routinely.

In considering the fit to system needs, it is also important to ensure there is a good fit to the parents' needs and concerns. Increasing evidence shows that parents make rational and rather predictable decisions about when not to attend community-based interventions (Dumas, Nissley-Tsiopinis, & Moreland, 2007). Finding predictors of successful engagement is more difficult, but it is likely that offering alternative delivery formats, including self-directed Internet- and DVD-based programs, based on parent needs assessments, will help to maximize population reach (Sanders et al., 2011).

Training of Clinicians

Ensuring adequate, appropriate training and technical assistance is essential to successful dissemination (Gotham, 2004). Making sure that adequate infrastructure is in place prior to training is important (Flay et al., 2005). This helps to ensure that practitioners have time and access to all the materials that they need to begin to practice their new skills immediately upon completing training. It also enables practitioners to become familiar with the application of the program to their setting and overcome any anxieties or confusion about the process of delivery. Where a program has an accreditation requirement, practitioners require the resources to implement the program in a timely manner to meet the required standards. Consultative support by the program disseminators ensures that new adopters take up the program in the most cost-effective manner by imparting knowledge and skills to managers and organizational representatives so that organizations are empowered to work independently and learn to celebrate their successes and problem solve issues internally. Building in supervisory structures and a culture of evaluation helps to promote reflective practice and good program fidelity while maintaining the most effective cost-benefit ratio. This kind of support can help practitioners have a positive view of the work they do with parents. Providing briefings and information for managers and administrators can help to make the organizational changes involved in implementation more comprehensible to these key staff who are essential to the effective service-wide implementation of the program, even though they may not be seeing families directly (Pentz, 2004).

A further consideration for training is staff turnover. Every Child Matters (2003) reported London staff vacancies as running at between 11% and 50% in some localities. Widespread adoption of a specific program across agencies makes areas less vulnerable to the impact of staff losses, and indeed newly appointed staff may already have the relevant training. It is probably only cost effective to establish an evidence-based program in an agency or locality that has the capacity to sustain the program over time.

An international study of the implementation of Triple P (Murphy-Brennan, 2007) highlights the cross-national difference that can exist in the level of prior training staff have received before they undertake Triple P training. In some countries, the workforce who are trained were predominantly graduates, often with postgraduate qualifications; in others, notably England and Scotland, there was a much higher percentage of staff with diploma-level qualifications. These differences need to be taken into account in designing the training and accreditation of staff, and in providing an appropriate level of supervision of practice. For staff who are not graduates with an appropriate discipline base, understanding the need for assessing client outcomes and evaluation generally may need greater emphasis.

A continuing dilemma for public health approaches to parenting is the requirement for programs on the one hand to be delivered with fidelity by well-trained and supported staff, while on the other the workforce available to implement parenting programs may have insufficient levels of training and experience. To resolve this dilemma considerable attention needs to be focused on developing a workforce with the necessary skills to deliver evidence-based programs. One response to this situation is the creation of the National Academy of Parenting Practitioners (UK), which is establishing more clearly articulated professional standards for the delivery of evidence-based parenting programs.

Strategies That Target Barriers to Adoption

In the process of implementation it is possible to encounter barriers at a number of levels, from the policy and managerial level to the individual practitioner and parent level. Barriers can interact across levels, and anticipation of these can assist the implementer in problem solving to ensure successful uptake. Below, we consider a number of different potential barriers that have been encountered in implementation and offer possible solutions, although assessment of local conditions and formulation of strategies will be essential. Table 11.1 summarizes potential solutions to barriers to implementation.

Concerns over durability. Environments characterized by short-term funding, and where staff are employed on short-term contracts to establish specific interventions, may raise anxieties that the initiative might cease to be funded in a short space of time. At a managerial level, it will be important to ensure that implementation is part of a long-term strategy, and that this is communicated effectively to funding bodies and to the workforce. For the staff delivering the intervention, putting systems in place to develop and enhance delivery of the intervention over time, with expected performance targets, will allow those who are trained to see that their input is expected, encouraged, and supported as part of a durable plan to reduce levels of child behavioral and emotional difficulties.

Innovation fatigue. Sometimes an agency may be required to implement several new and different programs or practices simultaneously, or in quick succession. This may influence the capacity of staff to engage with the program and to inform parents of what is available. Service leaders need to ensure that change is managed and innovations are planned in an integrated way to increase the likelihood that the introduction of new programs is welcomed. In an environment of financial uncertainty, it is unlikely that service managers will completely avoid some staff anxiety associated with an uncertain future. However, organization leaders through their positive outlook and modeling of how to accept change while maintaining a focus

TABLE 11.1 Potential Solutions to Barriers to Implementation

Implementation Issue	Potential Solutions
Concerns over durability	Planning and long-term decision making
	Cost–benefit analysis in planning
Innovation fatigue	Planning and long-term decision making
Ensuring the right people are trained	Careful selection of staff
	Ensuring managerial and supervisory frameworks are in place to facilitate delivery
Role and remit	Realistic expectations of staff
(i.e., the roles, and the expectations of the roles, held by the staff and practitioners involved in delivering Triple P)	Better coordinated management decision making and identification of appropriate staffing
	Deciding on what current activity needs to be replaced
	Novel ways of integrating parenting services (e.g., with school enrollment)
Understanding evidence-based practice	Careful selection of staff to be trained
	Training to ensure practitioners understand that this is good for families
	Demonstrating understanding of need for clear specification of goals and outcomes
	Performance monitoring
Research data collection	Research staff need to work with managers to ensure rationale and model are understood and data collection is supported
	Selection of realistic, brief measures
Teasing out the impact of intervention	Judicious selection of key programs for intervention
	Phased roll-outs
	Phasing in interventions in specific localities
Moving the focus from "problem families" to a population approach	Destigmatization of parenting advice
	Consultation, education, and training for practitioners
	Strategies for management of change of focus

on the organization's long-term goals and values can promote an organizational culture that accepts change as being inevitable and can have desirable outcomes.

Ensuring that the right people are trained. When policies are rolled out without sufficient consultation and agreement with staff, decisions may be made to send particular members of staff for training without adequate preparation or understanding of what will be required. In extreme cases this may result in staff attending training without understanding why they are there, or being trained and then not implementing the intervention, which represents a wasted resource. Careful planning is required at the managerial level to determine which staff should be trained and what the arrangements will be to free up time for them to implement their training in order to meet accreditation requirements and then begin to use the intervention on a regular basis. Integrating this into a clear supervisory framework will enhance implementation.

Role and remit. If a new program is not part of a clear, well-communicated plan, staff may be unsure whether it is their role to take on this specific kind of work, and whether time will be made available to undertake interventions, even if they have been sent for training. Managerial involvement in setting targets and goals for individual staff and managing their workload will help to ensure that training funds are well used and the desired outcomes are achieved. A memorandum of agreement can be useful between the funders and organizations to ensure that a sufficient number of programs are actually implemented with parents.

Understanding evidence-based practice. While the notion of evidence-based work is becoming the expected norm in service delivery, many practitioners who do not have a scientific background or sufficient prior training may not have a thorough grasp of the meaning of the concept. This may lead to a number of difficulties in implementation. It is possible, for example, that practitioners may depart significantly from the evidence-based protocol and make idiosyncratic modifications to the program. Practitioners who are not at ease with evidence-based practice may also not see the relevance or value of collecting and using questionnaire or observational data for families, whereas an experienced practitioner will know how valuable such measures are in identifying specific areas of difficulty to focus on. Experienced practitioners will also know how rewarding it can be for families to see that their scores on problem inventories have reduced. This understanding of the value of measurement as important feedback both for families and services is important for the establishment of effective evidence-based practice.

Research data collection. A more extreme form of the above problem can occur when practitioners are asked to contribute data on their practice to a research study on an evidence-based program, as may be the case when a new program is being rolled out. Practitioners may find the additional research consent procedures cumbersome, and there is a risk that they may not inform a research project of families taking up interventions. If evaluations of these kinds of public health-level interventions are to be well evaluated, it is necessary to be able to access data on change without having to utilize a system that is so time consuming for practitioners that data are lost (Spoth & Redmond, 2002). It is incumbent on researchers to work with service managers in undertaking careful planning of evaluation to minimize burden, and to combine this with sufficient training and information for practitioners to ensure that they understand the value of their contribution.

Teasing out the impact of intervention. Local services may have a number of different initiatives running in parallel, which makes it difficult to tease out a clear picture of change arising from a specific intervention. Adopting a population-level approach and minimizing the number of different programs in operation will help to clarify the contribution of that chosen approach. Planning phased rollouts of different programs at different times or across different sectors of a city or county, with a realistic timescale to see results, may help service managers to clarify the relative impact of different innovations.

Moving the focus from "problem families" to a population approach. Services that are accustomed to seeing parenting interventions as appropriate only for families showing marked levels of difficulties may struggle with the concept of a population-level approach, and the destigmatization of parenting advice that goes hand in hand with this. Consultation, education, and training are needed to shift perceptions away from a focus on families who experience the most extreme difficulties to a broader one, and to demonstrate the ways in which universal access to parenting interventions can have preventative value for families experiencing less serious difficulties, as part of a move toward a population-level, public health model.

OUTCOME EVALUATION

The evidence base for Triple P has been detailed elsewhere (e.g., Sanders, 1999; 2008). Triple P has featured prominently in four different meta-analyses, all of which have concluded that the intervention is effective in reducing behavior problems in children (e.g., de Graaf, Speetjens, Smit, de Wolff, & Tavecchio, 2008a, 2008b; Nowak & Heinrichs, 2008; Thomas & Zimmer-Gembeck, 2007), as well as systematic reviews of evidence-based programs for children (e.g., Eyberg et al., 2008). In addition, the program is featured as an evidence-based intervention for the prevention of violence on several independent lists of evidence-based programs including the National Institute of Clinical Excellence guidelines for the treatment of conduct disorder (NICE, 2006); the World Health Organization's recommended programs for global violence reduction (WHO, 2009), the United Nations' Task force on family based treatment for prevention of substance abuse (UNODC, 2009), Blueprints for Violence Prevention (www.colorado.edu/cspv/blueprints), the California Clearing House for Evidence-Based Social Work (www.cebc4cw.org), and the National Academy for Parenting Research (www.parentingresearch.org. uk). The evaluation of the Triple P system is a complex process. The different levels of the intervention with specific applications for different age groups, types of child problems, and delivery modalities have all been separately evaluated—mostly using randomized trial methodology. The rationale for this approach has been to determine that each program variant or delivery modality has specific positive effects that would justify incorporation into the multilevel system of intervention.

Triple P is the only parenting program to have implemented multiple levels of the same intervention concurrently to an entire population and shown population-level effects on rates of child maltreatment (e.g., Prinz, Sanders, Shapiro, Whitkaer & Lutzker, 2009; Sanders et al., 2008). The Triple P South Carolina Trial (Prinz et al., 2009) is a powerful and recent demonstration of the potential population-level effects of Triple P on child and parent factors. The South Carolina Trial randomized 18 moderate-sized South Carolina counties to conditions and assessed the effects at a population-level on indices of child abuse and neglect. The selected counties, ranging in population size from 50,000 to 175,000 per county, were matched in pairs based on child maltreatment prevalence rate, approximate size (population), and poverty level (proportion of households below the poverty line), and then assigned to a condition. The referent population in the 18 counties for the trial consists of the parents/caregivers in all households with one or more children in the birth to 7-year-old range. As part of the population approach, the trial involved several media and informational strategies such as local newspaper coverage of Triple P programming and dissemination in each county, public service radio spots about positive parenting and Triple P programming, and informational flyers and brochures distributed to community centers, advocacy organizations, and family households in the nine Triple P System counties.

The evaluation showed that after 3 years of implementation there were significantly lower rates of substantiated cases of maltreatment, hospitalization, and emergency room visits due to maltreatment-related injuries and out-of-home placements than in care-as-usual counties. This is the first study to document population-level effects on child maltreatment due to a parenting intervention.

In addition to population-level research, a large number of evaluation studies have been conducted using mixed research methods. These include single-subject research designs (e.g., Boyle et al., 2010); randomized trials with varying control conditions including waitlist controls, care as usual, and no treatment comparison conditions (e.g., Sanders et al., 2000); quasi-experimental evaluations (e.g., Zubrick et al., 1995); population-level trials using cluster randomized designs (e.g., Prinz et al., 2009); and independent meta-analyses (e.g., Nowak & Heinrichs, 2008). Studies generally show positive outcomes on child and parent outcome measures and have also been established in different cultures, service delivery contexts, sites and investigators. For example, Turner, Richards, and Sanders (2007) investigated the effects of a culturally tailored version of Triple P for indigenous parents in Australia. Extensive community consultation occurred in developing the tailored program. While program content was seen as appropriate, changes were made to the language and images used in program resources and the examples used to depict parenting strategies (e.g., culturally tailored video and workbook and presentation aids were developed). The structure of group sessions was also altered to allow more time to discuss the social and political context for parenting, develop trust, slow the pace of presentation, and share personal stories. Indigenous parents attending Group Triple P reported significant decreases in rates of problem child behavior in comparison to those in the waitlist condition, as well as a significant decrease in reliance on some dysfunctional parenting practices, and these gains were maintained at 6-month follow-up. The program resulted in high rates of consumer satisfaction, and there were generally positive comments about the cultural acceptability of the program content, resources, and format.

Triple P has an ongoing scientific agenda informed by an International Triple P Research Network (ITPRN). An annual scientific conference and scientific retreat is held to foster ongoing research and critical appraisal as well as international collaboration and independent program evaluations. An archive of all Triple P studies is hosted on a University of Queensland website (www.pfsc.uq.edu.au/evidence). There are many research groups around the world undertaking research using the Triple P model, including the University of Auckland (New Zealand) and the University of Manchester (United Kingdom). A commitment to ongoing research and development and critical appraisal is an integral part of the dissemination model that guides the ongoing development of the program. This model is outlined in Figure 11.1.

Conclusion

Our experience in implementing large-scale population-based parenting initiatives has convinced us of the necessity of such an approach if a population-level change in social, emotional, and behavioral problems in children and youth is to be achieved. The synergies created when multiple levels of an evidence-based intervention are concurrently offered in a geographical area hold great promise in producing change in important indicators of child well-being, such as rates of child maltreatment, hospitalizations and injuries, and out-of-home placements (e.g., Prinz et al., 2009). Large-scale implementation projects provide a rich source of information concerning ways of optimizing population-level outcomes. Over time responsivity to evidence-based practice will result in further tailoring of the program to new client populations, such as parents of children with a disability (Sanders, Mazzucchelli, & Studman, 2004; Whittingham, Sofronnoff, Sheffield, & Sanders, 2009) or health-related problems, such as obesity (West & Sanders, 2009). Ultimately, program developers need to take seriously and respond appropriately to field-based evidence so that all aspects of a program continue to evolve.

REFERENCES

American Psychological Association. (2009). *Effective strategies to support positive parenting in community health centers: Report of the Working Group on Child Maltreatment Prevention in Community Health Centers:* Washington, DC: Author.

Biglan, A. (1995). Translating what we know about the context of antisocial behavior into a lower prevalence of such behavior. *Journal of Applied Behavior Analysis, 28,* 479–492.

Boyle, C.L., Sanders, M.R., Lutzker, J.R., Prinz, R.J., Shapiro, C. & Whitaker, D.J. (2010). An analysis of training, generalization, and maintenance effects of primary care Triple P for parents of preschool-aged children with disruptive behavior. *Child Psychiatry and Human Development, 41,* 114–131.

Calam, R., Sanders, M. R., Miller, C., Sadhnani, V., & Carmont, S. A. (2008). Can technology and the media help reduce dysfunctional parenting and increase engagement with preventative parenting interventions? *Child Maltreatment, 13,* 347–361.

Connell, S., Sanders, M. R., & Markie-Dadds, C. (1997). Self-directed behavioral family intervention for parents of oppositional children in rural and remote areas. *Behavior Modification, 21,* 379–408.

de Graaf, I., Speetjens, P., Smit, F., de Wolff, M., & Tavecchio, L. (2008a). Effectiveness of the Triple P Positive Parenting Program on behavioural problems in children: A meta-analysis. *Behavior Modification, 32*, 714–735.

de Graaf, I., Speetjens, P., Smit, F., de Wolff, M., & Tavecchio, L. (2008b). Effectiveness of the Triple P Positive Parenting Program on Parenting: A meta-analysis. *Family Relations, 57*, 553–566.

Dumas, J. E., Nissley-Tsiopinis, J., & Moreland, A. D. (2007). From intent to enrollment, attendance and participation in preventive parenting groups. *Journal of Child and Family Studies, 16*, 1–26.

Every Child Matters. (2003). *Every Child Matters green paper.* Retrieved October 5, 2009, from http://publications.everychildmatters.gov.uk/eOrderingDownload/CM5860.pdf

Eyberg, S. M., Nelson, M. M. & Boggs, S. R. (2008). Evidence-based psychosocial treatments for children and adolescents with disruptive behaviour. *Journal of Clinical Child and Adolescent Psychology, 37*, 215–237.

Farquhar, J. W., Fortmann, S. P., Maccoby, N., Haskell, W. L., Williams, P. T, Flora, J. A., et al. (1985). The Stanford Five-City Project: Design and methods. *American Journal of Epidemiology, 122*, 323–334.

Flay, B. R., Biglan, A., Boruch, R. F., González Castro, F., Gottfredson, D., Kellam, S., et al. (2005). Standards of evidence: Criteria for efficacy, effectiveness and dissemination. *Prevention Science, 6*, 151–175.

Glasgow, R. E., Klesges, L. M., Dzewaltowski, D. A., Estabrooks, P. A., & Vogt, T. M. (2006). Evaluating the impact of health promotion programs: Using the RE-AIM framework to form summary measures for decision making involving complex issues. *Health Education and Research, 21*, 688–694.

Glasgow, R. E., Lichtenstein, E., & Marcus, A. C. (2003). Why don't we see more translation of health promotion research to practice? Rethinking the efficacy-to-effectiveness transition. *American Journal of Public Health, 93*, 1261–1267.

Gotham, H. J. (2004). Diffusion of mental health and substance use treatments: Development, dissemination and implementation. *Clinical Psychology: Science and Practice, 11*, 160–176.

Kaminski, J. W., Valle, L. A., Filene, J. H., & Boyle, C. L. (2008). A meta-analytic review of components associated with parent training program effectiveness. *Journal of Abnormal Child Psychology, 36*, 567–589.

Kazdin, A. E. (2005). *Parent management training: Treatment for oppositional, aggressive, and antisocial behavior in children and adolescents.* New York: Oxford University Press.

Mittlemark, M. B., Puska, P., O'Byrne, D., & Tang, K. C. (Eds.). (2005). *Health promotion: A sketch of the landscape.* Geneva: World Health Organization.

Murphy-Brennan, M. G. (2007). *Factors underlying the effective implementation of evidence-based programs.* Brisbane: University of Queensland.

National Institute of Clinical Excellence and Social Care. (2006). *Parent-training/education programmes in the management of children with conduct disorders.* London: Author.

National Research Council and Institute of Medicine. Committee on the Prevention of Mental Disorders and Substance Abuse among Children, Youth, and Young Adults: Research Advances and Promising Interventions. M. E. O'Connell, T. Boat, & K. E. Warner (Eds.), Board on Children, Youth, and Families, Division of Behavioral and Social Sciences and Education. (2009). *Preventing mental, emotional, and behavioral disorders among young people: Progress and possibilities.* Washington, DC: The National Academies Press.

Nowak, C., & Heinrichs, N. (2008). A comprehensive meta-analysis of Triple P-Positive Parenting Program using hierarchical linear modeling: Effectiveness and moderating variables. *Clinical Child and Family Psychology Review, 11,* 114–144.

Patterson, G. R., Reid, J. B., Jones, R. R., & Conger, R. E. (1975). *A social learning theory approach to family intervention: Volume I. Families with aggressive children.* Eugene, OR: Castalia Publishing Co.

Pentz, M. A. (2004). Form follows function: Designs for prevention effectiveness and diffusion research. *Prevention Science, 5,* 23–29.

Prinz, R. J., Sanders, M. R., Shapiro, C. J., Whitaker, D. J. & Lutzker, J. R. (2009). Population-based prevention of child maltreatment: The US Triple P system population trial. *Prevention Science, 10,* 1–12.

Risley, T. R., Clark, H. B., & Cataldo, M. F. (1976). Behavioral technology for the normal middle-class family. In E. J. Mash, L. A. Hamerlynck, & L. C. Handy (Eds.), *Behavior modification and families* (pp. 34–60). New York: Brunner/Mazel.

Sanders, M. R. (1999). The Triple P-Positive parenting program: Towards an empirically validated multilevel parenting and family support strategy for the prevention of behavior and emotional problems in children. *Clinical Child and Family Psychology Review, 2,* 71–90.

Sanders, M. R. (2008). The Triple P-Positive Parenting Program as a public health approach to strengthening parenting. *Journal of Family Psychology, 22,* 506–517.

Sanders, M., Calam, R., Durand, M., Liversidge, T., & Carmont, S. A. (2008). Does self-directed and web-based support for parents enhance the effects of viewing a reality television series based on the Triple P-Positive Parenting Programme? *Journal of Child Psychology and Psychiatry, 49,* 934–942.

Sanders, M. R., Cann, W., & Markie-Dadds, C. (2003). The Triple P-Positive Parenting Program: A universal population-level approach to the prevention of child abuse. *Child Abuse Review, 12,* 155–171.

Sanders, M. R., & Glynn, E. L. (1981). Training parents in behavioral self-management: An analysis of generalization and maintenance effects. *Journal of Applied Behavior Analysis, 14,* 223–237.

Sanders, M. R., Haslam, D., Calam, R., Southwell, C., & Stallman, H. M. (2011). Designing effective interventions for working parents: A web-based survey of parents in the UK workforce. *Journal of Children's Services, 6,*186–200.

Sanders, M. R., Markie-Dadds, C., Rinaldis, M., Firman, D., & Baig, N. (2007). Using household survey data to inform policy decisions regarding the delivery of evidence-based parenting interventions. *Child: Care, Health and Development, 33,* 768–783.

Sanders, M. R., Markie-Dadds, C., Tully, L. A., & Bor, W. (2000). The Triple P-Positive Parenting Program: A comparison of enhanced, standard, and self-directed behavioral family intervention for parents of children with early onset conduct problems. *Journal of Consulting and Clinical Psychology, 68,* 624–640.

Sanders, M. R., Markie-Dadds, C., & Turner, K. M. T. (1996). *Positive parenting.* Brisbane, Australia: Families International Publishing.

Sanders, M. R., Mazzucchelli, T. G., & Studman, L. (2004). Stepping Stones Triple P - The theoretical basis and development of an evidence-based positive parenting program for families with a child who has a disability. *Journal of Intellectual and Developmental Disability, 29*, 265–283.

Sanders, M.R. & Murphy-Brennan, M. (2010). Creating conditions for success beyond the professional training environment. *Clinical Psychology: Science & Practice, 17*, 31–35.

Sanders, M. R., & Prinz, R. J. (2008). Ethical and professional issues in the implementation of population-level parenting interventions. *Clinical Psychology: Science and Practice, 15*, 130–136.

Sanders, M. R., Ralph, A., Sofronoff, K., Gardiner, P., Thompson, R., Dwyer, S., et al. (2008). Every family: A population approach to reducing behavioral and emotional problems in children making the transition to school. *Journal of Primary Prevention, 29*, 197–222.

Singhal, A., Cody, M. J., Rogers, E. M., & Sabido, M. (Eds.). (2003). *Entertainment-education and social change: History, research and practice*. Mahwah, NJ: Lawrence Erlbaum.

Spoth, R. & Redmond, C. (2002). Project Family prevention trials based in community-university partnerships: Toward scaled-up preventive interventions. *Prevention Science, 3*, 203–221.

Thomas, R., & Zimmer-Gembeck, M. J. (2007). Behavioral outcomes of parent–child interaction therapy and Triple P—Positive Parenting Program: A review and meta-analysis. *Journal of Abnormal Child Psychology, 35*, 475–495.

Turner, K. M. T., & Sanders, M. R. (2006). Help when it's needed first: A controlled evaluation of brief, preventive behavioral family intervention in a primary care setting. *Behavior Therapy, 37*, 131–142.

Turner, K.M.T., Richards, M., &. Sanders, M.R. (2007). A randomised clinical trial of a group parent education program for Australian Indigenous families. *Journal of Pediatrics and Child Health, 43*, 429–437.

United Nations Office on Drugs and Crime (UNDOC), Vienna. (2009). *Guide to implementing family skills training programmes for drug abuse prevention*. New York: United Nations.

West, F., & Sanders, M. R. (2009). The Lifestyle Behaviour Checklist: A measure of weight-related problem behaviour in obese children. *International Journal of Pediatric Obesity, 1*, 1–8.

Whittingham, K., Sofronoff, K., Sheffield, J., & Sanders, M.R. (2009). Stepping Stones Triple P: An RCT of a parenting program with parents of a child diagnosed with an Autism Spectrum Disorder. *Journal of Abnormal Child Psychology, 37*, 469–480.

World Health Organization. (2009). *Preventing violence through the development of safe, stable and nurturing relationships between children and their parents and caregivers. Series of briefings on violence prevention: the evidence*. Geneva, Switzerland: Author.

Zubrick, S. R., Silburn, S. R., Garton, A., Burton, P., Dalby, R., Carlton, J., et al. (1995). *Western Australian Child Health Survey: Developing health and wellbeing in the nineties* (ISBN 0 642 20754 2). Perth, Western Australia: Australian Bureau of Statistics and the TVW Telethon Institute for Child Health Research.

Zubrick, S. R., Ward, K. A., Silburn, S. R., Lawrence, D., Williams, A. A., Blair, E., et al. (2005). Prevention of child behavior problems through universal implementation of a group behavioral family intervention. *Prevention Science, 6*, 287–304.

{12}

The Transport and Diffusion of Multisystemic Therapy

Sonja K. Schoenwald

Multisystemic Therapy (MST; Henggeler, Schoenwald, Borduin, Rowland, & Cunningham, 2009) is an intensive family- and community-based treatment originally developed for delinquent youth at imminent risk of incarceration or other restrictive out-of-home placement settings. Independent reviewers (see, e.g., Eyberg, Nelson, & Boggs, 2008; Hoge, Guerra, & Boxer, 2008; Waldron & Turner, 2008; Weisz, 2004), government reports (see, e.g., National Institute on Drug Abuse, 1999; National Institutes of Health, 2006; U.S. Public Health Service, 2001), and consumer groups (see, e.g., National Alliance for the Mentally Ill, 2003, 2008; National Mental Health Association, 2004) have identified MST as among the most effective treatments for serious antisocial behavior in adolescents, including chronic, violent, and substance-abusing delinquents.

Overview

MOTIVATION FOR THE DEVELOPMENT OF MULTISYSTEMIC THERAPY

A major impetus for the initial development of MST was the lack of empirical support for the treatments and social programs for delinquency that had permeated decades of juvenile justice practice and policy, and evidence that the emerging promise of treatments such as behavioral parent training for conduct problems in children did not appear to apply to adolescents (Henggeler, 1989). As MST development began in the late 1970s, published and ongoing correlational and longitudinal research showed delinquency was associated with multiple risk factors within and between the key systems in which children are embedded—family, peer, school, and neighborhood. Delinquency interventions, however, focused on one or a small set of these risk factors.

The extensive literature documenting the interplay of multiple risk factors across systems in the development of serious antisocial behavior and related problems in youth is consistent with Bronfenbrenner's (1979) theory of social ecology, the fundamental tenet of which is that individuals are embedded in multiple systems that have direct and indirect influences on behavior. That literature and social ecological theory formed the basis for the MST theory of change, which posited the necessity of addressing established risk factors across family and extrafamilial systems to reduce the serious antisocial behavior and related problems of adolescents.

MULTISYSTEMIC THERAPY CLINICAL AND SERVICE PARAMETERS

MST uses a short-term (3 to 5 months) intensive home- and community-based model of service delivery to implement comprehensive treatment that specifically targets factors in each youth's social ecology (family, peers, school, neighborhood, and community). Clinicians are organized into teams of two to four therapists and a clinical supervisor. MST therapists carry a caseload of four to six families at a time and vary the frequency and duration of treatment contacts to the circumstances, needs, and strengths of each family throughout the treatment episode. Nine treatment principles and a specified analytic process guide the clinical formulation process and MST assessment and intervention strategies. Interventions typically focus on improving caregiver discipline and monitoring practices, reducing family conflict, improving affective relations, decreasing youth association with deviant peers, increasing association with prosocial peers, improving school or vocational performance, and developing an indigenous support network of family, friends, and neighbors to support treatment progress and help the family sustain treatment gains in the long term. Specific treatment techniques are integrated into a social ecological framework for understanding behavior from those therapies that have the most empirical support, including behavioral and behavioral parent training, cognitive behavioral, and pragmatic family therapies.

MULTISYSTEMIC THERAPY QUALITY ASSURANCE/QUALITY IMPROVEMENT SYSTEM

The MST quality assurance and improvement (QA/QI) system is designed to support the sustainable implementation with fidelity of MST at multiple levels of the clinical context (Henggeler & Schoenwald, 1999). The development and refinement of this system was informed by procedures used to implement MST in randomized effectiveness trials, then-available theory and research on adopter-based models of the diffusion of innovation (Rogers, 2003) and technology transfer in behavioral health (Backer & David, 1995; Brown, 1995); and early experiences attempting the transport of MST. For example, case studies (Rogers, 2003) and research reviews (Brown, 1995) suggested proactive dissemination strategies could lead to the rejection, adoption, or adaptation of an innovation, pending the influence of characteristics of the innovation itself, end-users, and interface between innovators and end-users. A descriptive account of how MST and the QA/QI system might map onto such characteristics appears elsewhere (Schoenwald & Henggeler, 2002). In addition, organizational research—specifically on innovative organizations and organizational implementation of innovations—showed that organizational failure to implement an innovation properly was often mistaken for innovation failure (Klein & Sorra, 1996; Real & Poole, 2005). That literature suggested innovation-specific policies and procedures are needed to support adequate implementation (Klein & Knight, 2005).

The three broad components of the MST QA/QI system are (a) clinician training and ongoing support, (b) organizational support, and (c) implementation measurement and reporting. Each component is composed of several elements, described in this chapter. As illustrated in Figure 12.1, these elements are integrated into a feedback loop that includes data about MST implementation at the level of the family, therapist, supervisor, expert consultant, and organization operating the MST program. Optimizing youth outcomes is the focus of all elements of the system.

The MST QA/QI system is deployed through MST Services, LLC (MSTS) and its Network Partners (described subsequently). In 1996, following the trail blazed by other universities after federal legislation was enacted to increase the speed and reach of research innovations in the marketplace (the Bayh-Dole Act of 1980, Council on Government Relations, 1999), MSTS was licensed by the Medical

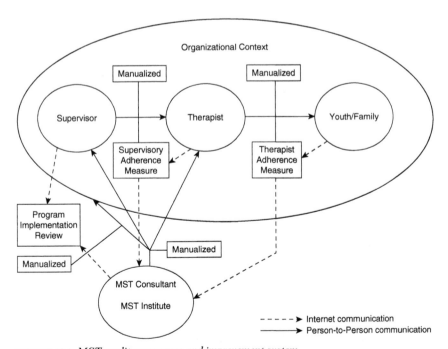

FIGURE 12.1 *MST quality assurance and improvement system.*
Reprinted with the permission of Guilford Press. From Henggeler, Schoenwald, Borduin, Rowland, and Cunningham (2009), *Multisystemic Therapy for Antisocial Behavior in Children and Adolescents, Second Edition,* © Guilford Press.

University of South Carolina (MUSC) to transfer MST-related technology to interested communities. Today, MSTS and its 21 Network Partners are the "purveyors" of MST (Fixsen, Naoom, Blase, Friedman, & Wallace, 2005), with the latter serving the majority of MST programs.

Circumstances Motivating the Transport of Multisystemic Therapy

INITIAL DEMAND FOR MULTISYSTEMIC THERAPY TRANSPORT

The transport of MST began as a function of demand from government agencies mandated to serve juvenile offenders and the organizations contracted by them to provide such treatment. Serving juvenile offenders was costly for these government agencies, as "service" consisted primarily of incarceration, residential treatment, and other out-of-home placements. Published evidence from randomized trials supported the long-term clinical and cost effectiveness of MST for the target population the government was mandated to serve. These mandates did not, however, require *effective* or *evidence-based* services to be provided.

KEY FEDERAL INITIATIVES

Two federal initiatives stimulated additional demand for MST. The Office of Juvenile Justice and Delinquency Prevention (OJJDP) and the Center for Mental Health Services (CMHS) of the Substance Abuse and Mental Health Services Administration (SAMHSA) funded initiatives for youth experiencing high rates of out-of-home placement and poor clinical, functional, and service system outcomes. OJJDP undertook four strategies to identify and support the broader use of *effective* juvenile justice prevention and intervention strategies. The strategies included (a) commissioning a comprehensive review of effective youth violence prevention and intervention programs by Delbert Elliott and his colleagues at the Center for the Study of the Prevention of Violence at the University of Colorado at Boulder (Elliott, 1998), and designating on the basis of that review the violence prevention programs with the best empirical evidence of effectiveness as Blueprints for Violence Prevention Model Programs (www.colorado.edu/cspv/blueprints); (b) through the Juvenile Accountability Block Grants (JABG) program (www.ojjdp.ncjrs.org/jabg/overview.html), issuing grants to states to reduce juvenile offending and requiring measurement of the effects of the grant-funded activities; (c) issuing a grant to help disseminate and evaluate the dissemination of the evidence-based Blueprints programs, which was subsequently amended to include evaluation of implementation and outcomes; and (d) providing seed funding to develop manuals and measures for key aspects of MST implementation, a rudimentary computerized fidelity and outcomes tracking system, and a pilot study of the feasibility of their use.

In the mid-1990s, expansion of the federal Comprehensive Community Mental Health Services for Children and Their Families Program increased the number of states receiving grants to develop systems of care (SOC) to improve the access, array, and child- and family-centered nature of community-based mental health services for youth with severe emotional disturbances (SEDs). Some state departments of mental health with SOC grants sought to import MST to treat youth with SEDs at imminent risk of placement. At the time, a randomized trial of an MST adaptation for youth in acute psychiatric crises was under way and yielding promising short-term results. The MST model developers and MSTS agreed to attempt the transport of MST to organizations serving the case mix of youth falling under the SOC umbrella. As the experience unfolded, it became clear that effective treatment for some youth in crisis would require the adaptations still being tested in the randomized trial. The longer-term outcomes of that trial were not yet known, however, and only the project staff had the expertise to train and support therapists. By mutual agreement, the model developers, MSTS, and several SOC sites discontinued the use of MST for this population or shifted the population served to juvenile offenders.

The SOC experience, among others, contributed to the creation by the MST developers and purveyors of a rubric identifying specific adaptations of MST for different populations (available online at www.mstservices.com). This rubric conveys and updates the status of the evidence base with respect to (a) the effectiveness of MST adaptations and (b) the transfer of training and clinical support expertise from the adaptation developers to purveyors needed to support community-based implementation. By virtue of this discernment process, and as reflected in the SAMHSA-sponsored National Registry of Evidence-Based Programs and Practices (NREPP; www.nrepp.samhsa.gov), adaptations of MST for specific populations tested in randomized trials are now identified in an easily accessible, public forum.

STATE INITIATIVES

State initiatives contributing to the diffusion of MST have taken various forms, several of which are presented here. In Washington and Florida, the legislatures identified juvenile crime and the associated community safety risks and costs as sufficiently onerous problems to warrant new legislation. In 1997, Washington legislated the use of research-based programs to reduce juvenile crime costs through the Community Juvenile Accountability Act. The Washington State Institute on Public Policy (WSIPP; www.wsipp.wa.gov) selected programs on the basis of a national research literature review and was also contracted to evaluate the performance of the programs as implemented in Washington. Counties chose the programs they wished to implement, and service funding was partially provided by the legislation, with the aforementioned JABG grants to states and Blueprints dollars contributing to the cause. Three counties established MST teams as a result of this initiative. In 2003, the Florida legislature undertook a statewide initiative to import evidence-based treatments for juvenile offenders and evaluate the effects of those treatments in Florida. The legislation was discharged through the state department of juvenile justice in a new program called Redirection. Redirection imported only models whose implementation and outcomes were favorable in Washington and other states; and MST and Functional Family Therapy (Sexton & Alexander, 2005) were the models imported.

In the intervening years, several states sought to import one or more evidence-based treatments and then to expand the reach of those treatments throughout the state. States differed in their approach to the task. The states' strategies can be conceptualized on a continuum from centralized to laissez-faire. Connecticut, for example, pursued a centralized approach to the import and expansion of MST. There, the Department of Children and Families, responsible for serving youth in state custody, initiated the import of MST as aftercare for juvenile offenders released from out-of-home placements. State-funded evaluations of MST were favorable, and these, along with political pressures to improve services for juvenile offenders not in state custody, prompted the Court Support Services Division of the judicial branch to support statewide expansion of MST. Today, the Department of Children and Families and Court Support Services Division directly reimburse contracted provider organizations for delivering MST to youth and families and jointly fund a Connecticut-based Network Partner organization to provide the training and quality assurance to all MST programs in the state.

Ohio provides an example in the middle of the continuum between centralized and laissez-faire strategies to take evidence-based treatments to scale. Although the import of MST was initiated in 1996 as a result of a governor's office initiative to improve and evaluate services for juvenile offenders, the growth of MST accelerated via the state's establishment in 1999 of Coordinating Centers of Excellence across all state departments (health, education, welfare, juvenile justice, mental health). The state provided infrastructure funds to support each Coordinating Center of Excellence, each of which established its own strategies for identifying practices it wished to import or develop. Within the Department of Mental Health, the Center for Innovative Practices was established to collaborate with local mental health boards (which control services and funds) and diverse stakeholders to identify and support a variety of clinical practices. As an MST Network Partner, the Center for Innovative Practices provides the QA/QI system to MST programs in Ohio.

Finally, Colorado presents an example of highly decentralized, non–publicly funded diffusion of MST. The first MST teams in Colorado were established with funding from the aforementioned federal JABG and Blueprints dissemination programs. The subsequent expansion of programs, however, was spearheaded by private provider organizations. Today, the MST Network Partner in Colorado, the Center for Effective Interventions, supports the majority of MST programs in Colorado, New Mexico, and neighboring states, but receives no state or county support or sponsorship for these activities. As occurs in Ohio and Connecticut, state and county agencies contract directly with provider organizations to serve youth and families with MST.

INTERNATIONAL PARALLELS

The continuum of centralized to laissez-faire dissemination of MST is also apparent among international sites. Space constraints prevent elaboration on this point, but interested readers can find details in recent publications (Ogden, Christiansen, Sheidow, & Hoth, 2008; Schoenwald, Heiblum, Saldana, & Henggeler, 2008). Norway provides an example of a highly centralized strategy, akin to that taken in Connecticut. A Norwegian government initiative launched in 1997 to provide evidence-based treatments to the nation's youth enabled counties and collaborating municipalities to select the treatments they wished to implement. In 1999, four counties launched MST teams; today, MST Norway, a Network Partner funded by the Norwegian government, supports MST programs in 17 of the 19 counties in Norway. Denmark is more similar to Ohio, in that the government provides infrastructure support to an umbrella agency, but the decision to start an MST program is locally made and funded. Finally, the Netherlands is more similar to Colorado, as private provider agencies are spearheading the import of MST and its dissemination.

Description of Multisystemic Therapy Programs

FUNDING

In 1994, South Carolina's state Medicaid, Juvenile Justice, and Mental Health agencies provided MST developers and researchers at MUSC a first opportunity to collaborate in crafting a strategy to transport MST using public financing strategies. This year-long process included collaboration in the development of a Medicaid standard that included medical necessity criteria, clinical standards, management standards, outcomes standards, and reimbursement levels and mechanisms that would neither reward "creaming" of youth and families to serve only those less complex problems nor truncate services to collect payment prior to treatment completion. Nebraska and New Mexico were among other states that pioneered the import of MST using Medicaid funds.

In South Carolina, the MST service reimbursement rate did not include the costs of training and consultation, as the latter occurred through a separate state contract to the Family Services Research Center (FSRC) to pilot operation of an MST training division for South Carolina service providers. Currently, payers (typically county or state agencies) vary with respect to the inclusion of the QA/QI costs as part of the service cost (i.e., per youth cost of providing care) or as separate expenses. In either case, inclusion of the QA/QI costs is reflected in estimates provided to communities interested in importing MST, and in costs compared in cost-effectiveness and cost-offset analyses (see, e.g., Aos, Miller, & Drake, 2006; Cartwright, Kitsantas, & Rose, 2009).

Because the sources of funding for MST programs vary within and across states, and because Medicaid coverage terms and reimbursement rates vary across states, the extent to which financing strategies for MST developed in one locale or state can generalize to another, or to other evidence-based treatments, is unclear. Examples of the funding mechanisms and strategies government agencies and private service provider organizations use to develop and sustain evidence-based treatment programs including MST are, however, described in a recent document authored by members of the National Implementation Research Network and MST Network Partners (George et al., 2008).

GOALS

MST was originally developed to treat delinquent youth, and the ultimate outcomes of the randomized trials for this population were to significantly reduce the short- and long-term rates and seriousness of youth criminal behavior and rates and length of incarceration and other restrictive out-of-home placements. Evidence from randomized trials supported the achievement of these goals, and of the MST theory of change, initially via evidence of significant condition differences favoring MST in such domains as family functioning and youth association with delinquent peers, and subsequently via formal mediation analyses, which also supported linkages between caregiver-reported therapist adherence and treatment-related change (Henggeler, Letourneau, et al., 2009; Huey, Henggeler, Brondino, & Pickrel, 2000; Schoenwald, Henggeler, Brondino, & Rowland, 2000). Accordingly, the outcomes typically sought by communities establishing MST programs for juvenile offenders include reductions in rearrest, out-of-home placements, and costs. The specific outcomes for which an MST program in a particular community is held accountable are detailed in the "MST Goals and Guidelines" document described subsequently.

NEEDS ASSESSMENT: ASSESSING AND CULTIVATING THE FIT OF MULTISYSTEMIC THERAPY AND THE COMMUNITY

MST program development is a process that begins with a community's initial expression of interest in MST and continues through the day a new MST program first treats a youth and family. The process typically unfolds in seven stages and can take a year, and sometimes longer, for the community and an MST purveyor to complete. Community key features of each stage are briefly summarized here. *Initial information collection* begins when someone representing an agency that funds services (e.g., juvenile justice, mental health, a behavioral health care system) contacts an MST purveyor to express interest in starting an MST program. Discussing a few key questions (e.g., intended type and size of target population) typically helps the interested party either eliminate MST from further consideration or take the next step, which is assessing the feasibility of an MST program in a particular locale. The *MST needs assessment* is designed to help communities determine whether the needs that prompted stakeholder interest in starting an MST program are likely to be met by MST, and whether an MST program is viable in a specific practice context. This process includes identification of a clearly defined target population in the community to be served by MST, identification of funding sources and a financial plan that can sustain the MST program, and cultivation of commitments from stakeholders to implement the program with fidelity.

Next, community representatives and the MST purveyor together make what is known as a *Go or No Go* decision that signals a commitment to conjointly take the next steps in the program development process to verify viability, but not necessarily to start an MST program. These steps include *MST critical issues sessions,* in which the MST purveyor and organizations planning to fund and implement MST specify how critical program components will be developed. Nearly a dozen issues (e.g., inclusion/exclusion criteria, discharge criteria, outcomes measurement) are discussed, and an individualized "MST Goals and Guidelines" document is developed that lays out how these issues will be addressed in a particular MST program serving a particular community. Next, a *Site Readiness Review Meeting* is scheduled to include the individuals who will be responsible for the day-to-day operations of the referral, funding, and service provider organizations that can affect how and when youth and families can receive MST (e.g., middle management or front-line staff from probation, public defenders, or the court). *Follow-up* conference calls and face-to-face meetings are scheduled as needed to align potentially conflicting organizational and service system procedures illuminated in the Site Readiness Review Meeting to support MST implementation. *Staff recruitment and orientation training* can begin before the Site Readiness Review Meeting and continues until all members of the new team are hired. Consultation from the MST purveyor is available regarding advertising, recruitment, and hiring of MST clinicians, given the workforce and job market in the particular locale. The 5-day Initial Orientation Training is the last step before the MST program opens its doors to youth and families.

TRAINING OF CLINICIANS

Providing a comprehensive and intensive treatment like MST to youths and families facing multiple stressors (including imminent risk of youth placement) day after day can be daunting to clinicians. Thus, multifaceted and ongoing training and clinical support is provided to them. The training and support structures and processes were designed to replicate those provided to therapists in randomized trials of MST. These include the following: (a) initial 5-day orientation training, (b) quarterly booster training, (c) weekly on-site supervision, and (d) weekly consultation with an MST expert (originally, the MST model developers and researchers).

Initial 5-Day Orientation Training

MST therapists, on-site supervisors, and other clinicians within the provider organization likely to participate in some aspect of treatment for youth in the program (e.g., a staff psychiatrist who might evaluate and prescribe medication for a youth or caregiver) participate in 5 days of initial orientation training. The first morning of the orientation week brings together the new MST team, interested members in the management and leadership of the organization starting the MST program, and key community stakeholders, including those who participated in the site assessment and program development process. The remainder of the orientation week focuses on the therapists and MST supervisor. The trainers—one of whom is the expert consultant who will provide ongoing training and consultation to the team—use didactic approaches to lay out the rationale for MST assessment and intervention strategies and experiential approaches to enable participants to observe and practice using such strategies in role-play situations. On-the-job training begins when therapists begin treating families and is supported via weekly on-site clinical and telephone expert consultation and quarterly booster training, described below. A written test of knowledge gained by therapists during the orientation week was administered in the early years of MST transport at the request of the agency funding the university-based training of practitioners. This evaluation was discontinued because it did not include observational assessment of MST skills and competencies and yielded a limited distribution of knowledge scores, and because the ongoing collection and reporting of therapist and supervisor adherence, program implementation, and youth outcomes in the QA/QI system enables tracking, troubleshooting, and support of therapist performance in the field.

Quarterly Booster Training

As therapists gain field experience with MST, the expert consultant working with the team conducts quarterly 1.5-day booster training sessions on site. The booster sessions are designed to enhance the knowledge and skills of team members to more effectively address clinical challenges they face over time (e.g., marital interventions, treatment of caregiver depression). The consultant and team use audio or video review and enactment (via role play) of particularly difficult cases to identify and problem solve barriers to progress and practice implementing needed intervention strategies. Therapists evaluate each booster, and consultants use this feedback to improve future booster experiences. Between booster sessions, the MST supervisor and consultant observe therapist implementation of the skills and strategies emphasized during the booster and identify and address barriers to such implementation (e.g., booster provided too few practice opportunities, use of strategies poorly monitored).

Supervision

The main objective of MST supervision is to help therapists use the clinical skills—conceptual and behavioral—needed to effectively implement MST in the field with each and every youth and family served. The MST team and supervisor meet as a group weekly. The supervisor follows a structured protocol for reviewing and addressing the issues in each case with the team; that protocol reflects the MST analytic process, which forms the basis for the MST Case Summary for Supervision and Consultation form completed by each therapist weekly, and by the supervisor and consultant prior to supervision and consultation, respectively. Additional group or individual supervision meetings can be convened to address a case crisis, when the need for field supervision emerges (i.e., supervisor accompanies the therapist), and to address the professional developmental needs of a therapist.

MST supervisors, like MST clinicians, are available 24 hours a day, 7 days a week, and many MST supervisors are recruited from the ranks of effective MST therapists. Supervisors of one team may also carry a reduced caseload of families, whereas supervisors of two or more teams typically do not. Training and support of MST supervisors occurs via several venues, which include review of the MST supervisory manual (Henggeler & Schoenwald, 1998); initial supervisor orientation training prior to or during the initial 5-day orientation training; and periodic conjoint review of supervisor work samples, including at least one audiotape of group supervision monthly. Booster sessions for MST supervisors are available and tailored to the opportunities and challenges awaiting supervisors with different levels of MST experience.

Consultation

The role of the MST expert consultant is to facilitate, within each MST team, the rapid development of the knowledge, skills, and competencies therapists and supervisors need to effectively implement MST with the diverse array of families they serve, and of the skills and processes needed to anticipate, identify, and address clinical, team-level, organizational, and systemic barriers to effective clinical implementation. The consultant provides the initial orientation training, weekly telephone consultation, and quarterly booster training to MST therapists and supervisors and supervisor orientation training and support to MST supervisors. The consultant provides 1 hour of phone time per week to consultation for each MST team.

The MST consultation manual (Schoenwald, 1998) outlines the knowledge base and skills individuals need to effectively execute their responsibilities. In contrast with the training context of most master's- and doctoral-level clinical training programs, the training context for MST involves on-the-job training of clinicians whose professional experience in mental health services predated their joining an MST program. MST consultants, therefore, aim to capitalize on and augment therapist practices to align them with MST as they teach and coach therapists in the conceptual and clinical strategies used in MST. Today, the majority of MST experts are individuals who were successful MST supervisors in communities that have sustained successful MST programs. The initial training process for consultants is codified in an on-the-job training manual and supported by seasoned consultants who serve as coaches in the training process. A full-time consultant can provide telephone consultation and accommodate the travel-associated orientation and booster training sessions for about 10 teams at a time, thereby affecting 30 to 40 therapists treating 360 to 480 families at a time!

Ongoing Organizational Support

Several strategies are used to support the implementation and outcomes of MST programs in the busy and diversified organizations that host MST programs, including an organizational manual for administrators, the program development process described previously, and ongoing organizational support. With respect to the latter, a semi-annual Program Implementation Review (PIR) is designed to enable the organization implementing MST, key stakeholders (including referral and funding sources), and the MST purveyor to examine together key program performance indicators derived from the Goals and Guidelines document for the MST program. In addition, web-based and telephone forums are available for peer learning among MST program directors. Finally, the MST consultant helps the team to address organizational and stakeholder barriers to the implementation of MST in specific cases during weekly consultation and at booster training sessions.

Implementation Measurement and Reporting

As depicted in Figure 12.1, feedback on the implementation of MST at multiple levels of the practice context is obtained from multiple respondents. Validated measures are used to assess therapist, supervisor, and consultant adherence. Caregiver reports of therapist adherence are obtained monthly, therapist reports of supervisor and consultant adherence are obtained semimonthly, and MST program performance is monitored on key program parameters every 6 months. Youth outcomes are measured using standardized discharge forms completed by therapists and official archival data (i.e., arrests, out-of-home placements) where such can be made available by service systems to the provider organizations. A web-based platform to support the reporting, scoring, and interpretation of therapist adherence, supervisor adherence, consultant adherence and youth outcomes is available via the MST Institute (www.mstinstitute.org). Details of the development and validation of the therapist, supervisor, and consultant measures are presented in a recent journal article (Schoenwald, 2008).

Strategies to Target Barriers to Adoption

To date, proactive dissemination efforts of MST—that is, efforts to inform the uninformed that MST may be an appropriate and effective treatment option for a target population of interest, or to persuade those informed but not yet using MST that this is the case—have not been undertaken by the MST model developers or purveyors. Such efforts have, however, been undertaken in the federal and state initiatives described in this chapter. To our knowledge, rigorous empirical evaluations have not been conducted of the impact of these federal and state initiatives on the rate of diffusion of MST and other evidence-based treatments encompassed by the initiatives, or on factors affecting rates of adoption and dis-adoption. Meanwhile, the focus of the model developers has been on supporting and evaluating the implementation and outcomes of MST in communities that sought out and chose to adopt MST. Thus, empirical evidence is scant regarding barriers to the adoption of MST for appropriate populations.

To the extent that insufficient capacity to meet demand could be construed as a barrier to adoption, two early MST transport strategies—moonlighting of MST researchers as trainers and establishment of a state-specific training division—were inadequate solutions, as neither could keep up with community demand for MST or serve adequately the fraction of communities served. The establishment of a university-licensed technology transfer company, and as or more important, of the Network Partner model to cultivate the indigenous expertise in nations, states, or regions interested in larger scale transport appear anecdotally to be addressing this barrier, in that the majority of new programs are established by these Network Partners, and not by MSTS.

EVALUATION

The positive and lasting effects of MST for delinquent youth demonstrated in randomized trials have been summarized in several independent scholarly reviews, meta-analyses, and government reports such as those cited at the beginning of the chapter. This section focuses on data obtained from evaluations conducted in communities that have imported MST.

Transportability Trials

Two groups of independent investigators have published the results of randomized trials examining the effectiveness of standard MST for juvenile offenders as transported from clinicians implementing the model under the supervision of the model developers and first -generation experts trained by them to clinicians supported by indigenous experts using the QA/QI system in distal and diverse clinical settings. In a four-site study in Norway, Ogden and colleagues found that MST significantly decreased youth symptoms and out-of-home placement and increased consumer satisfaction (Ogden & Hagen, 2006a; Ogden & Halliday-Boykins, 2004). In the United States, Timmons-Mitchell and colleagues (Timmons-Mitchell, Bender, Kishna, & Mitchell, 2006) found MST significantly improved youth functioning, decreased recidivism, and decreased substance use problems.

Quasiexperimental and Benchmarking Studies

Independent investigators have also conducted quasiexperimental studies to compare MST and other programs, and benchmarking studies to compare the results of

MST in usual care with those obtained in effectiveness trials. An example of the former is the comparison by Stambaugh and colleagues (2007) of the effectiveness of standard MST versus Wraparound in a SOC site. Wraparound is a widely disseminated family-based intervention for youth with serious emotional disturbance whose primary aim is to prevent out-of-home placements. Results at an 18-month follow-up showed that MST was significantly more effective than Wraparound at decreasing youth symptoms and, relative to Wraparound, decreased out-of-home placements by 54%.

Two MST benchmarking studies (i.e., studies comparing the strength of effects of community-based implementation with that of previous clinical trials) have recently been conducted. Ogden, Hagen, and Anderson (2007) found that MST outcomes (i.e., reducing antisocial behavior and out-of-home placement) in the second year of program operation matched or surpassed those achieved during the first year, when the aforementioned Norwegian clinical trial was conducted. Similarly, Curtis and colleagues (Curtis, Ronan, Heiblum, & Crellin, 2009) compared pre/post findings from MST programs in New Zealand with results from clinical trials conducted in the United States and found clinical outcomes were consistent with those achieved across previous MST studies.

Failures to Replicate

As can occur with individual clinical cases in treatment, transportability trials of MST have not always proven effective. Although neither published nor submitted for peer review, Leshied and Cunningham (2002) reported on a large four-site randomized trial comparing MST with usual services in Ontario, Canada, that began in the early years of MST transport. Short-term family- and youth-level outcomes were favorable for MST, but reductions in conviction rates were well below those found in published trials of MST. The quantity and quality of the adherence data collected at each site is largely unknown, but overall adherence was lowest in the site with the worst outcomes, a finding essentially replicated in Ogden's multisite trial in Norway and indicative that treatment fidelity is important to achieving youth outcomes.

Likewise, a more recent multisite trial conducted in Sweden (Sundell et al., 2008) has thus far failed to find outcomes favoring the MST condition. The length and intensity of MST in this study differed from that in U.S. studies, and treatment fidelity was very low across sites. Reductions in youth symptoms in the MST condition in Sweden were similar to those found in the Norwegian and U.S. trials in which MST outperformed usual care. Thus, the failure to attain MST effects in Sweden may reflect the relative strength of usual services (i.e., the comparison condition) there.

Finally, not all reviewers have viewed MST outcomes favorably. Disagreeing with the independent reviews and federal reports cited at the beginning of this chapter, Littell and colleagues (Littell, Popa, & Forsythe, 2005) concluded in their meta-analysis that MST was not significantly more effective than alternative services in reducing youth crime and out-of-home placement. This review relied heavily on an unpublished multisite Canadian study that revealed site effects (adherence and outcomes were better in some sites than others) in drawing its conclusions and included many methodological anomalies (see Ogden & Hagen, 2006b). The conclusions of the Littell review have not been replicated in other meta-analyses of MST (Aos et al., 2006; Curtis, Ronan, & Borduin, 2004).

State and Local Program Evaluations

Several states have conducted program evaluations to learn more about the parameters of MST implementation and effects in their locales. The methods and results of these evaluations are often reported in the internal reports of public agencies and rarely reported in peer-reviewed journals. In some states that pursued the larger scale transport of MST, the design and results of evaluations have been made available to the public. For example, a report from the Florida Redirection Project (which encompasses MST and Functional Family Therapy), based on over 2,000 youth and families served, showed the program reduced felony recidivism by 31% and saved millions of dollars in avoided residential placement (Office of Program Policy Analysis & Government Accountability, 2007). The Prevention Research Center at Pennsylvania State University (Chilenski, Bumbarger, Kyler, & Greenberg, 2007) evaluated outcomes of several MST programs that had served over 400 youth and families and found substantial reductions in substance use, delinquency, academic failure, truancy, and out-of-home placements. The Connecticut Center for Effective Practices conducted an extensive qualitative and quantitative evaluation of the MST programs in the state and found reductions in recidivism and out-of-home placement that appear to be sustained over time (Franks, Schroeder, Connell, & Tebes, 2008). Importantly, this evaluation also identified implementation challenges. For example, workforce issues were very difficult to resolve in light of the rapid expansion of MST statewide, and some stakeholders thought the promise of MST might have been oversold.

Empirical Support for Linkages among
Adherence and Outcomes

A prospective 45-site study of the transport and implementation of MST funded in 1999 by the National Institute of Mental Health has provided empirical support for linkages among adherence to MST at multiple levels of the practice context and youth outcomes in usual care settings. Specifically, caregiver ratings of therapist adherence predicted reductions in youth behavior problems at the end of treatment and through a 1-year posttreatment follow-up and criminal charges through 4 years posttreatment (Schoenwald, Sheidow, Letourneau, & Liao, 2003; Schoenwald, Carter, Chapman, & Sheidow, 2008; Schoenwald, Chapman, Sheidow, & Carter, 2009). Supervisor adherence predicted therapist adherence and reductions in youth behavior problems through 1 year posttreatment (Schoenwald, Sheidow, & Chapman, 2009) and long-term criminal charges (Schoenwald., 2008). The effects of consultant adherence on therapist adherence and youth outcomes were assessed in two samples of therapists, consultants, and families, one of which was drawn from the MST Transportability Study. Linkages were found among consultant competence, focus on MST procedures, therapist adherence, and youth outcomes (Schoenwald, Sheidow, & Letourneau, 2004).

In addition, experimental studies have evaluated the effects of varying the intensity of quality assurance strategies on the implementation of a new evidence-based treatment protocol by therapists already practicing MST (Henggeler, Sheidow, Cunningham, Donohue, & Ford, 2008) and of an organizational and community intervention on the implementation and outcomes of MST (Glisson & Schoenwald, 2005). Results of the latter are not yet available, while results of the former suggest more rather than less intensive support is needed to implement a new evidence-based treatment protocol even among therapists already trained in MST.

Conclusion

The initial transport and early diffusion of MST began by virtue of stakeholder and community demand, or "pull," rather than "push" strategies. The OJJDP-supported Blueprints initiative, Connecticut initiative, and Norwegian initiative are, however, important examples of push strategies—strategies designed to increase awareness of, and interest in adopting, MST and other evidence-based treatments for specific target populations. The continued diffusion of MST has generated data from randomized trials, multisite studies of treatment transport, and local evaluations that suggest MST implementation and outcomes are favorable in many communities. Results of these studies also illuminate contextual factors that may affect implementation and outcomes. Similar data are not yet available with respect to factors that affect the diffusion of MST or illuminate the interaction of diffusion rates with the quality and outcomes of MST implementation. The design and evaluation of proactive dissemination strategies remains on the horizon, to be undertaken in future collaborations with stakeholders operating, supporting, and researching the implementation, impact, and dissemination of MST and other evidence-based treatment programs in usual care.

Author Note

Preparation of this manuscript was supported by grants 1 P20 MH0784458–01A2 (M. Atkins, University of Illinois-Chicago, PI) and 1P30MH074678–01A2 (J. Landsverk, Rady Children's Hospital, San Diego, PI) from the National Institute of Mental Health and by the Annie E. Casey Foundation The views presented here are those of the authors alone and do not necessarily reflect the opinions of the Annie E. Casey Foundation.

The author is a board member and stockholder in MST Services, LLC, which has the exclusive licensing agreement through MUSC for the transfer of MST technology.

REFERENCES

Aos, S., Miller, M., & Drake, E. (2006). *Evidence-based public policy options to reduce future prison construction, criminal justice costs, and crime rates.* Olympia, WA: Washington State Institute for Public Policy.

Backer, T.E., & David, S.L. (1995). Synthesis of behavioral science learnings about technology transfer. In T.E. Backer, S.L. David, & G. Soucy (Eds.), *Reviewing the behavioral science knowledge base on technology transfer* (pp. 262–279). (NIDA Research Monograph 155, NIH Publication No. 95–4035). Rockville, MD: National Institute on Drug Abuse.

Bronfenbrenner, U. (1979). *The ecology of human development: Experiments by design and nature.* Cambridge, MA: Harvard University Press.

Brown, B. S. (1995). Reducing impediments to technology transfer in drug abuse programming. In T. E. Backer, S. L. David, & G. Soucy (Eds.). (1995). *Reviewing the behavioral science knowledge base on technology transfer* (pp. 169–185). (NIDA Research Monograph 155, NIH Publication No. 95–4035). Rockville, MD: National Institute on Drug Abuse.

Cartwright, W. S., Kitsantas, P., & Rose, S. R. (2009). A demographic-economic model for adolescent substance abuse and crime prevention. *Journal of Comparative Social Welfare, 25*, 157–172.

Chilenski, S. M., Bumbarger, B. K., Kyler, S., & Greenberg, M. T. (2007). *Reducing youth violence and delinquency in Pennsylvania: PCCD's research-based programs initiative.* Prevention Research Center for the Promotion of Human Development, University Park, PA: The Pennsylvania State University.

Council on Government Relations. (1999). *The Bayh-Dole Act: A guide to the law and implementing regulations.* Washington, DC: Author.

Curtis, N. M., Heiblum, N., Ronan, K. R., & Crellin, K. (2009). Dissemination & effectiveness of multisystemic treatment in New Zealand: A benchmarking study. *Journal of Family Psychology, 23*, 119–129.

Curtis, N. M., Ronan, K. R., & Borduin, C. M. (2004). Multisystemic treatment: A meta-analysis of outcome studies. *Journal of Family Psychology, 18*, 411–419.

Elliott, D. S. (Series Ed.). (1998). *Blueprints for violence prevention.* Boulder, CO: Institute of Behavioral Science, Regents of the University of Colorado.

Eyberg, S. M., Nelson, M. M., & Boggs, S. R. (2008). Evidence-based treatments for child and adolescent disruptive behavior disorders. *Journal of Clinical Child and Adolescent Psychology, 36*, 418–429.

Fixsen, D. L., Naoom, S. F., Blase, K. A., Friedman, R. M., & Wallace, F.(2005). *Implementation research: A synthesis of the literature* (FMHI Publication #231). Tampa, FL. University of South Florida, Louis de la Parte Florida Mental Health Institute, The National Implementation Research Network.

Franks, R. P., Schroeder, J. A., Connell, C. M., & Tebes, J. K. (2008). *Unlocking doors: Multisystemic Therapy for Connecticut's high-risk children and youth—An effective home-based alternative treatment.* Farmington, CT: Connecticut Center for Effective Practice, Child Health and Development Institute of Connecticut.

George, P., Blase, K. A., Kanary, P. J., Wotring, J., Bernstein, D., & Carter, W. M. (2008). *Financing evidence-based programs and practices: Changing systems to support effective service.* Denver, CO: The Child and Family Evidence-Based Practices Consortium.

Glisson, C., & Schoenwald, S. K. (2005). The ARC organizational and community intervention strategy for implementing evidence-based children's mental health treatments. *Mental Health Services Research, 7,* 243–259.

Henggeler, S. W. (1989). *Delinquency in adolescence.* Newbury Park, CA: Sage Publications.

Henggeler, S. W., Letourneau, E. J., Chapman, J. E., Borduin, C. M., Schewe, P. A., & McCart, M. R. (2009). Mediators of change for multisystemic therapy with juvenile sexual offenders. *Journal of Consulting and Clinical Psychology, 77,* 451–462.

Henggeler, S. W., & Schoenwald, S. K. (1998). *The MST supervisory manual: Promoting quality assurance at the clinical level.* Charleston, SC: The MST Institute.

Henggeler, S. W., & Schoenwald, S. K. (1999). The role of quality assurance in achieving outcomes in MST programs. *Journal of Juvenile Justice and Detention Services, 14,* 1–17.

Henggeler, S. W., Schoenwald, S. K., Borduin, C. M., Rowland, M. D., & Cunningham, P. B. (2009). *Multisystemic therapy for antisocial behavior in children and adolescents* (2nd ed.). New York: Guilford Press.

Henggeler, S. W., Sheidow, A. J., Cunningham, P. B., Donohue, B. C., & Ford, J. D. (2008). Promoting the implementation of an evidence-based intervention for adolescent marijuana abuse in community settings: Testing the use of intensive quality assurance. *Journal of Clinical Child & Adolescent Psychology, 37,* 682–689.

Hoge, R. D., Guerra, N. G., & Boxer, P. (Eds.). (2008). *Treating the juvenile offender.* New York: Guilford Press.

Huey, S. J., Henggeler, S. W., Brondino, M. J., & Pickrel, S. G. (2000). Mechanisms of change in multisystemic therapy: Reducing delinquent behavior through therapist adherence and improved family and peer functioning. *Journal of Consulting and Clinical Psychology, 68,* 451–467.

Klein, K. J., & Knight, A. P. (2005). Innovation implementation: Overcoming the challenge. *Current Directions in Psychological Science, 14,* 243–246.

Klein, K. J., & Sorra, J. S. (1996). The challenge of innovation implementation. *Academy of Management Review, 21,* 1055–1080.

Leshied, A., & Cunningham, A. (2002, February). *Seeking effective interventions for serious young offenders: Interim results of a four-year randomized study of multisystemic therapy in Ontario, Canada.* London: Centre for Children & Families in the Justice System.

Littell, J. H., Popa, M., & Forsythe, B. (2005). *Multisystemic therapy for social, emotional, and behavioral problems in youth aged 10–17.* Campbell Collaborative Library. Retrieved from http://www.campbellcollaboration.org/Library

National Alliance for the Mentally Ill. (2003, Fall). *NAMI beginnings.* Arlington, VA: Author.

National Alliance for the Mentally Ill. (2008, Winter). Medicaid coverage of multisystemic therapy. In *NAMI beginnings.* Arlington, VA: Author.

National Institute on Drug Abuse. (1999). *Principles of drug addiction treatment: A research-based guide* (NIH Publication No. 99–4180). Rockville, MD: National Institute on Drug Abuse.

National Institutes of Health. (2006). National Institutes of Health State-of-the-Science Conference Statement: Preventing violence and related health-risking, social behaviors in adolescent, October 13–15, 2004. *Journal of Abnormal Child Psychology, 34,* 457–470.

National Mental Health Association. (2004). *Mental health treatment for youth in the juvenile justice system: A compendium of promising practices.* Alexandria, VA: Author.

Office of Program Policy Analysis & Government Accountability. (2007, February). *Redirection pilots meet and exceed residential commitment outcomes; $5.8 million saved.* Tallahassee, FL: Florida Legislature.

Ogden, T., Christensen, B., Sheidow, A. J., & Holth, P. (2008). Bridging the gap between science and practice: The effective nationwide transport of MST programs in Norway. *Journal of Child and Adolescent Substance Abuse, 17*, 93–109.

Ogden, T., & Hagen, K. A. (2006a). Multisystemic therapy of serious behaviour problems in youth: Sustainability of therapy effectiveness two years after intake. *Journal of Child and Adolescent Mental Health, 11*, 142–149.

Ogden, T., & Hagen, K. A. (2006b). Virker MST? Kommentarer til en systematisk forskningsoversikt og meta-analyse av MST. *Nordisk Sosialt Arbeid, 26*, 222–233.

Ogden, T., Hagen, K. A., & Anderson, O. (2007). Sustainability of the effectiveness of a programme of multisystemic treatment (MST) across participant groups in the second year of operation. *Journal of Children's Services, 2*, 4–14.

Ogden, T., & Halliday-Boykins, C. A. (2004). Multisystemic treatment of antisocial adolescents in Norway: Replication of clinical outcomes outside of the US. *Child & Adolescent Mental Health, 9*, 77–83.

Real, K., & Poole, M. S. (2005). Innovation implementation: Conceptualization and measurement in organizational research. *Research in Organizational Change and Development, 15*, 63–134.

Rogers, E. M. (2003). *Diffusion of innovations* (5th ed.). New York: The Free Press.

Schoenwald, S. K. (1998). *Multisystemic therapy consultation manual.* Charleston, SC: The MST Institute.

Schoenwald, S. K. (2008). Toward evidence-based transport of evidence-based treatments: MST as an example. *Journal of Child and Adolescent Substance Abuse, 17*, 69–91.

Schoenwald, S. K., Carter, R. E., Chapman, J. E., & Sheidow, A. J. (2008). Therapist adherence and organizational effects on change in youth behavior problems one year after Multisystemic Therapy. *Administration and Policy in Mental Health and Mental Health Services Research, 35*, 379–394.

Schoenwald, S. K., Chapman, J. E., Sheidow, A. J., & Carter, R. E. (2009). Long-term youth criminal outcomes in MST transport: The impact of therapist adherence and organizational climate and structure. *Journal of Clinical Child and Adolescent Psychology, 38*, 91–105.

Schoenwald, S. K., Heiblum, N., Saldana, L., & Henggeler, S. W. (2008). The international implementation of multisystemic therapy. *Evaluation & The Health Professions [Special issue]: International Translation of Health Behavior Research Innovations, Part I,* 211–225.

Schoenwald, S. K., & Henggeler, S. W. (2002). Mental health services research and family-based treatment: Bridging the gap. In H. Liddle, G. Diamond, R. Levant, J. Bray, & D. Santiseban (Eds.), *Family psychology intervention science* (pp. 259–282). Washington, DC: American Psychological Association.

Schoenwald, S. K., Henggeler, S. W., Brondino, M. J., & Rowland, M. D. (2000). Multisystemic therapy: Monitoring treatment fidelity. *Family Process, 39*, 83–103.

Schoenwald, S. K., Sheidow, A. J., & Chapman, J. E. (2009). Clinical supervision in treatment transport: Effects on adherence and outcomes. *Journal of Consulting and Clinical Psychology, 77*, 410–421.

Schoenwald, S.K., Sheidow, A.S., & Letourneau, E.J. (2004). Toward effective quality assurance in evidence-based practice: Links between expert consultation, therapist fidelity, and child outcomes. *Journal of Child and Adolescent Clinical Psychology*, *33*, 94–104.

Schoenwald, S. K., Sheidow, A. J., Letourneau, E. J., & Liao, J. G. (2003). Transportability of Multisystemic Therapy: Evidence for multi-level influences. *Mental Health Services Research, 5*, 223–239.

Sexton, T. L., & Alexander, J. F. (2005). Functional Family Therapy for externalizing disorders in adolescents. In J. L. Lebow (Ed.), *Handbook of clinical family therapy* (pp. 164–194). Hoboken, NJ: John Wiley & Sons, Inc.

Stambaugh, L. F., Mustillo, S. A., Burns, B. J., Stephens, R. L., Baxter, B., Edwards, D., et al. (2007). Outcomes from wraparound and multisystemic therapy in a center for mental health services system-of-care demonstration site. *Journal of Emotional and Behavioral Disorders, 15*, 143–155.

Sundell, K., Hansson, K., Lofholm, C. E., Olsson, T., Gustle, L-H., & Kadesjo, C. (2008). The transportability of Multisystemic Therapy to Sweden: Short-term results from a randomized trial of conduct-disordered youths. *Journal of Family Psychology, 22*, 550–560.

Timmons-Mitchell, J., Bender, M. B., Kishna, M. A., & Mitchell, C. C. (2006). An independent effectiveness trial of multisystemic therapy with juvenile justice youth. *Journal of Clinical Child and Adolescent Psychology, 35*, 227–236.

U.S. Public Health Service. (2001). *Youth violence: A report of the Surgeon General.* Washington, DC: Author.

Waldron, H. B., & Turner, C. W. (2008). Evidence-based psychosocial treatments for adolescent substance abuse. *Journal of Clinical Child and Adolescent Psychology, 37*, 238–261.

Weisz, J.R. (2004). *Psychotherapy for children and adolescents: evidence-based treatments and case examples.* New York, NY: Cambridge University Press.

{13}

Dissemination and Implementation of Evidence-Based Psychological Interventions
CURRENT STATUS AND FUTURE DIRECTIONS
R. Kathryn McHugh and David H. Barlow

In the United States, fewer than one third of adults with a psychological disorder receive treatment (Kessler, Demler, et al., 2005), with even lower rates of treatment receipt among children (e.g., Collins, Westra, Dozois, & Burns, 2004). Rates of untreated mental illness are even higher in developing countries, with annual rates of treatment as low as less than 2% (Wang et al., 2007). Although there is a trend for increasing rates of treatment receipt, this has not been associated with decreases in disability, implying that even among those receiving treatment, many are not receiving effective care (see Insel, 2009). This is not a problem of the existence of effective treatment, but rather a problem of the availability of effective treatment. As Berwick argued: "In health care, invention is hard, but dissemination is even harder" (2003, p. 1970).

The dissemination and implementation (D&I) of psychological interventions has been a particular challenge. Despite concurrent advances in effective pharmacological and psychological treatments for psychological disorders, the dissemination of psychotropic medication has far outpaced that of psychological interventions. Antidepressant medications became the most commonly prescribed class of medication in the United States in 2005 (Cherry, Woodwell, & Rechtsteiner, 2007; Olfson & Marcus, 2009), with an estimated 10% of the population—or over 27 million people—receiving these medications annually. There is also evidence for a concurrent decrease in the utilization of psychological treatments in recent years (e.g., Marcus & Olfson, 2010). This has occurred against the backdrop of the identification of psychological treatments as front-line treatments for most psychological disorders, favorable evidence for their cost effectiveness, and evidence suggesting that patients prefer psychological to pharmacological interventions (see Chapter 1, this volume).

Evidence highlighting the lack of access to evidence-based psychological interventions (EBPIs) from large-scale reports from the Institute of Medicine (2001), U.S. Surgeon General (U.S. Department of Health and Human Services, 2001), and the President's New Freedom Commission on Mental Health (2003) as well as empirical studies (e.g., Becker, Zayfert, & Anderson, 2004; Crow, Mussell, Peterson, Knopke, & Mitchell, 1999; Goisman, Warshaw, & Keller, 1999; Haas & Clopton, 2003; Mussell et al., 2000; Santa Ana et al., 2008; Stewart & Chambless, 2007) has resulted in an urgent call for the increased availability of these interventions. This urgency is evident in the initiation of mandates and other incentives for the provision of evidence-based services by government, third-party payers, and accrediting agencies. For example, the American Academy of Sleep Medicine has mandated the availability of cognitive behavioral therapy (CBT)—a front-line treatment for insomnia (Schutte-Rodin, Broch, Buysse, Dorsey, & Sateia, 2008)—at accredited sleep centers (see Lamberg, 2008). In 2003, the Oregon State Senate passed legislation initiating a funding shift requiring that 25% of mental health treatment funding be dedicated to EBPIs by 2007, 50% by 2009, and 75% by 2011 across state agencies including corrections, children's services, mental health, and addiction. There clearly has been a call to action from numerous sources to address this problem; however, meeting this urgent need is a major challenge.

Successful D&I is a challenge in any field. Among the most commonly cited examples of this is the dissemination of nutritional interventions to prevent scurvy among British sailors in the 1600s. An experiment conducted in 1601 demonstrated strong evidence that a small daily dose of lemon juice prevented scurvy (at the time, the most common cause of death among sailors); however, this research had no impact on practice. Over 100 years later in 1747, a similar experiment replicated these results with similarly minimal impact on practice. It was not until 1795 that the British Navy implemented this intervention and until 1865 that it was also implemented for trade sailors (see Mosteller, 1981). Thus, from identification of this evidence-based treatment to implementation was an astounding 264 years. Although 17 years has been a widely cited estimate of the lag between publication and implementation of research findings in health care (Balas & Boren, 2000), the time to implementation may actually be quite a bit longer than that, if implementation is even achieved (Trochim, 2010). At this time, the field faces a major challenge that will require commitment of various stakeholder groups to advance understanding of the best practices for improving this lag from discovery to routine practice.

This volume has highlighted some of the leading efforts that are under way to increase access to EBPIs. These state-of-the-art programs have begun to make significant advances toward addressing this public health problem, and as data collection continues, these programs have enormous potential to advance the field. At this very early stage in the practice and research of targeted, intensive D&I efforts in mental health, there are numerous important areas for further research and important future directions for the field. Below, we highlight 10 areas that we think will be of particular importance in the next several years as the field aims to address the challenge of improving access to effective care and reducing the burden of mental illness.

Future Directions in the Dissemination and Implementation of Evidence-Based Psychological Interventions

1. GREATER ATTENTION TO DISSEMINATION AND IMPLEMENTATION SCIENCE

Recognition of the need for evidence-based procedures for the transport of evidence-based interventions has led to increased attention to dissemination and implementation science (Eccles et al., 2009; Stirman, Crits-Christoph, & DeRubeis, 2004). These areas of research examine the processes for the transmission of information and the adoption and utilization of innovations in practice settings. The director of the National Institute of Mental Health (NIMH) in the United States highlighted as a core objective for funding to "strengthen the public health impact of NIMH-supported research. . . . Translational research will focus not only on 'bench to bedside,' but also on 'bedside to practice' as the institute focuses on increasing its public health impact, addressing disparities in mental health care, and reducing the burden of mental illness" (Insel, 2009, p. 132).

Among the earliest aims of D&I research is the establishment of common terminology and conceptual models to guide the field. Inconsistent use of terminology has been a particular limitation of research efforts to date (see Chapter 2, this volume). The field has begun to approach a greater consensus on such issues recently and numerous models and frameworks of D&I have emerged with the potential to facilitate systematic research in this area (see Chapter 2, this volume), such as the Texas Christian University Program Change Model (Simpson & Flynn, 2007) and the Addiction Technology Transfer Center (ATTC) Network Technology Transfer Model (ATTC Network Technology Transfer Workgroup, 2011). A limitation of some of the major D&I efforts already under way is that many developed quickly in response to urgent requests precluding consultation and collaboration among programs about best practices (McHugh & Barlow, 2010). Recently, efforts have been initiated to expedite the research and practice of D&I by enhancing collaboration and communication. For example, the annual National Institutes of Health conference on the Science of Dissemination and Implementation (which conducted its fourth annual conference in 2011) and the Seattle Implementation Research Conference, partially funded by the National Institute of Mental Health, are providing a forum for stakeholders to collaborate and communicate research findings.

D&I research will necessarily be both translational and multidisciplinary in nature (Thornicroft, Lempp, & Tansella, 2011). Given that D&I is not a problem unique to health care, there is much to be gained from collaboration with other fields facing similar challenges. For example, marketing and organizational behavior perspectives may be applicable to efforts in mental health care (see Chapter 2, this volume). Also, models of clinician training increasingly draw from adult learning theories (see Chapter 3, this volume). Collaboration among disciplines to take a multiple-perspective approach to this complex challenge will facilitate more rapid advancement of D&I science.

The advancement of this research agenda will also require a commitment of research funding to accompany the commitment of public and private funding afforded to the public health efforts reviewed in this volume. Although recent years have begun to see a proliferation of D&I research, this research agenda is in its relative infancy. Opportunities are beginning to become available through mechanisms such as the National Institutes of Health Clinical and Translational Science Awards and program announcements calling for grant submissions in the area of D&I; however, the availability of funding for D&I research will continue to be critical to establishing effective methods for transporting EBPIs to service provision settings.

2. STANDARDIZATION OF PROCEDURES FOR OUTCOMES ASSESSMENT

Another critical element of advancing understanding of effective D&I procedures is the use of outcomes assessment. Consistency and standardization of measurement will enhance the ability to compare across studies and applied efforts to more rapidly advance D&I science. Tracking of outcomes has numerous benefits including treatment planning for individual patients, identification of need areas, and evaluation of treatment effectiveness. An example of the benefits of standardizing outcomes assessment is found in efforts by specialty cystic fibrosis clinics in response to calls from policymakers and payers to monitor outcomes (Gawande, 2004, 2007). Initially, providers were reluctant to make these data public and had insisted on anonymity. But examination of the data surprisingly identified that one clinic was consistently outperforming others with exceptional functional and health outcomes. Providers then requested that the exceptional clinic be identified, so that they could learn from the policies and practices of the leading clinic and then implement these procedures themselves. In this case, consistent outcomes assessment facilitated communication and more rapid advancement of practice as well as the ability to identify problem and strength areas. These benefits would not have been possible without a level of standardization of assessment and communication among sites. Similarly, Lambert and colleagues (2003) have shown that providing periodic feedback on patient progress to clinicians during the course of treatment improves treatment outcomes.

Elsewhere, we have presented a proposal for comprehensive standards for assessment and training in psychological interventions (McHugh & Barlow, 2010). These standards include outcomes to evaluate the success of D&I efforts with respect to proximal (i.e., training) as well as distal (i.e., patient symptoms and functioning) outcomes. Evaluation of D&I program outcomes will also aid in the identification of what elements contribute to the effectiveness of these programs and to determine the most cost-effective combination of these strategies. For example, although many of the leading efforts in this area utilize similar procedures, it is unclear whether all of them are necessary for success or what combination may ultimately prove most effective.

Assessment in service provision settings also contributes to the establishment of an evidence base for interventions. This can be particularly beneficial relative to issues of generalizability and feasibility that can inform decisions about what interventions to disseminate in what setting. Outcomes assessment in D&I programs is consistent with concepts such as practice-based evidence (see Horn & Gassaway, 2010) and community-based participatory research (see Becker, Stice, Shaw, & Woda, 2009), which involve evaluation of interventions in naturalistic settings and emphasize collaboration among stakeholders. These approaches have particular promise relative to traditional investigator-driven research for evaluating the generalizability of treatments in service provision settings and the identification of predictors of who will respond to what treatment.

3. BETTER COLLABORATION BETWEEN "RESEARCH AND PRACTICE"

Involvement of consumers is a central tenet of product development for market goods and services (Hayes, Barlow, & Nelson-Gray, 1999). Sobell (1996) drew the parallel between such models and the development of EBPIs: "Many innovative companies get their best product ideas by listening to what their customers say. If scientists want to see their science translated into widescale practice, they too need to listen to their customers—the practitioners" (p. 301). Weisz and colleagues further emphasized the bi-directional benefits of such collaboration: "Clinical researchers may have a great deal to learn from practicing clinicians, just as clinicians may learn useful new approaches from the research community. If the obstacles to researcher-clinician collaboration can be overcome, both groups may profit, and to the ultimate benefit of the children and families who seek help" (Weiss, Donenberg, Han, & Weiss, 1995, p. 699). As long as the research versus practice and academic setting versus real-world setting dichotomies continue to dominate our language and conceptualization of the clinical research process, the barriers to successful implementation will likely remain too large to overcome.

Research on treatment development and testing must consider how services are provided outside of the specialty clinics often associated with academic centers. Although many have argued for the importance of effectiveness research (e.g., Carroll & Rounsaville, 2003), such studies continue to be underrepresented relative to efficacy studies. This is even reflected in the selection of evidence-based interventions for inclusion in "best practice" or empirically-supported treatment lists, which focus on evidence for efficacy rather than effectiveness or transportability (Barlow, Levitt, & Bufka, 1999). Similarly, service delivery and treatment efficacy/effectiveness research agendas have progressed independently with little overlap, communication, or collaboration (Southam-Gerow, Ringeisen, & Sherrill, 2006).

In addition to better collaboration after interventions have been developed, the consideration of factors relating to transportability *at the very earliest stages of treatment development* will be necessary to advancing this research agenda efficiently. The focus on internal validity and efficacy has been necessary for the rapidity of advancements in treatment development in recent years; however, at this time, there is a need for more emphasis on factors related to transportability. By increasing the bi-directionality of communication between service provision settings and academic research settings, feasibility, generalizability, cost effectiveness, and compatibility can be emphasized to facilitate the development and modification of treatments better suited for implementation in service provision settings. Better transportability should yield easier D&I through reducing barriers related to fit and clinician acceptability.

4. TRANSDIAGNOSTIC TREATMENTS

Treatment development and efficacy testing has focused largely on single-disorder approaches. Although this has yielded highly efficacious treatments well targeted to specific symptom clusters, the dissemination and implementation of single-diagnosis treatments on a large scale is not feasible. Given the intensity of effort needed to adequately train clinical providers in any one treatment (see Chapter 3, this volume), training providers in the multiple treatments needed to capture the range of presentations seen in their clinical practice is unrealistic. Even at a specialty treatment center for anxiety disorders, a clinical provider would presumably need to receive training in six or seven discrete protocols to capture the range of anxiety disorders (assuming that the provider is trained in only one of the available treatments per disorder). Moreover, comorbidity has been demonstrated to be the rule rather than the exception, with estimates of close to 50% or more of those with a psychological disorder meeting criteria for two or more diagnoses (e.g., Brown, Campbell, Lehman, Grisham, & Mancill, 2001; Demyttenaere et al., 2004; Kessler, Chiu, Demler, Merikangas, & Walters, 2005).

Transdiagnostic treatments are an alternative to single-diagnosis treatments. Several types of transdiagnostic approaches have been developed, including theory-driven protocol-based modular treatments addressing higher order factors common across classes of disorders, such as emotional disorders (Barlow et al., 2011) or eating disorders (Fairburn, Cooper, Shafran, & Wilson, 2008). These approaches have in common a distillation of principles that overlap across available treatments or overlapping clinical features across disorder presentations (e.g., emotion dysregulation) to provide an intervention that can be flexibly applied to a range of disorders and comorbidities. In addition, more pragmatic modular treatments (e.g., Chorpita, 2007) and principle- or component-based treatments (e.g., Chorpita & Daleiden, 2009) that may be tailored to a variety of individual presenting problems have been developed. A major benefit of these treatments is the potential to dramatically reduce the training needs of clinical providers.

Another particular benefit of transdiagnostic treatments is the potential to be more adaptable to individual cases (McHugh, Murray, & Barlow, 2009). The degree to which an innovation can be adapted is an important predictor of utilization (Rogers, 2003). Moreover, there has been a recent emphasis on the importance of flexible application of EBPIs that maintains fidelity to the treatment model but also maximizes fit to the individual (Kendall, Gosch, Furr, & Sood, 2008). Overly rigid clinician adherence to an intervention may negatively impact patient understanding and learning retention—a rarely evaluated but potentially important mediator of outcome (McHugh et al., 2009). Transdiagnostic treatment approaches allow for greater flexibility that may enhance adaptability and acceptability to clinicians.

5. STEPPED-CARE MODELS AND HETEROGENEITY OF DELIVERY METHODS

Even if training efforts successfully doubled or tripled the number of EBPI providers available, significant need for services would remain. Kazdin and Blase (2011) estimated that in the United States there are approximately 75 million people in need of services and only 700,000 mental health professionals (or 107 people per provider). This does not include those with subsyndromal conditions which are also associated with high levels of distress and disability (e.g., Andrea, Bültmann, van Amelsvoort, & Kant, 2009; Fullana et al., 2009). However, a large portion of individuals who could benefit from mental health services do not require a high-intensity course of psychological treatment with a highly trained provider. Many individuals can benefit from lower intensity options, such as guided self-help (e.g., Furmark et al., 2009; Striegel-Moore et al., 2010). Stepped-care approaches include several levels of intervention delivery, which are targeted to the level of care needed. Thus, this approach aims to offer lower intensity interventions to individuals who may benefit from them and target higher intensity services to those with greater severity or those who do not respond to a lower level of care. In the context of the discrepancy between the available workforce (particularly those trained in EBPIs) and patient need, such an approach may allow much greater access to effective services and may also yield substantial cost savings by reserving high-intensity (and high-cost) services for those with a greater level of severity.

This model is currently being utilized in the United Kingdom as part of the Improving Access to Psychological Therapies (IAPT) Program in the National Health Service (NHS). The IAPT program is a large initiative to increase availability of EBPIs for depression and anxiety funded by the NHS that utilizes a stepped-care approach based on the identification of appropriate levels of care during the initial assessment. Preliminary outcomes have suggested high feasibility and excellent outcomes with respect to numbers of clinicians trained, patient access to treatment, and symptom and functional outcomes (see Chapter 4, this volume).

6. INTEGRATION OF MENTAL HEALTH
CARE IN PRIMARY CARE

Two major challenges to the successful D&I of EBPIs are the identification of the need for services and logistical barriers to service receipt. Better integration of mental health care into primary care settings has great promise for addressing these challenges. Assessment of need for mental health services in primary care is being implemented on a large scale in the United Kingdom, but is in much earlier stages in the United States.

Several programs have shown success for using primary care as a point of intervention for EBPIs. Collaborative care models have been implemented and have demonstrated excellent outcomes for both depression (Gilbody, Bower, Fletcher, Richards, & Sutton, 2006; Unützer et al., 2002) and anxiety (Craske et al., 2011; Roy-Byrne et al., 2010). These models utilize a care manager who works with primary care physicians and psychiatrists/psychologists to coordinate mental health care and aid the patient in identifying and selecting treatment options. For example, the Coordinated Anxiety Learning and Management (CALM) program involves the integration of assessment and treatment of anxiety disorders in primary care settings (see Sullivan et al., 2007). Interventions for anxiety include evidence-based psychological therapy and pharmacotherapy. The program utilizes anxiety clinical specialists (typically with a social work or nursing degree) as care managers who are responsible for assessment and coordination of treatment. Patients are then educated about treatment options, including medication and clinician-assisted computer-based CBT. Ongoing assessment is conducted to determine whether the treatment plan should be modified (i.e., adjuncts added) in the case of insufficient treatment response. The CALM program has demonstrated improvement over treatment as usual for the treatment of a range of anxiety disorders (Craske et al., 2011). The program has also been associated with favorable patient satisfaction (Stein et al., 2011).

Systemic changes in primary care will be challenging given the heterogeneity of these settings and health care systems, particularly in the United States; however, the incorporation of better screening and referral may dramatically improve the ability to identify and intervene and may lead to earlier detection of psychological disorders.

7. INFORMATION TECHNOLOGY

There are numerous benefits to the use of information technology (IT) in mental health care, including flexibility of use, potential to increase service availability (e.g., when barriers to seeing a face-to-face provider exist), and compatibility with the use of technology in patients' daily lives. The field has just begun to tap the potential uses of IT for advancing access to EBPIs. Several types of applications of IT have been explored including assessment, treatment, prevention, and training.

IT can simplify the delivery of these mental health care practices, reducing the burden on clinical providers.

IT also has the potential to fundamentally change the way in which interventions are delivered. The typical means of delivering EBPIs is in the face-to-face individual or group weekly therapy hour. Given its portability, technology applications can deliver interventions more regularly and as needed in "real time." For example, mobile phones and portable computers have been used to deliver ecological momentary interventions (i.e., "in the moment" interventions) for a range of psychological and behavioral health symptoms, such as anxiety, smoking cessation, and physical activity (see Heron & Smyth, 2010).

The success of IT for delivering treatment has been significant (for review see Andrews, Cuijpers, Craske, McEvoy, & Titov, 2010; Newman, Szkodny, Llera, & Przeworski, 2011); however, this research agenda is still in a relatively early stage. At this time, these interventions are typically recommended as lower intensity interventions that may be best utilized in adjunctive or stepped-care models (National Institute for Health and Clinical Excellence, 2006), but as these technologies continue to be refined, they may demonstrate increasing promise for more moderate and severe mental illness. In fact, technology has been successfully incorporated into stepped-care (e.g., Clark et al., 2009) and collaborative care (e.g., Sullivan et al., 2007) programs.

Although the potential for leveraging technology is substantial, there are a number of cautionary points. For example, issues with security, confidentiality, regulation of practice (e.g., licensure) across geographical locations, and risk management all remain concerns. As these advances continue, the consideration of ethical, legal, and professional challenges unique to technology will be of particular importance.

8. SOLVING THE SUSTAINABILITY PROBLEM

One of the greatest D&I challenges is sustaining the utilization of EBPIs once initial implementation has been achieved. For example, handwashing practices—a simple and critical practice for reducing infection in hospital settings—have proven exceptionally difficult to sustain despite successes with initial implementation (see Gawande, 2007). Numerous interventions, ranging from education, to the utilization of new technologies (e.g., water-less sanitizers), to monitoring of individual behaviors, to public reporting of infection rates, have often failed to lead to sustained change in practice. Although there is increasing evidence that successful implementation can be achieved with targeted intervention (such as the efforts described in this volume), the ultimate success of these D&I efforts relies on maintenance of implementation over time. Understanding predictors of maintenance and identification of procedures to facilitate sustainability (e.g., ongoing monitoring and feedback systems, "booster" trainings) are essential research questions at this time (Gallo & Barlow, 2011).

Funding is a particular challenge to sustainability. At this time, significant public and private funds are being dedicated to the D&I of EBPIs; however, it is safe to assume that such resources will not always be available. Innovative strategies for maintaining resources to support ongoing training and consultation and other implementation costs will be of particular importance. Strategies such as university–clinic collaborations may be one way to maintain funding streams over time. It is also important to note that economic analysis in the United Kingdom suggested that a large-scale effort to increase access to EBPIs for depression and anxiety would basically pay for itself in terms of the costs offset by achieving positive outcomes (Centre for Economic Performance's Mental Health Policy Group, 2006), an assertion with increasing evidence. Similarly, others have argued that effective treatment would likely be associated with lower cost than untreated depression (Simon et al., 2001). This is not surprising given data suggesting that psychological disorders are enormously costly to society due to costs associated with health care utilization and lost productivity (e.g., Greenberg et al., 1999, 2003; Smit et al., 2006). Advocacy for funding efforts that will lead to both initial and maintained success will be critical, especially once early implementation successes are achieved.

9. DISSEMINATION AND IMPLEMENTATION EFFORTS AS A MECHANISM FOR TARGETING MENTAL HEALTH CARE DISPARITIES

Disparities in both health and health care remain substantial. In mental health care, discrepancies in the availability and quality of care among groups are significant (e.g., Alegria et al., 2008; U.S. Department of Health and Human Services, 2001). Factors such as race (Wells, Klap, Koike, & Sherbourne, 2001), socioeconomic status (Newacheck et al., 2003), and geographical location (McGuire, Alegria, Cook, Wells, & Zaslavsky, 2006) are all associated with disparities in care. For example, receipt of psychological care among Caucasian patients in primary and specialty care settings is estimated to be almost double that of other racial groups (Lasser, Himmelstein, Woolhander, McCormick, & Bor, 2002). Even greater disparities in receipt of evidence-based care have been noted (U.S. Department of Health and Human Services, 2001; Wang, Berglund, & Kessler, 2000; Young, Klap, Sherbourne, & Wells, 2001).

As D&I efforts seek to improve access to care, particular attention must be paid to existing care disparities. As innovations are disseminated, there is a risk of further widening of social gaps as "the rich get richer" (Rogers, 2003; Sandler, 2007). This can happen both at the provider and patient level. For example, service provision settings with sufficient financial resources to provide training opportunities for providers may be able to more quickly implement EBPIs and also have the resources to better sustain such changes. Patients with financial resources to seek specialty care have an advantage over those who are uninsured or unable to pay privately for services. These benefits continue to accrue as these patients presumably are able to more quickly return to functioning (if treatment is effective), thus continuing to maintain and build resources for the future.

Rogers (2003) highlighted three primary reasons for such social impact of innovation dissemination including differences in resources for adoption, access to information about innovations, and access to information via peer networks. D&I efforts occur in the context of existing social disparities and thus must consider these gaps to prevent them from widening. In fact, D&I efforts may serve as an opportunity to reduce these gaps through targeted efforts to reduce barriers to the receipt of effective care among certain groups; however, this will require specific attention to these issues in the design and implementation of these efforts.

10. USE OF DIRECT-TO-CONSUMER MARKETING EFFORTS

Much attention in D&I efforts has focused on clinical providers and systems as the consumers of evidence-based care. However, there are also potential benefits to targeting patients in such efforts. We have recently articulated the benefits of "direct-to-patient" dissemination efforts (Santucci, McHugh, & Barlow, in press). The potential benefits are twofold. First, such efforts may enhance adoption of self-help interventions (e.g., bibliotherapy, certain types of computerized therapies). Second, they may also yield pull demand for interventions: as patients become more aware of the benefits of EBPIs, they will begin requesting them from providers, thus potentially enhancing the demand among clinicians and clinical systems to offer them.

Targeting information to patients may also serve to reduce barriers to accessing care. A large study in the United States suggested that patient perceptions/attitudes about treatment were much greater barriers to receipt and completion of treatment than logistical/structural barriers, such as financial factors (Mojtabai et al., 2011). Of those with a diagnosable psychological disorder who did not seek treatment, 45% endorsed a low perceived need for treatment as a barrier to care. Even among those who did perceive a need, 73% reported that they wanted to manage the illness on their own. Interestingly, more than 16% of those who perceived a need for services did not think that services would be effective (among those with a severe disorder, this number increased to 26%). Although these findings do not mitigate the importance of targeting structural barriers to access—particularly among certain groups (e.g., uninsured, racial/ethnic minorities)—it highlights the importance of also targeting patient perceptions as critical to improving access to care. Interventions to improve mental health literacy and to facilitate patient understanding about the availability and effectiveness of treatment will be important to enhancing treatment access.

Conclusion

Research efforts have yielded much success with respect to the development of psychological interventions that are efficacious, effective, and cost effective and have the potential to alleviate the suffering of those with mental illness. The next major challenge of the field is to connect these advances to the ultimate marker of success: the public health impact of these interventions on a wide scale. Although attention to dissemination and implementation is increasing, the centrality of public health impact was eloquently stated by Lightner Witmer in the earliest stages of modern clinical psychology. Witmer argued that: "the pure and the applied sciences advance in a single front. What retards the progress of one, retards the progress of the other; what fosters one, fosters the other. But in the final analysis the progress of psychology, as of every other science, will be determined by the value and amount of its contributions to the advancement of the human race" (Witmer, 1907/1996, p. 2491). Much like Witmer's early observation, the impact of the successes in intervention development yielded by basic and clinical research will be truly felt in its ability to change the impact of mental illness on individuals, families, and societies.

REFERENCES

Addiction Technology Transfer Center Network Technology Transfer Workgroup. (2011). Research to practice in addiction treatment: Key terms and a field driven model of technology transfer. *Journal of Substance Abuse Treatment, 41*, 169–178.

Alegría, M., Chatterji, P., Wells, K., Cao, Z., Chen, C. N., Takeuchi, D., et al. (2008). Disparity in depression treatment among racial and ethnic minority populations in the United States. *Psychiatric Services, 59*, 1264–1272.

Andrea, H., Bültmann, U., van Amelsvoort, L. G., & Kant, Y. (2009). The incidence of anxiety and depression among employees-the role of psychosocial work characteristics. *Depression and Anxiety, 26*, 1040–1048.

Andrews, G., Cuijpers, P., Craske, M. G., McEvoy, P., & Titov, N. (2010). Computer therapy for the anxiety and depressive disorders is effective, acceptable and practical health care: A meta-analysis. *PLoS One, 5*, e13196.

Balas, E. A., & Boren, S. A. (2000). *Yearbook of medical informatics: Managing clinical knowledge for health care improvement.* Stuttgart, Germany: Schattauer Verlagsgesellschaft mbH.

Barlow, D. H., Farchione, T. J., Fairholme, C. P., Ellard, K. K., Boisseau, C. L., Allen, L. B., et al. (2011). *Unified protocol for the transdiagnostic treatment of emotional disorders: Therapist guide.* New York: Oxford Press.

Barlow, D. H., Levitt, J. T., & Bufka, L. F. (1999). The dissemination of empirically supported treatments: A view to the future. *Behaviour Research and Therapy, 37*, S147–S162.

Becker, C. B., Stice, E., Shaw, H., & Woda, S. (2009). Use of empirically supported interventions for psychopathology: Can the participatory approach move us beyond the research-to-practice gap? *Behaviour Research and Therapy, 47*, 265–274.

Becker, C. B., Zayfert, C., & Anderson, E. (2004). A survey of psychologists' attitudes towards and utilization of exposure therapy for PTSD. *Behaviour Research and Therapy, 42*, 277–292.

Berwick, D. M. (2003). Disseminating innovations in health care. *Journal of the American Medical Association, 289*, 1969–1975.

Brown, T. A., Campbell, L. A., Lehman, C. L., Grisham, J. R., & Mancill, R. B. (2001). Current and lifetime comorbidity of the DSM-IV anxiety and mood disorders in a large clinical sample. *Journal of Abnormal Psychology, 110*, 585–599.

Carroll, K. M., & Rounsaville, B. J. (2003). Bridging the gap: A hybrid model to link efficacy and effectiveness research in substance abuse treatment. *Psychiatric Services, 54*, 333–339.

Centre for Economic Performance's Mental Health Policy Group. (2006). *The depression report: A new deal for depression and anxiety disorders.* London: London School of Economics and Political Science.

Cherry, D. K., Woodwell, D. A., & Rechtsteiner, E. A., (2007). *National Ambulatory Medical Care Survey: 2005 summary* (Advance data from Vital and Health Statistics No. 387). Hyattsville, MD: National Center for Health Statistics.

Chorpita, B. F. (2007). *Modular cognitive-behavioral therapy for childhood anxiety disorders.* New York: Guilford Press.

Chorpita, B. F., & Daleiden, E. L. (2009). Mapping evidence-based treatments for children and adolescents: Application of the distillation and matching model to 615 treatments from 322 randomized trials. *Journal of Consulting and Clinical Psychology, 77*, 566–579.

Clark, D. M., Layard, R., Smithies, R., Richards, D. A., Suckling, R., & Wright, B. (2009). Improving access to psychological therapy: Initial evaluation of two UK demonstration sites. *Behaviour Research and Therapy, 47*, 910–920.

Collins, K. A., Westra, H. A., Dozois, D. J. A., & Burns, D. D. (2004). Gaps in accessing treatment for anxiety and depression: Challenges for the delivery of care. *Clinical Psychology Review, 24*, 583–616.

Craske, M. G., Stein, M. B., Sullivan, G., Sherbourne, C., Bystritsky, A., Rose, R. D., et al. (2011). Disorder-specific impact of coordinated anxiety learning and management treatment for anxiety disorders in primary care. *Archives of General Psychiatry, 68*, 378–388.

Crow, S., Mussell, M. P., Peterson, C., Knopke, A., & Mitchell, J. (1999). Prior treatment received by patients with bulimia nervosa. *International Journal of Eating Disorders, 25*, 39–44.

Demyttenaere, K., Bruffaerts, R., Posada-Villa, J., Gasquet, I., Kovess, V., Lepine, J. P., et al. (2004). Prevalence, severity, and unmet need for treatment of mental disorders in the World Health Organization World Mental Health Surveys. *Journal of the American Medical Association, 291*, 2581–2590.

Eccles, M. P., Armstrong, D., Baker, R., Cleary, K., Davies, H., Davies, S., et al. (2009). An implementation research agenda. *Implementation Science, 4*, 18.

Fairburn, C. G., Cooper, Z., Shafran, R., & Wilson, G. T. (2008). Eating disorders: A transdiagnostic protocol. In D. H. Barlow (Ed.), *Clinical handbook of psychological disorders: A step-by-step treatment manual* (4th ed., pp. 578–614). New York: Guilford Press.

Fullana, M. A., Mataix-Cols, D., Caspi, A., Harrington, H., Grisham, J. R., Moffitt, T. E., et al. (2009). Obsessions and compulsions in the community: Prevalence, interference, help-seeking, developmental stability, and co-occurring psychiatric conditions. *American Journal of Psychiatry, 166*, 329–336.

Furmark, T., Carlbring, P., Hedman, E., Sonnenstein, A., Clevberger, P., Bohman, B., et al. (2009). Guided and unguided self-help for social anxiety disorder: Randomised controlled trial. *British Journal of Psychiatry, 195*, 440–447.

Gallo, K. P., & Barlow, D. H. (2011). *Factors involved in clinician adoption and nonadoption of evidence based interventions in mental health.* Manuscript submitted for publication.

Gawande, A. (2004, December 6). The bell curve. *The New Yorker,* (80). Retrieved from Academic OneFile via Gale.

Gawande, A. (2007). *Better: A surgeon's notes on performance.* New York: Metropolitan Books.

Gilbody, S., Bower, P., Fletcher, J., Richards, D., & Sutton, A. J. (2006). Collaborative care for depression: A cumulative meta-analysis and review of longer-term outcomes. *Archives of Internal Medicine, 166,* 2315–2321.

Greenberg, P. E., Kessler, R. C., Birnbaum, H. G., Leong, S. A., Lowe, S. W., Berglund, P. A., et al. (2003). The economic burden of depression in the United States: How did it change between 1990 and 2000? *Journal of Clinical Psychiatry, 64,* 1465–1475.

Greenberg, P. E., Sisitsky, T., Kessler, R. C., Finkelstein, S. N., Berndt, E. R., Davidson, J. R., et al. (1999). The economic burden of anxiety disorders in the 1990s. *Journal of Clinical Psychiatry, 60,* 427–435.

Goisman, R. M., Warshaw, M. G., & Keller, M. B. (1999). Psychosocial treatment prescriptions for generalized anxiety disorder, panic disorder and social phobia, 1991–1996. *American Journal of Psychiatry, 156,* 1819–1821.

Haas, H. L., & Clopton, J. R. (2003). Comparing clinical and research treatments for eating disorders. *International Journal of Eating Disorders, 33,* 412–420.

Hayes, S. C., Barlow, D. H., & Nelson-Gray, R. O. (1999). *The scientist practitioner: Research and accountability in the age of managed care* (2nd ed.). Needham Heights, MA: Allyn & Bacon.

Heron, K. E., & Smyth, J. M. (2010). Ecological momentary interventions: Incorporating mobile technology into psychosocial and health behaviour treatments. *British Journal of Health Psychology, 15,* 1–39.

Horn, S. D., & Gassaway, J. (2010). Practice based evidence: Incorporating clinical heterogeneity and patient-reported outcomes for comparative effectiveness research. *Medical Care, 48,* S17–S22.

Insel, T. R. (2009). Translating scientific opportunity into public health impact: A strategic plan for research on mental illness. *Archives of General Psychiatry, 66,* 128–133.

Institute of Medicine. (2001). *Crossing the quality chasm: A new health system for the 21st century.* Washington, DC: Author.

Kazdin, A. E., & Blase, S. L. (2011). Rebooting psychotherapy research and practice to reduce the burden of mental illness. *Perspectives on Psychological Science, 6,* 32–37.

Kendall, P. C., Gosch, E., Furr, J. M., & Sood, E. (2008). Flexibility with fidelity. *Journal of the American Academy of Child and Adolescent Psychiatry, 47,* 987–993.

Kessler, R. C., Chiu, W. T., Demler, O., Merikangas, K. R., & Walters, E. E. (2005). Prevalence, severity, and comorbidity of 12-month DSM-IV disorders in the National Comorbidity Survey Replication. *Archives of General Psychiatry, 62,* 617–627.

Kessler, R. C., Demler, O., Grank, R. G., Olfson, M., Pincus, H. A., Walters, E. E., et al. (2005). Prevalence and treatment of mental disorders, 1990 to 2003. *New England Journal of Medicine, 352,* 2515–2523.

Lamberg, L. (2008). Despite effectiveness, behavioral therapy for chronic insomnia still underused. *Journal of the American Medical Association, 300,* 2474–2475.

Lambert, M. J., Whipple, J. L., Hawkins, E. J., Vermeersch, D. A., Nielsen, S. L., & Smart, D. W. (2003). Is it time for clinicians to routinely track patient outcome? A meta-analyses. *Clinical Psychology: Science and Practice, 10,* 288–301.

Lasser, K. E., Himmelstein, D. U., Woolhander, S. J., McCormick, D., & Bor, D. H. (2002). Do minorities in the United States receive fewer mental health services than whites? *International Journal of Health Services, 32*, 567–578.

Marcus, S. C., & Olfson, M. (2010). National trends in the treatment for depression from 1998 to 2007. *Archives of General Psychiatry, 67*, 1265–1273.

McGuire, T. G., Alegria, M., Cook, B. L., Wells, K. B., & Zaslavsky, A. M. (2006). Implementing the Institute of Medicine definition of disparities: An application to mental health care. *Health Services Research, 41*, 1979–2005.

McHugh, R. K., & Barlow, D. H. (2010). Dissemination and implementation of evidence-based psychological interventions: A review of current efforts. *American Psychologist, 65*, 73–84.

McHugh, R. K., Murray, H. W., & Barlow, D. H. (2009). Balancing fidelity and adaptation in the dissemination of empirically-supported treatments: The promise of transdiagnostic interventions. *Behaviour Research and Therapy, 47*, 946–953.

Mojtabai, R., Ofson, M., Sampson, N. A., Jin, R., Druss, B., Wang, P. S., et al. (2011). Barriers to mental health treatment: Results from the National Comorbidity Survey Replication. *Psychological Medicine, 41*, 1751–1761.

Mosteller, F. (1981). Innovation and evaluation. *Science, 211*, 881–886.

Mussell, M. P., Crosby, R. D., Crow, S. J., Knopke, A. J., Peterson, C. B., Wonderlich, S. A., et al. (2000). Utilization of empirically supported psychotherapy treatments for individuals with eating disorders: A survey of psychologists. *International Journal of Eating Disorders, 27*, 230–237.

Newacheck, P. W., Hung, Y. Y., Park, M. J., Brindis, C. D., & Irwin, C. E. (2003). Disparities in adolescent health and health care: Does socioeconomic status matter? *Health Services Research, 38*, 1235–1152.

Newman, M. G., Szkodny, L. E., Llera, S. J., & Przeworski, A. (2011). A review of technology-assisted self-help and minimal contact therapies for drug and alcohol abuse and smoking addiction: Is human contact necessary for therapeutic efficacy? *Clinical Psychology Review, 31*, 178–186.

National Institute for Health and Clinical Excellence. (2006). *Computerized cognitive behaviour therapy for depression and anxiety* (Technology Appraisal 97). London: Author. Retrieved April 28, 2011, from http://guidance.nice.org.uk/TA97

Olfson, S. C., & Marcus, M. (2009). National patterns in antidepressant medication treatment. *Archives of General Psychiatry, 66*, 848–856.

President's New Freedom Commission on Mental Health. (2004). *Achieving the promise: Transforming mental health care in America.* Retrieved May 7, 2008, from http://www.mentalhealthcommission.gov/reports/FinalReport/toc.html

Rogers, E. M. (2003). *Diffusion of innovations.* (5th ed.). New York: Free Press.

Roy-Byrne, P., Craske, M. G., Sullivan, G., Rose, R. D., Edlund, M. J., Lang, A. J., et al. (2010). Delivery of evidence-based treatment for multiple anxiety disorders in primary care: A randomized controlled trial. *Journal of the American Medical Association, 303*, 1921–1928.

Sandler, J. (2007). Community-based practices: Integrating dissemination theory with critical theories of power and justice. *American Journal of Community Psychology, 40*, 272–289.

Santa Ana, E. J., Martino, S., Ball, S. A., Nich, C., Frankforter, T. L., & Carroll, K. M. (2008). What is usual about "treatment-as-usual"? Data from two multisite effectiveness trials. *Journal of Substance Abuse Treatment, 35*, 369–379.

Santucci, L. C., McHugh, R. K., & Barlow, D. H. (in press). Direct-to-consumer marketing of evidence-based psychological interventions: Introduction to a special series. *Behavior Therapy.* doi:10.1016/j.beth.2011.07.003

Schutte-Rodin, S., Broch, L., Buysse, D., Dorsey, C, & Sateia, M. (2008). Clinical guidelines for the evaluation and management of chronic insomnia in adults. *Journal of Clinical Sleep Medicine, 4,* 487–504.

Simpson, D. D., & Flynn, P. M. (2007). Moving innovations into treatment: A stage-based approach to program change. *Journal of Substance Abuse Treatment, 33,* 111–120.

Simon, G. E., Barber, C., Birnbaum, H. G., Frank, R. G., Greenberg, P. E., Rose, R. M., et al. (2001). Depression and work productivity: The comparative costs of treatment versus nontreatment. *Journal of Occupational and Environmental Medicine, 43,* 2–9.

Smit, F., Cuijpers, P., Oostenbrink, J., Batelaan, N., de Graaf, R., & Beekman, A. (2006). Costs of nine common mental disorders: Implications for curative and preventive psychiatry. *Journal of Mental Health Policy and Economics, 9,* 193–200.

Sobell, L. C. (1996). Bridging the gap between scientists and practitioners: The challenge before us. *Behavior Therapy, 27,* 297–320.

Southam-Gerow, M. A., Ringeisen, H. L., & Sherrill, J. T. (2006). Integrating interventions and services research: Progress and prospects. *Clinical Psychology: Science and Practice, 13,* 1–8.

Stein, M. B., Roy-Byrne, P. P., Craske, M. G., Campbell-Sills, L., Lang, A. J., Golinelli, D., et al. (2011). Quality of and patient satisfaction with primary health care for anxiety disorders. *Journal of Clinical Psychiatry, 72,* 970–976.

Stewart, R. E., & Chambless, D. L. (2007). Does psychotherapy research inform treatment decision in private practice? *Journal of Clinical Psychology, 63,* 267–281.

Stirman, S. W., Crits-Christoph, P., & DeRubeis, R. J. (2004). Achieving successful dissemination of empirically supported psychotherapies: A synthesis of dissemination theory. *Clinical Psychology: Science and Practice, 11,* 343–359.

Striegel-Moore, R. H., Wilson, G. T., DeBar, L., Perrin, N., Lynch, F., Rosselli, F. et al. (2010). Cognitive behavioral guided self-help for the treatment of recurrent binge eating. *Journal of Consulting and Clinical Psychology, 78,* 312–321.

Sullivan, G., Craske, M. G., Sherbourne, C., Edlund, M. J., Rose, R. D., Golinelli, D., et al. (2007). Design of the Coordinated Anxiety Learning and Management (CALM) study: Innovations in collaborative care for anxiety disorders. *General Hospital Psychiatry, 29,* 379–387.

Thornicroft, G., Lempp, H., & Tansella, M. (2011). The place of implementation science in the translational medicine continuum. *Psychological Medicine, 41,* 2015–2021.

Trochim, W. M. (2010, March). *Translation won't happen without dissemination and implementation: Some measurement and evaluation issues.* Paper presented at the 3rd annual National Institutes of Health Conference on the Science of Dissemination and Implementation. Bethesda, MD.

Unützer, J., Katon, W., Callahan, C. M., Williams, J. W., Hunkeler, E., Harpole, L., et al. (2002). Collaborative care management of late-life depression in the primary care setting: A randomized controlled trial. *Journal of the American Medical Association, 288,* 2836–2845.

U.S. Department of Health and Human Services. (1999). *Mental health: A report of the Surgeon General.* Rockville, MD: Author.

U.S. Department of Health and Human Services. (2001). *Mental health: Culture, race, and ethnicity, supplement to mental health: A report of the Surgeon General.* Rockville, MD: Author.

Wang, P. S., Aguilar-Gaxiola, S., Alonso, J., Angermeyer, M. C., Borges, G., Bromet, E. J., et al. (2007). Use of mental health services for anxiety, mood, and substance disorders in 17 countries in the WHO world mental health surveys. *Lancet, 370,* 841–850.

Wang, P. S., Berglund, P. A., & Kessler, R. C. (2000). Recent care of common mental disorders in the United States. *Journal of General Internal Medicine, 15,* 284–292.

Wells, K., Klap, R., Koike, A., & Sherbourne, C. (2001). Ethnic disparities in unmet need for alcoholism, drug abuse and mental health care. *American Journal of Psychiatry, 158,* 2027–2032.

Weisz, J. R., Donenberg, G. R., Han, S. S., & Weiss, B. (1995). Bridging the gap between laboratory and clinic in child and adolescent psychotherapy. *Journal of Consulting and Clinical Psychology, 63,* 688–701.

Witmer, L. (1907/1996). Clinical psychology. *American Psychologist, 51,* 248–251.

Young, A. S., Klap, R., Sherbourne, C. D., & Wells, K. B. (2001). The quality of care of depressive and anxiety disorders in the United States. *Archives of General Psychiatry, 58,* 55.

{INDEX}

Page ranges in emboldened type indicate chapters. Italicized page numbers indicate a figure or table. 'n' following a page number indicates a footnote. EBP = evidence-based practice.